AF110525

# CASES IN SIMULATED DISASTER MEDICINE

"This book is an essential resource that will be extremely helpful to support any medical professional who may be planning to respond to a disaster. The thoughtfully developed cases are incredible tools that help learners think through their response options (as well as the pitfalls they may encounter) before they need to act in a real-world situation. The cases cover a wide range of scenarios, from natural to human-caused disasters, and are structured to support safe and constructive discussions and learning. Learning using the simulations in this book could be considered a must-do before anyone's first time in the field or for anyone responsible for leading medical disaster planning and response."

**Paul D. Biddinger,** MD FACEP
Chief Preparedness and Continuity Officer, Mass General Brigham
Chief, MGB Division of Emergency Preparedness
Ann L. Prestipino MPH Endowed Chair in Emergency Preparedness
Director, Center for Disaster Medicine
Director, Harvard T. H. Chan School of Public Health Emergency Preparedness Research, Evaluation, and Practice (EPREP) Program

"This book offers an unparalleled contribution to medical education, particularly in preparing healthcare professionals for the unique and often overwhelming challenges of disaster response. This comprehensive resource stands out by providing vivid, ready-to-teach cases that directly simulate rarely encountered, high-stakes scenarios, encompassing everything from natural disasters like volcanic eruptions and tsunamis to complex human-made crises such as chemical exposures and bioterrorism attacks.

A scalable and customizable design ensures its utility across all learning environments, from novices to seasoned practitioners, fostering hands-on, experiential learning that aligns perfectly with how emergency medicine physicians and other learners acquire and retain critical knowledge. Emphasizing critical decision-making and resource allocation in overwhelming, resource-limited situations, it uniquely equips learners with the knowledge and skills to navigate complexities where good decisions can mean the difference between life and death for large numbers of patients."

**Selim Suner** MD, MS, FACEP
Professor of Emergency Medicine, Surgery, and Engineering
Brown University

# CASES IN SIMULATED DISASTER MEDICINE

Edited by

**ANDREW MILSTEN**
University of Massachusetts Medical Center

**JOHN BROACH**
University of Massachusetts Medical Center

CAMBRIDGE
UNIVERSITY PRESS

CAMBRIDGE
UNIVERSITY PRESS

Shaftesbury Road, Cambridge CB2 8EA, United Kingdom

One Liberty Plaza, 20th Floor, New York, NY 10006, USA

477 Williamstown Road, Port Melbourne, VIC 3207, Australia

314–321, 3rd Floor, Plot 3, Splendor Forum, Jasola District Centre, New Delhi – 110025, India

103 Penang Road, #05–06/07, Visioncrest Commercial, Singapore 238467

Cambridge University Press is part of Cambridge University Press & Assessment, a department of the University of Cambridge.

We share the University's mission to contribute to society through the pursuit of education, learning and research at the highest international levels of excellence.

www.cambridge.org
Information on this title: www.cambridge.org/9781009279017

DOI: 10.1017/9781009279024



When citing this work, please include a reference to the DOI 10.1017/9781009279024

First published 2026

Cover images courtesy of Andrew Milsten

*A catalogue record for this publication is available from the British Library*

*A Cataloging-in-Publication data record for this book is available from the Library of Congress*

ISBN 978-1-009-27901-7 Paperback

# Contents

# Contributors

James Aiken MD, MHA FACEP, Clinical Professor of Emergency Medicine, Emergency Medicine Residency Program, Louisiana State University Health Sciences Center, New Orleans

Rashed Al Remeithi MD, Emergency Medicine Resident, Sheikh Shakhbout Medical City, Abu Dhabi, United Arab Emirates

Sukhshant Atti MD, FACEP, Assistant Professor, Department of Emergency Medicine, University of Alabama at Birmingham; Associate Director, Alabama Poison Information Center

Lauren Bacon MD, MBA, Assistant Professor of Emergency Medicine, Emergency Department, University of Connecticut Health

Paul Baker MBChB, FRCS, Clinical Lead for Burns, New Zealand National Burn Centre; Consultant Plastic and Reconstructive Surgeon, Auckland Regional Centre for Plastic Reconstructive & Hand Surgery; Honorary Senior Lecturer, Waipapa Taumata Rau – The University of Auckland; New Zealand Vice President Australia and New Zealand Burn Association (ANZBA)

Jennifer Carey MD, Associate Professor, Department of Emergency Medicine, University of Massachusetts Chan Medical School

Matthew Carlisle MD, Department of Medicine, Section of Emergency Medicine, Louisiana State University Health Sciences Center New Orleans

Guy Carmelli MD, MSEd, Assistant Professor, Emergency Medicine, University of Massachusetts Chan Medical School

C. Clare Charbonnet MD, Disaster Medicine Fellow, Department of Emergency Medicine, UMass Memorial Medical Center

Michael De Luca MD, MS, Adjunct Assistant Professor, School of Medicine, Georgetown University

Colleen M. Donovan MD, Associate Professor, Emergency Medicine, Simulation & Clinical Skills Director, Rutgers-Robert Wood Johnson Medical School

Romeo Fairley MD, MPH, University of Texas Health San Antonio

Denise Fernandez MD, Assistant Professor, Department of Emergency Medicine, and Medical Toxicology Division Chief, Rutgers Robert Wood Johnson Medical School

Emerson Franke MD, FACEP, FAEMS, FAAEM, Associate Simulation Director, Rutgers Health/ RWJBarnabas Health Community Medical Center

Jonathan Gammel MD, Assistant Professor, Department of Emergency Medicine, University of Massachusetts

Jennifer E. Geller MD, General Surgery Resident Physician, Department of Surgery, Thomas Jefferson University Hospital

Alexander Hart MD, Department of Emergency Medicine, Hartford Hospital, University of Connecticut School of Medicine

Christopher Hayden MD, Louisiana State University

Kyle Herbert MD, MBMS, CPT (USAR), Department of Emergency Medicine, Disaster and Operational Medicine Section, George Washington-Medical Faculty & Associates

Jordan Hitchens DO, Medical Director, Disaster Preparedness & Emergency Management, New York City Health + Hospitals/South Brooklyn Health, Ruth Bader Ginsburg Hospital

Ameer F. Ibrahim MD, MS, FACEP, Assistant Professor of Emergency Medicine, Department of Emergency Medicine, University of Massachusetts Chan Medical School

Cody Johnson MD, GW Maritime Medical Access, George Washington University Medical Faculty Associates

Ziad Kazzi MD, FAAEM, FACEP, FACMT, FAACT, Professor of Emergency Medicine, Emory University

Michelle B. Locke MBChB, MD, FRACS (Plastics), Plastic & Reconstructive Surgeon, Auckland Regional Centre for Plastic, Reconstructive & Hand Surgery; Associate Professor, Waipapa Taumata Rau – The University of Auckland

Cassandra Mackey MD, FACEP, Simulation Lead, Department of Emergency Medicine; Assistant Professor, University of Massachusetts Chan Medical School

Emily Marx MD, Emergency Medicine Physician, Sinai Chicago

Meghan Maslanka MD, Clinical Assistant Professor, Emergency Medicine, Louisiana State University; Deputy Medical Director, New Orleans EMS; Director of Emergency Management, University Medical Center New Orleans

Mary G. McGoldrick MD, Rutgers Robert Wood Johnson Medical School

Andrew Milsten MD, MS, FACEP, Professor, Department of Emergency Medicine, Director, Disaster Medicine & Emergency Management Fellowship, University of Massachusetts Medical School, University of Massachusetts Memorial Medical Center

Natalie Moore MD, MPH, Assistant Professor, Fellowship Director, International Disaster Emergency Medicine, University of Connecticut School of Medicine

James P. Phillips MD, Associate Professor, Emergency Medicine, and Section Chief of Disaster and Operational Medicine, School of Medicine and Health Sciences, George Washington University

Liam Porter MD, Clinical Assistant Professor, Florida International University

Lekha Reddy MD, Rutgers Robert Wood Johnson Medical School

Morgan Ritz MD, MPH, CPH, Assistant Clinical Professor of Emergency Medicine, Baylor Scott & White Health-Temple Emergency Medicine, Emergency Ultrasound, Disaster Medicine, Baylor College of Medicine-Temple

David Ruby MD, FACEP, Director of Emergency Medicine Simulation/Attending Physician, Hartford Hospital

Daniel Saltzman DO, FACEP, Assistant Professor, Emergency Medicine, University of Massachusetts Chan Medical School

Ritu Sarin MD, MScDM, FACEP, Faculty, BIDMC Fellowship in Disaster Medicine, Department of Emergency Medicine, Beth Israel Deaconess Medical Center, Boston, MA

Natalie Sullivan MD, George Washington University

Matthew A. Tovar MD, LT, MC, USN, Department of Emergency Medicine, Navy Medical Center

Larissa H. Unruh MD, MPH, Director of Education and Training Director, National Center for Disaster Medicine and Public Health

Michael Weiner MD, Department of EMS and Disaster, University of Massachusetts Memorial Medical Center

Jorge Yarzebski EMT-P, Simulation Educator iCELS Healthcare Simulation Lab, University of Massachusetts Chan Medical School; Critical Care Transport Flight Paramedic, Lifeflight

SECTION 1

# INTRODUCTORY CHAPTERS

CHAPTER 1

# Introduction to Simulation

Cassandra Mackey and Jennifer Carey

---

**Case 1:** You are the only physician on site working in a small community emergency department. Your local emergency medical services reports that there is an apartment fire with many critically ill and potentially unstable patients. The prehospital emergency medical team is unable to immediately transport victims directly to the burn center so all patients will be coming to your small emergency department. How do you handle multiple victims without overwhelming resources in your small hospital?

**Case 2:** You are called to the scene of a bombing as the medical director to assist in triaging patients. You decide who gets transported, who gets treated on scene, and who does not get any treatment. This is your first bombing. How do you know what to do?

---

## WHY SIMULATION?

Adults as opposed to children learn best by using life experiences and applying knowledge.[1] Adults, due to life experience, have habits that form and seek to find knowledge through self-directed learning.[2] Emergency medicine physicians as learners are generally people who "learn by doing." The best way to educate these learners is to take advantage of these two facts.[3] In order to learn and retain information, learning must be purposeful and effortful, and the individual must strive to achieve success. Learning that is easy and is oftentimes forgotten.[4]

The idea of simulated practice was developed using the principles of adult learning theory. Simulation is used in medical education to enhance real patient experiences with created scenarios designed to mimic real clinical encounters[5]; a way to provide hands-on practice of situations and procedures prior to being called upon to act in real situations or on live patients. The cornerstone of medical education historically relied on classroom lectures and multiple-choice exams. However, this may not translate as relevant to clinical practice, particularly in situations where there is not always a "correct" answer.[6] Simulation provides experiential learning, scenarios, and cases mimicking real-life situations, which leads to better knowledge acquisition that is more easily called upon in real life situations.[4]

Using simulation-based-education, participants can learn practical material that is relevant to current everyday or future patient encounters. Instead of sitting in a lecture imagining how to place a central line, students have an opportunity to get hands-on experience with the procedure, learn techniques, and discuss indications without taking away from patient safety or patient care.[5] In addition, simulation-based education allows for real-time feedback. As stated by Matlala et al., "simulation is a technique, not a technology, to replace or amplify real experiences with guided experiences, often immersive in nature, that evoke or replicate substantial aspects of the real world in a fully interactive fashion."[7]

## HISTORY OF SIMULATION AND BASIC SIMULATION TOOLS

Simulation-based medical education has been around since at least the seventeenth century when birthing mannequins were used.[8] Simulation has been employed by other professions; notably, simulation was introduced in the early 1900s for pilot training and continues to be a fundamental part of instruction as it is required for licensure. There is documentation from the 1950s and 1960s of using a cardiovascular simulator for the evaluation of prosthetic aortic valves leading to the first mannequin-based system developed by Denson and Abrahamson and later by Gaba and DeAnda.[5] A life-sized doll, Laerdal's Resusci Anne, was the next creation, followed by incorporation of computer algorithms into mannequins as patient simulators by Sim One.[9] Since that time, technology has continued to advance allowing more realistic experiences for learners including new technology incorporating virtual reality into simulations. They are designed to create safe environments to practice a wide variety of medical scenarios and procedures.

The tools necessary to run current simulations are instructors, mannequins, or standardized patients or a combination of both. Mannequins can be used for "high-fidelity" simulation scenarios when they incorporate computer algorithms and practical components or as "low fidelity" using parts or components to practice focused learning and procedural skills. Research has shown that hands-on simulation-based education improves learner's education and patient outcomes.[10–16] Ideally, instructors should be simulation-trained educators who have the knowledge base to create well-designed scenarios and provide feedback to enhance learners' knowledge.

## CONCLUSION

Simulation is utilized for learners to be prepared for real-life scenarios in team settings or individually. The cases presented, such as multiple burn victims or bomb victims, illustrate real-life scenarios that are rarely encountered by most medical professionals. Though an individual may not have encountered these cases previously, the knowledge and practice in simulated scenarios may lead to quick recall, which could improve patient outcomes and survival. In a disaster situation, one may need to reorganize treatment priorities, shifting from providing maximal care for everyone to offering lifesaving care only, doing the best with the available resources. Simulation of these challenging situations will prepare the learner for situations not frequently encountered but during which good decision making can mean the difference between life and death for large numbers of patients.

## REFERENCES

1. Curry RH, Hershman WY, Saizow RB. Learner-centered strategies in clerkship education. *Am J Med.* 1996;100(6):589–595. doi:10.1016/s0002-9343(97)89424-7.
2. Kaufman DM. Applying educational theory in practice. *BMJ.* 2003;326(7382):213–216. doi:10.1136/bmj.326.7382.213.
3. David TJ, Patel L. Adult learning theory, problem-based learning, and paediatrics. *Arch Dis Child.* 1995;73(4):357–363. doi:10.1136/adc.73.4.357.
4. Brown PC, Roediger HL, McDaniel MA. *Make It Stick: The Science of Successful Learning.* Cambridge: Harvard University Press; 2014.
5. McLaughlin S, Fitch MT, Goyal DG, et al. Simulation in graduate medical education 2008: a review for emergency medicine. *Acad Emerg Med.* 2008;15(11):1117–1129. doi:10.1111/j.1553-2712.2008.00188.x.
6. Elstein AS. Beyond multiple-choice questions and essays: the need for a new way to assess clinical competence. *Acad Med.* 1993;68(4):244–249. doi:10.1097/00001888-199304000-00002.
7. Matlala S. Educators' perceptions and views of problem-based learning through simulation. *Curationis.* 2021;44(1):e1–e7. doi:10.4102/curationis.v44i1.2094.

8. Mulligan T, Winters ME, Mattu A, Martinez JP, Rogers RL, eds. *Practical Teaching in Emergency Medicine*. 2nd ed. Chichester: Wiley Blackwell; 2012.
9. Sinz EH, Taekman JM New educational technology. *Int Anesthesiol Clin*. 2008;46(4):137–150. doi:10.1097/aia.0b013e3181817b1a.
10. Barsuk JH, Ahya SN, Cohen ER, McGaghie WC, Wayne DB. Mastery learning of temporary hemodialysis catheter insertion by nephrology fellows using simulation technology and deliberate practice. *Am J Kid Dis*. 2009;54(1):70–76. doi:10.1053/j.ajkd.2008.12.041.
11. Barsuk JH, Cohen ER, Feinglass J, McGaghie WC, Wayne DB. Use of simulation-based education to reduce catheter-related bloodstream infections. *Arch Intern Med*. 2009;169(15):1420–1423. doi:10.1001/archinternmed.2009.215.
12. Barsuk JH, McGaghie WC, Cohen ER, Balachandran JS, Wayne DB. Use of simulation-based mastery learning to improve the quality of central venous catheter placement in a medical intensive care unit. *J Hosp Med*. 2009;4(7):397–403. doi:10.1002/jhm.468.
13. Grantcharov TP, Kristiansen VB, Bendix J, et al. Randomized clinical trial of virtual reality simulation for laparoscopic skills training. *Br J Surg*. 2004 Feb;91(2):146–150. doi:10.1002/bjs.4407.
14. McGaghie WC, Issenberg SB, Petrusa ER, Scalese RJ. Effect of practice on standardised learning outcomes in simulation-based medical education. *Med Educ*. 2006;40(8):792–797. doi:10.1111/j.1365-2929.2006.02528.x.
15. . Revisiting "A critical review of simulation-based medical education research: 2003–2009." *Med Educ*. 2016;50(10):986–991. doi:10.1111/medu.12795.
16. Ten Eyck RP, Tews M, Ballester JM. Improved medical student satisfaction and test performance with a simulation-based emergency medicine curriculum: a randomized controlled trial. *Ann Emerg Med*. 2009;54(5):684–691. doi:10.1016/j.annemergmed.2009.03.025.

CHAPTER 2

# Disaster Simulation

## The Best Way to Prepare for the Worst

David Ruby

Disaster simulation is a useful tool for medical provider preparation, education, and training. Simulation has been used to help integrate prehospital responder protocols with the ED disaster plan by allowing the ED providers and first responders to work together.[1] In addition, it can be used for identifying preparedness gaps in hospitals so that these gaps can be addressed in order to improve overall disaster preparedness.[2]

When writing a disaster case, it is important to follow the same principles that guide the writing of all simulation cases. Each case starts with educational objectives, which act as the scaffolding for building the case scenario. These objectives can include testing a specific operational system or highlighting medical learning objectives. As an example, a case could be written to test the ED protocols for mass casualty incidents (MCIs). A similar case aimed at ED residents might have more specific educational objectives such as learning the blast injury classification and treatment of these injuries. If the disaster simulation is being incorporated into a disaster exercise, then it is important to remember that sizable drills will likely have learners from multiple disciplines, therefore requiring multiple learning objectives.

The degree of fidelity of the simulation and the attention paid to scenario realism should be an important consideration when planning an event. In addition, the location of the simulation should be determined as should the number of anticipated victims. The latter decision should be made based on the expected learners, overall goals of the simulation, equipment available, personnel available, presence of volunteers as patients, and cost (among other considerations).

This chapter focuses on large MCI scenario/drills. Decreasing the fidelity (blow-up mannequins or tabletop aspects) can be useful as it increases the efficiency of the simulation and decreases the resource requirements although it does sacrifice learner immersion in the scenario. To increase the fidelity of the simulation, live actors and high-fidelity mannequins can be used, which more fully capture the learner's attention and provoke more genuine reactions from them. Virtual reality is also a growing option, with evidence that it can be as effective as mannequin-based disaster simulation,[3] although this can be challenging to implement on a large scale.

Scenario selection should be based on a realistic number of expected casualties from a given event. Some simulations may have only one or a few patients if the concepts being taught relate to detailed patient management of complex illness (i.e. a patient with viral hemorrhagic fever) but due consideration should be paid to the nonmedical aspects of such a presentation. In the case of a highly infectious disease, for example, risk communication within the institution, management of potentially exposed family or others, etc. should be considered. For MCI simulations, knowledge of local response capacity is important to gauge the number and complexity of victims that would overwhelm usual operational plans. For many large hospital EDs, 20–25 patients presenting in an hour on top of usual volume is sufficient but more or fewer should be chosen depending upon the goals of the exercise. The case scenario should start with an inciting event or background information that may or may not include a complete picture of what has occurred. For example, if the scenario is a train derailment, most relevant information might be known by responders and thus relayed to hospital staff. In the case of a covert bioterrorism attack, many details may be unknown at the time of first patient contact and, instead, the scenario may simply include a large number of patients with unusual or characteristic symptoms that should lead the learners to suspect that an abnormal event has occurred.

For an MCI scenario, there should be a realistic spread between green, yellow, red, and black tagged victims; not all patients in the case need to be critically ill and depending upon the goals of the simulation, the type of patients can be modulated to meet the objectives. Some can be used as distractors or subtle cases to test the learner's abilities to diagnose further. A victim's condition can change over the course of the scenario, going from a green tagged to a red tagged person as their condition worsens. In addition, consider if you want any nonlive actor cases (such as mannequins), as these can portray more possible conditions. An operator is required for high-fidelity mannequins, which can be a potential drawback.

Having a planned surprise twist built into the scenario is another option, which changes the dynamic of the case and can enhance the educational value of the simulation. This could be something that causes an additional influx of patients, removes resources, or even incapacitates the providers. This can further test the learners' abilities to adapt and respond, as well as allow additional services to take part in the case. For example, an active shooter during the case can create new victims, test the learners' knowledge of what to do in such a situation, and provide a logical entry for the local police to be part of the case.

Once the case is complete, having a set of debriefing points is vital to ensuring proper delivery of the information related to the simulation. Although it is important to have debriefing points that cover all the objectives, it is also important to realize that each iteration of the case will have potentially different responses by the learners, which could create new discussion points that need to be addressed.

Once the case is written and designed, it is important to take inventory of available space, resources, and personnel when designing the actual simulation. Knowing how many patient rooms you can provide will help ensure the case is confined to a particular space. Procedural capability will need to be analyzed, including available task trainers and procedure kits for the learners. If there are mannequin patients involved, there will need to be an inventory of what kinds of mannequins are available and how many. Foot traffic is also a major consideration, to ensure that each provider, victim, and actor have an appropriate path through the case, as well as ensuring the case does not interfere with other hospital operations and regular daily foot traffic if the simulation is occurring in active patient care areas. As part of this, having a staging area for the victims will be important to ensure they are not obstructive and that they get sent into the case in a timely fashion.

When planning the case, having a proper start and finish is critical. It is common to have to brief the participants on the rules of the simulation, as well as provide an introduction to the case. Make sure to have a set of ground rules that will be communicated to the learners before beginning the case. This gives you more control over the case, allows for customization, and helps ensure the safety of all participants. In addition, having a specific set of triggers that will advance the case will ensure that it adheres to the expected timeline. One method of pacing the simulation is controlling the influx of patients that learners have to deal with at a given time.

To further control the case, the timing of the patient arrivals should be determined in advance. Determine how much time you have for the drill (including debriefing and cleanup/turnover if it will be running more than once). Use this information combined with the number of patients in the drill to determine an optimal rate of patient arrivals.

When planning a large case, it will be important to create a list of roles. Be aware that these roles should be both for case creation and in-case support. Jobs that will be needed include event coordination, patient pool organization, sim room coordinators, moulage team and leadership, actor orientation and check-ins, mannequin operators, foot traffic control, and special effects technicians. The full list of roles is unique to each drill, but it will be important to ensure each aspect of the preparation and execution of the drill has oversight.

You should maintain control over the flow in a case, so that the desired timeline is followed and maintained. Most cases follow a similar general timeline of briefing, case start, trigger events, case end, and debriefing. It is advised that each event has a specific time attached to it. The usual flow is to give the learners an initial briefing of the case, then allowing them five minutes to organize themselves. Trigger events may occur based on the number of patients who have been sent into the drill or based on the progress toward learning objectives that the learners are making. The trigger for concluding the simulation should be established in advance with the simulation director announcing an end to the case at the appropriate time.

If you are planning a twist event during a case, it will be important to pay special attention to the timing and when this change is due to occur. For example, if you are planning an active shooter scenario where the shooter makes an entrance, you must have the entry point and timing determined ahead of time. If you wish to display their motive, you must ensure it is written properly into the case. If you are going to have any moulage during the case, you must figure out the physical flow of people who will get the victims to be moulaged out of the case discretely, as well as back into the case and in position just as discretely. These sorts of movements can be disguised with proper planning of routes and distractors (loud patients, choreographed fights, etc.). It is a good idea to have a group of people who are working behind the scenes specifically devoted to the twist to ensure it is timed and executed properly.

When recruiting volunteers for the case, make sure to draw on all available sources. Volunteers are the lifeblood of simulated MCI drills. Many live actors may be needed to handle the number of moving parts in a large MCI scenario. Look for groups of people with some medical training first, as this will make orientation to the case much easier on the day of the drill. Students in healthcare fields (medical, nursing, radiology, and respiratory therapy students), colleagues in your department, EMS workers, and first responders are all good choices. Determine the number of victims in the case, and then try to exceed that number in terms of volunteers to ensure that the drill can run despite some cancellations.

To ensure smooth running of the simulation, plan for dedicated time on the day of the event before the actual simulation to adequately prepare. Volunteer preparation can be extensive and ample time should be dedicated to moulage, volunteer preparation, and time for questions and concerns. Depending upon the size of the simulation, allow at least three to four hours of preparation time on the day of the event to ensure that all runs smoothly. As the time for the drill approaches, the volunteers will need to be gathered and oriented on the overall flow of the case, as well as brought to the entry point.

While the volunteers are being prepped and moulaged, test any special effects. Be sure to account for the fact that smoke machines can set off fire alarms and that some people are sensitive to strobe lights. Sound effects should be tested for volume, and props should be double checked. There should also be clear, wearable markings for staff who are not part of the case, so the learners can identify them. There needs to be a safety word that, when utilized, stops the scenario. Furthermore, having appropriate signage, contacting local police and fire, and establishing strict safety protocols are necessary.

Throughout the day, it will be important to ensure the staff members can communicate with each other, with radios being a good option. There should be multiple channels for different groups of staff to ensure proper communication between the event coordinator and other members of the team. For example, if there is moulage during the case, the moulage team may need their own channel.

To ensure all trigger events go smoothly, the event coordinator should have a channel to the patient pool coordinator and should frequently check in with them to know how many patients have been sent into the case. Special effects teams should have a channel as well, to ensure that the effects are timed properly with the case.

Once the simulation is complete, a thorough debriefing is required. Debriefing is an optimal way to deliver the intended learning points while ensuring a higher rate of retention due to inclusion of the learners. Since these are simulation cases, it is important to be aware that, although each case has planned debriefing points, each group of learners will approach the drill differently and will require custom debriefing points that will need to be addressed as well.

Each case can be enhanced by having special guests to aid in the debriefing. EMS, fire department, and police officers are common choices based on the case and offer alternate points of view that the learners may not have considered.

During the debrief, it is also important to allow the learners to give feedback, especially while the case is fresh in their minds. This allows for the ability to improve upon each successive case. While the debrief is happening, the area where the drill is taking place can be turned over and reset or cleaned if there are no further drills that day.

Disaster simulation is a small, but growing field within the overall world of medical simulation, and has tremendous potential to provide preparedness to first responder agencies, medical residencies, hospital systems, and other entities involved in disaster response.[4] With proper preparation and execution, any institution can run a successful scenario and drill and take advantage of the benefits they provide.

## REFERENCES

1. Alexander AJ, Bandiera GW, Mazurik L. A multiphase disaster training exercise for emergency medicine residents: opportunity knocks. *Acad Emerg Med.* 2005;12:404–409. doi:10.1197/j.aem.2004.11.025.
2. Bennett RL. Chemical or biological terrorist attacks: an analysis of the preparedness of hospitals for managing victims affected by chemical or biological weapons of mass destruction. *Int J Environ Res Public Health.* 2006 Mar;3(1):67–75. doi:10.3390/ijerph2006030008. PMID: 16823078; PMCID: PMC3785681.
3. Smith S, Farra SL, Hodgson E. Evaluation of two simulation methods for teaching a disaster skill. *BMJ Simul Technol Enhanc Learn.* 2020 May 18;7(2):92–96. doi:10.1136/bmjstel-2019-000572. PMID: 35520385; PMCID: PMC8936753.
4. Gable BD, Misra A, Doos DM, et al. Disaster day: a simulation-based disaster medicine curriculum for novice learners. *J Med Educ Curric Dev.* 2021 Jun 8;8:23821205211020751. doi:10.1177/23821205211020751. PMID: 34164580; PMCID: PMC8191058.

CHAPTER 3

# Simulation Debriefing

Jorge Yarzebski and Jordan Hitchens

Debriefing is an intentional, facilitator-led, analytical discussion following an event that aims to integrate lessons learned to improve future practice. In simulation-based education a facilitator leads a reflective process aiming to assimilate preexisting thoughts, feelings, knowledge, and emotions with lessons learned during the simulation. The goal is to either bolster existing beliefs or enhance and improve knowledge, skills, and attitudes. In the debriefing process, simulation facilitators seek to uncover the driving forces behind the actions seen in the simulation.[1] Effective debriefings have their foundation in the prebrief phase, where facilitators show great intentionality in creating a supportive environment for learning that is then guided by unyielding curiosity throughout the debrief.

## HISTORY OF DEBRIEFING

Debriefing was first practiced during World War II by S.L.A. Marshall, who served as Chief Combat Historian of the armed forces. The debriefing process used by Marshall consisted of a fact-based technical debrief immediately following combat events. The debriefing sessions occurred in small, safe, and supportive groups of peers and were described to be beneficial for the soldiers involved.[2]

In 1983, the Critical Incident Stress Debriefing (CISD) model was created by Jeffrey Mitchell, PhD in Baltimore, MD, which remains the gold standard for cognitive debriefing today. Norwegian psychologist Alte Dyregrov expanded the concept and coined the term psychological debriefing in 1989, defining it as debriefing that takes place 48–72 hours post event to assist in emotional processing.[3] The Multiple Stressor Debriefing Model is a four-step model developed in 1991 by Armstrong et al. specifically for disaster responders.[4] The previously described models were designed to distill information learned from battle and to mitigate the effects of trauma experienced in real life events. The main goal of a critical or traumatic incident debrief is to recover from the experience and return to the front lines as quickly as possible.

Simulation debriefing combines adult learning principles and a rich history of military and psychological debriefing. Most agree that debriefing is the most important part of simulation-based education where learners make sense of what just occurred and connect outcomes to thoughts, knowledge, and actions that occurred during the event. Effective debriefing is a skill that is acquired over time, requiring practice, debriefing the debriefing, and repetition. Debriefers should engage in regular quality assurance of their debriefing skills, which includes self-reflection and peer-to-peer debriefing.

Simulation-based debriefing practices have entered the clinical setting. The supportive, team-focused analysis, conversational structure of simulation debriefing, use of open-ended discussion and reflection are effective in boosting healthcare worker wellness and mitigating burnout.[5] Despite the success of debriefing in high-reliability organizations such as aviation, clinical debriefing occurs at a lower rate than in other high-stake and high-performing industries.[6,7] Debriefings should not only be reserved for negative outcomes and near misses, but they should also be incorporated into regular practice and can be used to celebrate successes as they are used to change or improve actions.

## WHY DEBRIEFING IS IMPORTANT

There are multiple reasons why debriefing is important. In the setting of simulation, debriefing is often described as the "heart and soul" and the "lynchpin" of the simulation process.[8] The reflection that occurs during a debriefing directly after or in some cases during a simulation is thought to be where most of the learning and retention occurs. The debriefing process in simulation-based activities is a critical element to experiential learning. Adult learners encode long-term memory more effectively when they are active participants in educational activities. Active participation not only involves the act of the simulation but also the assimilation of lessons learned through facilitator-guided reflective discussions after the event. Facilitators serve as unobstructive guides in a debriefing session, introducing the debrief; promoting a supportive environment; guiding discussions based on learner reactions, observed actions, and reflection; and connecting outcomes with program goals and objectives.

It is also useful to debrief after real-world critical incidents (i.e. disasters, cardiac arrest resuscitations, trauma response, etc.). Studies confirm that debriefing has a positive effect on clinical outcomes.[10] As concerns continue to rise regarding the well-being of medical providers, it is important to also conduct research on the effects of debriefing on providers of clinical medicine. This research is less explicit, but what is clear is that disaster workers, along with military personnel, emergency medical providers, and police officers are at risk for posttraumatic stress disorder (PTSD).[11]

The well-being of providers is an important topic, especially in recent years due to the COVID pandemic.[12–14] Debriefing is thought to be a way to combat severe symptoms of PTSD associated with traumatic events, such as working through a pandemic, disaster response to weather events, or complex humanitarian crises. It also is thought to contribute to career longevity for those continually exposed to traumatic events.[15]

A core component of simulation-based education is the simulation facilitator. Facilitators are individuals who help bring about an outcome (such as learning, productivity, or communication) by providing indirect, guidance, or supervision.[10] Facilitators are not required to be subject matter experts (SMEs) in the simulation's topic; they should, however, possess understanding of simulation-based education pedagogy and debriefing techniques. These individuals are responsible for introducing the simulation, assisting its flow, ensuring a supportive environment for learning is maintained and leading a debrief. Often, facilitators are colearners rather than leaders, using curiosity to help learners reach learning objectives. In cases where a facilitator is not knowledgeable in the topic being simulated, they can be paired with an SME to help fill the knowledge gap. Debriefing skills develop over time and require feedback and practice. It is important to note that it is easy to facilitate ineffective debriefings, which can cause significant harm to learners and clinicians participating in academic or clinical debriefings.

## PREBRIEFING

Essential to a good debrief session is a great prebrief. The prebrief is the time preceding the simulation where facilitators introduce the simulation, its purpose, and learning objectives and attend to logistical details such as confidentiality, fidelity, and context. Social agreements are proposed where facilitators outline expected behavior and request confidentiality as it relates to case content and learner performance. Facilitators use this time to create a supportive environment with the intent of promoting psychological safety. It is important to establish this intentionality as there are learners who may never feel safe despite the best conditions for learning. Stating "This is a safe environment" should be done with caution or even avoided. Rather, "Our intent is to create a safe and supportive environment for learning, meaning you are free to be yourselves without fear of consequence" is an example of a statement that captures the spirit of the intent to promote psychological safety. To aid in the creation of a supportive environment, facilitators and learners alike should maintain a mental stance of human nature. In simulation, the Basic Assumption™ refers to this stance where facilitators state "Everyone participating in this simulation is intelligent, capable, cares about doing their best and wants to improve."[15] Holding learners in positive regard further enhances the supportive learning environment. Developing this mental stance is cathartic and challenges you to go beyond the Basic Assumption™ forming a core belief that respects individuals, welcomes diversity (of people and experience), and trusts that learners want to improve, which primes learners and facilitators alike for simulation and debriefing.

## DEBRIEFING SIMULATED DISASTERS

Simulation is a learner-centered approach to education and in the same vein, debriefing is learner centered with a calculated balance between team and individual performance. Simulation design is informed by the learning objectives or the desired results for the learning activity. It is important to clearly define the objectives and design of the simulation before implementation. These learning objectives can be cognitive, procedural, and nontechnical. The debrief connects the simulation experience to the objectives and allows facilitators to explore the thoughts that drove action during the simulation. Several debriefing models exist. The level of learner, experience of the facilitators, and goals of the simulation may guide which debriefing construct is used. Generally, there may be two situations in which disaster medicine providers may encounter the need for debriefing; after simulated experiences and after real-world responses. Whether simulated or real world, the goal is to improve and learn from the experience, and though that could also be a goal of the debriefing process or practice, the main goal of a critical or traumatic incident debrief is to recover from the experience.

There are multiple types of debriefing constructs and a variety of well-accepted tools and outlines to guide the process. Experienced debriefers may be facile enough to switch between styles based on the situation; there are, however, common elements to the debriefing process that should be followed. Prior to beginning the debrief, the facilitator will announce, "The simulation has ended, we will now debrief the simulation." This defined break in the action helps the learners shift their focus and mentally prepare for the debriefing phase of simulation. The debrief may occur in the same room as the simulation or in a defined debriefing space. Separating learners from the simulation suite may help ease tension and will allow simulation technicians to reset for the next case.[16] The facilitator then sets expectations for the duration of the debrief and the ground rules for debriefing and reestablishes learners' mental stance. In terms of ground rules, it is important for learners to speak for themselves using "I" statements and to be respectful as learners may share personal reflections of the event. Facilitators are encouraged to allow time for reflection to identify emotions that were elicited during the event and to clarify what happened during the simulation by providing a succinct synopsis. This summary helps demystify the simulation as some learners may have perceived the event from a different lens. There is a paucity of empirical evidence that suggests which is the best debriefing strategy for each situation. Regardless of the strategy, facilitators must approach debriefing with curiosity and through a lens that holds the learners in high regard. To focus the facilitator, the "Plus/Delta" or +/Δ is a tool where the facilitator uses two columns to take field notes during the simulation. The + side features successes in the simulation, and the Δ column denotes areas for improvement. The observations serve as launching points for conversations. Simulations, especially disaster simulations often elicit significant emotional reactions. It is important to reflect and acknowledge emotions prior to continuing a debrief. Multiphase debriefing constructs such as Debriefing with Good Judgment (Reaction, Analysis, Summary) and GAS (Gather, Analyze, Summarize) ask learners to share their emotions, reactions, and analysis of events.[15,16] Both constructs allow learners space to reflect on the simulation, seeking initial reactions and gathering feedback on the event. In the second phase, an analysis of the reactions seeks to understand what led to the actions seen in the simulation. Finally, in the summative phase, facilitators connect outcomes to objectives and outline the lessons learned in the simulation.

Facilitating debriefs can be intimidating and complex. Learner reactions, knowledge and experience level can play roles during the debrief. To lessen the cognitive load on the facilitator, the use of a structured debriefing process is recommended. Promoting Excellence and Reflective Learning in Simulation (PEARLS) is a blended multiphase approach that uses plus/delta in combination with reaction, description, analysis, and summary (Table 3.1).[17]

PEARLS uses the Advocacy/Inquiry (A/I) conversational technique to explore the "frames" of the learner. Frames are the lived experiences, knowledge, thoughts, and essence that comprise learners as humans. In this concept, it is believed that frames guide the actions that lead to results. Using A/I a facilitator can gain a better understanding of why the learner acted or communicated as was observed in the simulation. Through debriefing, frames can be supported or altered. Using the A/I approach, the facilitator advocates for their point of view and provides a rationale before asking the learner their thoughts. An example of this conversational method is "I noticed you continued to care for the contaminated patient without donning personal protective equipment. I suggest wearing gloves, eye protection, and a respirator before caring for these patients. I'm concerned because you may become a second victim and if injured, you will not be able to care for those in need. What was on your mind as you cared for that patient?" A/I promotes psychological safety by adding transparency to the exchange between facilitator and learner. The learner is not left in limbo wondering what the facilitator is expecting for an answer; rather, they receive an upfront assessment from the facilitator with an opportunity to share how they arrived at their thought process (frame). The opposite, less-supportive question is "What was wrong with your assessment and care of the patient?" This line of

**Table 3.1** The structure of PEARLS

| | **Objective** | **Task** | **Sample** |
|---|---|---|---|
| Set the stage | Create a supportive/ safe context | State the goal of debriefing and articulate your mental stance | "We will spend the next 20 minutes debriefing the case. As a reminder, please speak with 'I' sentences and remember everyone is trying their best." |
| Reactions | Explore feelings | Solicit reactions | "How are you feeling right now?" "Take a minute to reflect on the simulation and how you feel." |
| Descriptions | Clarify facts | Develop a shared mental model | Ask for a succinct synopsis of the case |
| Analysis | Explore performance domains | Decision-making, technical and nontechnical skills | Use Advocacy/Inquiry |
| Application/ summary | Identify takeaways | Learner and instructor centered | What are some takeaways? The key learning points are ... |

questioning places the learner in a defensive position, rather than adding to their learning; the learner questions "What is the right answer, what does the instructor want me to say?" In the final stage of PEARLS, facilitators identify key takeaways from the debriefing. These can be shared by the learners; in addition, the facilitator can directly state the key learning points.

## DEBRIEFING REAL-LIFE INCIDENTS: CRITICAL INCIDENT STRESS DEBRIEFING

The most used approach to debriefing is the CISD method published in 1983 by Dr. Mitchell. Though this is the best-known approach, it is worth noting that the literature is controversial regarding its efficacy.[18–20] Although there is not unanimous acceptance of the process, attempts made to cohesively approach debriefing have failed to garner widespread approval by medical societies. CISD is a facilitator-led approach to enable participants to review the facts, thoughts, impressions, and reactions after a critical incident. Its main aim is to reduce stress and accelerate normal recovery after a traumatic event by stimulating group cohesion and empathy. Because CISD is the most used type of cognitive debriefing, a summary is provided here.

The objectives of CISD are:

1. Mitigate the impact of a traumatic incident
2. Facilitate normal recovery process and offer adaptive functions in psychologically healthy people who are distressed by an unusually disturbing event
3. Screen and identify members who might benefit from additional support services or a referral for professional care[21]

A brief overview of the seven steps of CISD follows.

### Introduction

- Team members introduce themselves and describe the process.
- Create outline, guideline, and what to expect during the CISD.
- Invite and motivate the participants to engage actively in the process.

### Facts

- Only brief overviews of the facts are requested. Excessive detail is discouraged.
- Serves as an introduction to the event.
- The usual question is, "Can you give our team a brief overview of what happened in the situation?"

### Thoughts

- The thought phase is a transition from the cognitive domain toward the affective domain. It is easier for people to speak of their thoughts than to focus immediately on the most painful aspects of an event.
- The typical question in this phase is, "What was your first thought or your most prominent thought once you realized you were thinking?"

### Reactions

- The reaction phase is the heart of a critical incident stress debriefing.
- Comprises the affective or emotional domain.
- Focus on the impact of the event on the participants.
- The trigger question is, "What is the worst thing about this event for you personally?"

### Symptoms

- Ask "How has this tragic experience shown up in your life?" or "What cognitive, physical, emotional, or behavioral symptoms have you been dealing with since this event?"

**Teaching**
- Normalize the symptoms brought up by participants.
- Provide explanations of the participants' reactions.
- Provide stress management information.

**Reentry**
- The participants may ask questions or make final statements, provide a summary.
- Final explanations, information, action directives, guidance, and thoughts are presented to the group.
- Provide follow-up opportunities.[22,23]

## DEFINING THE RECOMMENDED APPROACH TOWARD DEBRIEFING

Many debriefing models are focused on a technical debrief, otherwise known as a "hotwash." A technical debrief is solution oriented and focuses on the honest facts of the event. There are psychological, emotional, and cognitive aspects of an event may benefit from debriefing as well. The term preferred to describe the psychosocial and emotional debrief is conceptual debrief. It is important to distinguish between these two types of debriefs because it is important to establish a clear objective and goal for each debriefing session.

A technical debrief is characteristic of:

- Short, succinct, goal-oriented session
- Based on factual, objective information
- Occurs directly after event
- Goal to mitigate, adapt, improve, and learn

A conceptual debrief is characterized by the following:

- Occurs 48–72 hours after event
- Concentrates on emotional and psychological well-being
- Mental health professional could be available
- Goal is to focus on recovery

## RECOMMENDATIONS FOR DEBRIEFING

For the purposes of real-life events, it is recommended, based on the literature, to practice a multistep approach for debriefing that is reflective of the situation. It is recommended to use a combined technical and conceptual approach to debriefing with the dual focus of learning from the event and speeding recovery as both response performance and the recovery of those involved are critically important.

Similar to simulated learning it is important to establish a safe zone for both learning, and for sharing difficulties, emotions, thoughts, and concerns.[24] Maintaining the Basic Assumption™ helps promote a safe zone for debriefing. Further, this concept that every team member is always trying their best, is also an essential part of effectively functioning in a high-stress environment that involves working as a team.

Initial technical debriefing can be focused on how not to repeat efforts that did not meet expectations. The technicalities and logistics of the efforts for the event that day should be addressed and corrected in situ and in real time so as not to repeat efforts that did not function effectively. This activity is the primary goal of the technical debrief.

The preference is to open the entire debriefing process with a statement that connects a technical and conceptual debrief. This could be "How did that feel?" This helps to validate the initial emotional response and encourage open discussion which, in turn, can defuse some of the emotional complexity of being in a stressful or traumatic situation, whether simulated or real. An alternative opening to the debriefing process can include a check-in question such as, "How are you doing?" The initial emotional check-in is also tied with the idea of establishing a safe zone for sharing and the idea of participants feeling comfortable with participation.

Next, open-ended questions such as "What went well today? What could be better? How do we improve this?" can help facilitate open discussion. Plus-Delta approach as previously described is an adaptation of the US Army's After-Action Review.[25] It is meant to be a succinct and straightforward approach that addresses the need for change and review, while also recognizing the positive aspects of the experience.

A facilitator will ask these questions of the team. The objective of asking these questions is to focus on improvement and learning. The technical debrief can be brief or last up to an hour but should be focused and solution oriented. The technical debrief should occur directly after or even during the event. A conceptual debriefing will concentrate on the psychological and emotional well-being of the responders.[26]

The literature regarding the clinical benefit for psychological debriefing is controversial and not all positive.[21–23] There are also certain limitations related to psychological debriefing.[24] It is also very important to remember the purpose of psychological debriefing – namely to support successful processing of the event by responders.

Several components of a successful debriefing are widely agreed upon. First, the participants should always be peers, and the group should be limited to only those who actively participated in the event. In addition, the research underscores the importance of ongoing support. The psychological debriefing is not meant to be a single-session debriefing without further check-ins. Psychological debriefing is meant to be just one prong of a comprehensive approach to managing psychological stress.

Though research does not show an improvement in the symptoms of PTSD in the long term, one interesting aspect regarding the data is that there was a positive impact in the short-term recovery of participants and their symptomatology on an immediate level.[18,26] This may have a positive impact on the ability of the disaster responder to recover enough to keep functioning which is valuable.

## CONCLUSION

Debriefing is a complex and highly debated topic. The most important aspects of debriefing are to design the debrief around the goals for the session, to take a multipronged approach, and to offer continued access to resources and support. Paramount in a successful debrief is the promotion of a supportive environment to reflect, learn, and share. The safe space is intended to be free of consequence where participants are asked to be themselves and to take risk as they reflect and the academic event or real-life disaster.

Although further research and practice on a combined and multipronged debriefing approach are required, debriefing serves a purpose both in the process of learning and improvement in skills and also in the process of recovery in disaster response. with a goal to assimilate knowledge and future events. Debriefing is a vulnerable time for learners and disaster participants. As a facilitator, respect the trust given to you by learners and disaster participants, lean in with curiosity, and maintain a core belief and Basic Assumption™ of your colleagues.

## REFERENCES


1. Lioce L, Lopreiato J, Anderson M, et al., eds.; Terminology and Concepts Working Group. *Healthcare Simulation Dictionary*. 3rd ed. Rockville, MD: Agency for Healthcare Research and Quality; 2025. AHRQ Publication No. 24-0077. www.ahrq.gov/patient-safety/resources/simulation/terms.html. Accessed April 7, 2025.
2. Marshall SLA. *Island Victory: The Battle of Kwajalein Atoll*. Lincoln: University of Nebraska Press; 1944.
3. Dyregrov A. Caring for helpers in disaster situations: psychological debriefing. *Disaster Manage*. 1989;2(1):25–30.
4. Armstrong K, O'Callahan W, Marmar CR. Debriefing Red Cross disaster personnel: the multiple stressor debriefing model. *J Trauma Stress*. 1991;4(4):581–593.
5. Arriaga AF, Szyld D, Pian-Smith MCM. Real-time debriefing after critical events: exploring the gap between principle and reality. *Anesthesiol Clin*. 2020 Dec;38(4):801–820. doi:10.1016/j.anclin.2020.08.003. Epub 2020 Oct 13. PMID: 33127029; PMCID: PMC7552980.
6. Seaman DF, Fellenz RA. *Effective Strategies for Teaching Adults*. Columbus, OH: Merrill; 1989.
7. Rall M, Manser T, Howard SK. Key elements of debriefing for simulator training. *Eur J Anaesthesiol*. 2000;17:516–517. doi:10.1046/j.1365-2346.2000.00724-1.x.
8. Gardner R. Introduction to debriefing. *Semin Perinatol*. 2013 Jun;37(3):166–74. doi:10.1053/j.semperi.2013.02.008. PMID: 23721773.
9. Kolb DA. *Experiential Learning: Experience as the Source of Learning and Development*. Upper Saddle River, NJ: Pearson FT Press; 2014.
10. Fanning R, Gaba DM. The role of debriefing in simulation-based learning. *Simul Healthc*. 2007 Summer;2(2):115–125. doi:10.1097/SIH.0b013e3180315539.
11. Ursano RJ, Fullerton CS, Vance K, et al. Posttraumatic stress disorder and identification in disaster workers. *Am J Psychiatry*. 1999;156:353–359.
12. Elhadi M, Msherghi A, Elgzairi M, et al. The mental well-being of frontline physicians working in civil wars under coronavirus disease 2019 pandemic conditions. *Front Psychiatry*. 2021 Jan 14;11:598720. doi:10.3389/fpsyt.2020.598720. PMID: 33542695; PMCID: PMC7852461.
13. Chang J, Ray JM, Joseph D, Evans LV, Joseph M. Burnout and post-traumatic stress disorder symptoms among emergency medicine resident physicians during the COVID-19 pandemic. *West J Emerg Med*. 2022 Feb 28;23(2):251–257. doi:10.5811/westjem.2021.11.53186. PMID: 35302461; PMCID: PMC8967473.
14. Marco CA, Larkin GL, Feeser VR, Monti JE, Vearrier L; ACEP Ethics Committee. Post-traumatic stress and stress disorders during the COVID-19 pandemic: survey of emergency physicians. *J Am Coll Emerg Physicians Open*. 2020 Nov 2;1(6):1594–1601. doi:10.1002/emp2.12305. PMID: 33392568; PMCID: PMC7771764.
15. Rudolph JW, Simon R, Dufresne RL, Raemer DB. There's no such thing as "nonjudgmental" debriefing: a theory and method for debriefing with good judgment. *Simul Healthc*. 2006 Spring;1(1):49–55. doi:10.1097/01266021-200600110-00006. PMID: 19088574.
16. Phrampus P, O'Donnell J. Debriefing using a structured and supported approach. In: Levine A, DeMaria S, Schwartz A, Sim A, eds. *The Comprehensive Textbook of Healthcare Simulation*. New York: Springer; 2013:73–85.
17. Eppich W, Cheng A. Promoting Excellence and Reflective Learning in Simulation (PEARLS): development and rationale for a blended approach to healthcare simulation debriefing. *Simul Healthc*. 2015;10(2):106–115. doi:10.1097/SIH.0000000000000072.
18. Mitchell JT. When disaster strikes . . . the critical incident stress debriefing process. *JEMS*. 1983 Jan;8(1):36–39. PMID: 10258348.
19. Sawyer T, Deering S. Adaptation of the US Army's after-action review for simulation debriefing in healthcare. *Simul Healthc*. 2013 Dec; 8(6):388–397. doi:10.1097/SIH.0b013e31829ac85c.
20. Scott SD, Hirschinger LE, Cox KR, et al. The natural history of recovery for the healthcare provider "second victim" after adverse patient events. *Qual Saf Health Care*. 2009 Oct;18(5):325–330. doi:10.1136/qshc.2009.032870. PMID: 19812092.

21. Bisson JI, Jenkins PL, Alexander J, et al. Randomised controlled trial of psychological debriefing for victims of acute burn trauma. *Br J Psychiatry*. 1997 Jul;171:78–81.
22. Hobbs M, Mayou R, Harrison B, et al. A randomised controlled trial of psychological debriefing for victims of road traffic accidents. *BMJ*. 1996 Dec 7;313:1438–1439.
23. Rose S, Bisson J, Wessely S. *Psychological Debriefing for Preventing Post-Traumatic Stress Disorder*. Oxford: Update Software; 2002. Cochrane Library issue 2.
24. Wessely S, Deahl M. Psychological debriefing is a waste of time. *Br J Psychiatry*. 2003 Jul;183(1):12–14. doi:10.1192/bjp.183.1.12.
25. McFarlane AC. The longitudinal course of posttraumatic morbidity: the range of outcomes and their predictors. *J Nerv Ment Dis*. 1988 Jan;176:30–39.
26. Griffiths JA, Watts R. *The Kempsey and Grafton Bus Crashes: The Aftermath*. East Lismore, Australia: Instructional Design Solutions; 1992.

SECTION 2

# GEOPHYSICAL NATURAL DISASTERS

CASE 1

# Options for Delayed Extraction Following an Earthquake

Michael Weiner and C. Clare Charbonnet

DISASTER PRINCIPLES

- National disaster response
- Disaster Medical Assistance Teams (DMAT)
- National response framework
- Incident Command System (ICS) basics
- Crisis standards of care
- Medical surge capability
- Field operations and logistics
- Mass-casualty care in the field
- Field stabilization, treatment, and transport
- EMS disaster operations
- Search and rescue
- Structural collapse
- Earthquakes
- Crush syndrome

## 1. SCENARIO OVERVIEW

a. This is a standardized patient scenario with options for wound care/hemorrhage task trainer or mannequin based on desired complexity. It takes place at an apartment complex in a major metropolitan area in Southern California following a massive earthquake that occurred at 5:43 AM. There has been sweeping devastation to housing and infrastructure including local highways across ten counties.
b. Jackson Thompson is a 42-year-old male with a history of hypertension who lives on the second floor of a six-story apartment building that was not built to code. Mr. Thompson was sleeping when the apartment building collapsed during the event. A heavy structural steel girder is lying across his right thigh. He is lying prone on top of other debris on the floor, intermittently propping himself up on his arms.
c. Four hours after the building's collapse, search and rescue workers reach Mr. Thompson. He complains of severe pain in his RLE and lightheadedness. He is unable to move his RLE.
d. Learner(s) is/are physician member(s) of a 28-person Federal Emergency Management Agency (FEMA) Type 3 Urban Search and Rescue (USAR) task force. They are deployed in the area for search and rescue operations. In-hospital learners (e.g. medical students, residents, nursing students, etc.) can be paired with prehospital learners (e.g. paramedics, firefighters, etc.).

e. Learners should focus on situational awareness and medical care. Their first action on scene must be to express concern about scene safety. Their option for creating a safe scene is to verbalize that they, as the USAR team, are shoring up all hazards prior to attempting extrication. If this statement is not made out loud, then the first person who attempts extrication becomes a victim.
f. Learners can assume that other appropriate incident command assets are within earshot or can be hailed on the radio (including an on-scene incident commander and a transportation officer). They may also assume that once extrication and transport are initiated, that appropriate safe transport of the patient will occur.

## 2. TEACHING OBJECTIVES AND DISCUSSION POINTS

### Situational Awareness

a. Verbalize concern for scene safety.
b. Use appropriate PPE.
c. Establish roles for different people on scene including potentially establishing on-scene incident command.
d. Exhibit strong interpersonal communication with team members on scene.
e. Call for additional support rapidly including extrication and transportation personnel.
f. Provide routine situation updates to incident command.
g. Communicate with receiving facilities such as a casualty collection point, Disaster Medical Assistance Team field hospital, ED, etc.

### Clinical and Medical Management

a. Evaluate the patient's initial clinical stability in the context of anticipated prolonged extrication.
b. Demonstrate appropriate management of a crush victim including medically assisted extrication, hemorrhage control, crush syndrome prevention/treatment, irrigation and decontamination, and splinting.

## 3. SUPPLIES

a. Rubble including large "steel girder" to place on the prone patient's right leg
b. Audio of sounds from the scene (e.g. yelling, alarms, creaking structural elements, etc.)
c. PPE including gloves, facemask, eye protection, helmets, and high-visibility vests
d. Stethoscope
e. Sphygmomanometer
f. Pulse oximeter
g. Nasal end-tidal capnography sensor
h. Two-way radios
i. Glucometer
j. Monitor with 3-lead ECG (and preprinted 3-lead ECG that shows peaked T waves)
k. IV start kits
l. Normal saline (4 L) with IV tubing
m. Three 3 g IV syringes of calcium gluconate
n. Sodium bicarbonate (either three 50 mEq in one 50 mL ampule or 1 L bags of D5 with 150 mEq)
o. Regular insulin (10 units)
p. Dextrose 50% (two 25 g in one 50 mL ampule)
q. Any reasonable quantities of IV narcotics and IV antiemetics

r. Airway equipment
   i. Portable oxygen tank with nasal cannula, nonrebreather mask, and bag-valve mask
   ii. Laryngoscope and blade
   iii. Endotracheal tube with stylet and syringe
   iv. Rapid-sequence intubation (RSI) medications
   v. In-line end-tidal capnography
s. Wound care
   i. Tourniquet
   ii. Distilled water
   iii. Povidone-iodine
   iv. Alcohol wipes
   v. Suture material and instruments
   vi. Bandaging, gauze, elastic rolls, tape
   vii. Cravats, flexible splints, safety pins
   viii. Wound care/hemorrhage task trainer (if planning to have learners demonstrate local wound evaluation, tourniquet placement, medical assistance with extrication, or field amputation)
   ix. Optional: electrical bone saw or manual Gigli saw

## 4. MOULAGE

a. Standardized patient (or high-fidelity mannequin) trapped within the building has severe swelling and bruising on his right thigh. His clothing can be torn randomly and scattered with small amounts of blood and debris. If possible, his right leg distal to the steel girder should be cold.
b. Blood will simulate arterial bleeding that will occur from the patient's RLE that will occur once the patient is extricated.

## 5. IMAGES AND LABS

a. Three-lead ECG that shows peaked T waves

## 6. ACTORS AND THEIR ROLES

a. Patient: standardized patient, who may be supplemented by high-fidelity mannequin. Either of these options should be supplemented with a wound care/hemorrhage control task trainer.
b. Team leader: member of the medical response team who takes command of shoring up hazards on the scene, stabilizing the patient, extricating the patient, and coordinating transport for the patient.
c. Physician learners: team members performing stabilization.
d. EMS learners: team member performing stabilization
e. Optional EMS: a facilitator who is embedded in the scenario, prompting learners during the case
f. Receiving ED physician: a facilitator who receives report and prompts learners to perform any missed critical actions.

## 7. CRITICAL ACTIONS

a. Inquire about scene safety.
   i. Consider including unstable structural components requiring shoring before scene is safe. This may require involvement of an USAR technical specialist.

   ii. If the team fails to verbalize the need to shore up unsafe structural elements before a rescue attempt is made, the person attempting the rescue is pinned beneath additional falling rubble and becomes a victim.
   iii. Don appropriate PPE.
b. Obtain a history.
   i. Make contact and introduce team to patient.
   ii. Ascertain approximately how long the patient has been pinned.
c. Perform an exam.
   i. Perform complete physical exam to evaluate patient for traumatic injuries. Given location of girder, learners will ideally ask about pelvic stability.
   ii. Then perform a focused physical exam of RLE. Learners should ask questions to assess for limb ischemia, neurologic status, compartment syndrome, open or closed fractures, degloving, and arterial bleeding.
d. Assess for and manage life threats.
   i. Verbalize assessing patient's airway, breathing, circulation, disability, and exposure.
   ii. Place patient on the monitor.
   iii. Obtain a finger-stick blood glucose.
   iv. Manage crush syndrome (traumatic rhabdomyolysis, metabolic acidosis, hyperkalemia, dysrhythmias, and hypotension) through aggressive resuscitation and hyperkalemia cocktail.
      1. Learners should know or be taught that calcium's action on the myocardium lasts only 30–60 minutes. Therefore, redosing this medication may be necessary in prolonged extrications.
      2. Learners may want to use albuterol as a potassium shifter. If so, they should know or be taught that high doses (i.e. 10–20 mg) are needed to have any effect and will cause significant tachycardia.
e. Perform extrication versus amputation (with option for cardiac arrest)
   i. Scenario 1: extrication
      1. USAR technical specialist advises that safe extrication will require another 1-2.
      2. Provide initial patient stabilization, basic wound care, and management of crush syndrome. (If facilitators believe crush syndrome is not being adequately treated, they can proceed to scenario 2, in which patient decompensates and/or codes.)
      3. Perform right calf fasciotomies.
      4. Patient remains stable enough for extrication to proceed.
      5. With assistance from USAR technical specialist, extricate patient with stabilized limb.
      6. Once patient is extricated, right leg will hemorrhage from midthigh. Tourniquet must be placed.
      7. Consider antibiotics, analgesia, and tetanus prophylaxis.
   ii. Scenario 2: amputation
      1. USAR technical specialist advises that extrication from beneath the offending structural elements is not possible in the foreseeable future. (Alternatively, extrication is initiated but then learners are informed that patient has become unstable.)
      2. Consent patient for amputation.
      3. Intubate and then perform amputation (otherwise, call incident command to dispatch a surgeon and have learner assist).
   iii. Optional confounder: either of the scenarios with cardiac arrest from crush syndrome

1. Cardiac arrest will occur either after amputation or after release of limb from entrapment. Return of spontaneous circulation occurs only after administration of 6 grams of calcium gluconate and two 50 mL ampules of sodium bicarbonate.
2. If this confounder is used, supplies will need to include ACLS drugs.

f. Disposition patient
   i. Determine that patient should be evacuated to a trauma center. Facilitators can prompt learners about types of destinations and resources at each. Travel times are significant during disaster due to road damage or closure. Normal receiving hospitals may be damaged or on diversion.

## 8. TIMELINE WITH TRANSITION POINTS

### Time: Two Minutes – Prebrief

a. You are (a) physician member(s) of a standard Type 3 USAR team. You are located in Southern California. It's Tuesday morning in June. A magnitude 7.8 earthquake struck the area at 5:43 AM while most people were home asleep. There has been widespread damage to a lot of structures including lots of dense housing complexes and elevated highways. Rescue operations have been ongoing for most of the morning. It's now about 9:30 AM, and your team has been dispatched to an apartment complex that collapsed during the quake.
b. You are sweeping the complex when you hear someone calling for help from inside the rubble. As you scale the rubble, you see Mr. Jackson Thompson waving from within the flattened structure. He is alert and oriented, and he tells you he's in severe pain. Something has pinned his right leg and he cannot climb out to you.
c. Anticipated questions
   i. Shoring up the area to safely approach this patient?
      1. There will be experts from our USAR team who can make the approach safe and assist with an extrication if instructed to do so.
   ii. Transportation?
      1. Incident command has been setup one block over, where the fire chief is overseeing rescue of civilians from three neighboring buildings. A representative of the incident command staff will be available via radio.

### Time: Zero – Arrival on Scene

a. Summary of initial presentation: A middle-aged man is frantically waving and calling for help. He is visible between large pieces of debris near the outer perimeter of the flattened structure. He is alert, oriented, and obviously in severe pain. He tells you his right leg is pinned and he cannot crawl out.
b. Critical actions: scene safety. Order technical specialist to shore up area to ensure safe approach to patient. Verbalize donning PPE.

### Time: Two Minutes – Patient Contact and History

a. Standardized patient: "Oh man, I didn't think anyone would come. I'm Jackson, please help me. I'm in so much pain and my arms are so tired. My leg hurts so much."
b. HPI: Patient was asleep in bed when he felt the room shaking. He tried to get to into a doorway but the room collapsed around him before he could get that far.
c. PMH: HTN

d. PSH: appendectomy at age 16
e. Allergies: NKDA
f. Meds: losartan
g. Place patient on monitor.
   i. BP 100/60, HR 115, RR 18, $SpO_2$ 94%
   ii. If asked, FSBS 222 mg/dL

## Time: Two–Four Minutes – Physical Exam

a. Trauma primary: airway intact, symmetric bilateral breath sounds, cool dry skin with 4-second capillary refill and 1+ radial pulses. Moving both upper extremities and left lower extremity spontaneously. RLE pinned.
b. General: anxious and in severe pain. Dressed in pajama pants. Alert and oriented to person, place, time, and event.
c. Skin: pale, dry, with scattered abrasions and small lacerations on face and neck and exposed forearms.
d. HEENT: scattered abrasions on face, PERRL, EOMI, no proptosis, midface is stable, no oral trauma
e. Neck: no midline tenderness, no tracheal deviation, no crepitus
f. Chest: no clavicular or chest deformities or tenderness
g. Heart: tachycardia, regular, without murmurs or rubs or gallops
h. Lungs: symmetric bilateral breath sounds, no wheezing
i. Abdomen: soft, nontender, nondistended without ecchymoses
j. Pelvis: stable
k. Bilateral upper extremities and left lower extremity are without bony deformities or pulsatile bleeding.
l. RLE
   i. Severe tenderness at midthigh where leg is pinned beneath steel girder
   ii. Small amount of drying tacky blood on the side of the pajama pants at sight of girder. No pulsatile bleeding.
   iii. Angular deformity at midshaft of femur beneath the girder
   iv. Edema and markedly decreased sensation distal to pinned section
   v. If asked, very weak ankle plantar and dorsiflexion
   vi. If asked, no palpable dorsalis pedis pulse
   vii. If asked, firm calf compartments

## Time: 4–10 Minutes – Field Management

a. New VS: BP 95/68, HR 118, RR 20, $SpO_2$ 94%
b. Contact incident command on scene to coordinate emergency transport once patient is extricated.
c. Obtain peripheral IV access. Bolus at least 1 L NS immediately.
d. If they wish, learners can choose to analyze ECG morphology on monitor (or printed-out 3-lead ECG) to assess for hyperkalemia.
e. Treat crush syndrome with large volumes of IVF, repeated doses of calcium every 30–60 minutes, multiple ampules of bicarbonate or a bicarbonate infusion, as well as hyperkalemia doses of insulin and dextrose.
   i. New VS
      1. If appropriately resuscitated: BP 118/72, HR 105, RR 16, $SpO_2$ 95%
      2. If incompletely resuscitated: BP 88/58, HR 126, RR 24, $SpO_2$ 92%
f. Make the decision to extricate patient's pinned limb (including performing fasciotomies) or to perform the field amputation.

g. Scenario 1: extrication
   i. Advise team that this process will take one to two hours. Prompt them to consider what they need to do for this patient to keep him stable in the meantime and reduce likelihood of renal failure or fatal dysrhythmias.
   ii. Perform right calf fasciotomies. Provide appropriate analgesia and sedation.
   iii. Splint RLE in preparation for extrication.
   iv. If crush syndrome is inadequately managed, patient becomes unstable.
   v. Once extrication occurs, an arterial bleed is identified at sight of open femur fracture. Learners must place tourniquet promptly or patient becomes unstable.
   vi. Facilitator has option for patient to code following extrication regardless of resuscitation efforts.
   vii. Perform additional wound care as indicated as well as analgesia, antibiotics, tetanus.
h. Scenario 2: amputation
   i. Determine if learners will perform amputation or if they will contact incident command to dispatch a surgeon (who can arrive in 35 minutes).
   ii. Brief patient on situation. Consent for intubation and field amputation.
   iii. Perform RSI. Confirm tube placement with on-hand equipment.
   iv. Apply tourniquet and perform amputation.
   v. If crush syndrome is inadequately managed, patient can become unstable.
   vi. Facilitator has option for patient to code following extrication regardless of resuscitation efforts.
   vii. Additional wound care as indicated as well as analgesia, antibiotics, tetanus.

### Time: 10+ Minutes – Transport and Final Considerations

a. Choose disposition facility.
   i. Local hospitals are damaged but are able to take some patients following a discussion with on-scene providers.
   ii. The nearest facility is one to two hours away by ground and has a staffed and functioning emergency department with X-ray capability. It has very limited surgical and advanced imaging capabilities. It also does not have hemodialysis capabilities.
   iii. Surgery-capable and undamaged facility with dialysis is 3-4 hours away by ground.
   iv. The conversation should prompt learners to consider everything that this patient will require: advanced imaging, orthopedic surgery, acute care/trauma surgery, hemodialysis, and likely ICU depending on scenario.
b. Learners must give report to receiving facility.
   i. Facilitators acting as receiving ED physicians can prompt long-term thinking by asking what specialists the learners think should be consulted (e.g. nephrology for emergent dialysis, trauma surgery for fasciotomies, vascular for arterial repair, etc.).

## BIBLIOGRAPHY

Health and Medical Response System. *Response Teams Description Manual.* Washington, DC: US Department of Health and Human Services; 1999, May. www.odmt.org/docs/DMAT_OPS_NDMS.pdf. Accessed April 2, 2025.

Schultz CH, Schlesinger SA. Earthquakes. In: Koenig KL, Schultz CH, eds. *Koenig and Schultz's Disaster Medicine: Comprehensive Principles and Practices*, 2nd ed. New York: Cambridge University Press; 2016:642–660.

CASE 2

# Covered in Oil

## HAZMAT Injuries after a Refinery Collapse

Liam Porter

DISASTER PRINCIPLES

- Disaster Medical Assistance Teams (DMATs)
- Field operations and logistics
- Mass-casualty care in the field
- Field stabilization, treatment, and transport
- EMS disaster operations
- Earthquakes
- Information management/communications
- Organizational preparedness and resiliency
- Business continuity
- Hospital preparedness
- Decontamination in the field
- Structural collapse
- Chemical safety
- Decontamination

## 1. SCENARIO OVERVIEW

Four days ago, a 9.1 earthquake caused moderate to severe damage to a city's infrastructure. Your Disaster Medical Assistance Team (DMAT) was deployed and set up medical tents two days ago. You and the team have been treating patients and assisting with local Urban Search and Rescue operations when available. While you are working, you get word that a local petroleum refinery that was damaged in the initial earthquake has collapsed. The factory had been cleared of injured people yesterday, but a number of workers were on site today surveying the damage. During the collapse, several tanks containing gasoline and other petroleum products ruptured. The patients are coated in oil. They are approximately 15 minutes away. The vast majority are uninjured but require decontamination.

One patient develops pulmonary complications shortly after arrival. Initially his vitals will be normal but gradually he will become more tachypneic and hypoxic. If ordered, an X-ray will show pulmonary edema and congestion. Patient will gradually decompensate unless BiPAP or intubation is performed. He will require transport to a local hospital for stabilization and admission. All other patients will be uninjured and after decontamination, can be safely discharged or observed depending on the setup.

Learner(s) is/are a physician or team at the triage/emergency tent of a DMAT field hospital.

*Number of patients is flexible depending on participants. Minimum of two or three if possible. If large-scale event planned, mass casualty incident triage system can be incorporated.*

## 2. TEACHING OBJECTIVES AND DISCUSSION POINTS

**Clinical and Medical Management**

- Appropriate decontamination of patients exposed to hydrocarbons
- Appropriate management of patient with hydrocarbon skin exposure
- Appropriate management of pulmonary complications of hydrocarbon exposure

**Communication and Teamwork**

- Work as a team to appropriately manage a patient with hydrocarbon exposure
- Appropriate and timely discussion with receiving hospital for transfer

## 3. SUPPLIES

- IV fluids
- Blankets
- Standardized patient (SP) or mannequin with moulage described in the next section
- Airway management equipment (intubation equipment, BiPAP if available, NRB/NC) and meds
- Decontamination equipment and setup

## 4. MOULAGE

- Black or brown oily material applied to skin and clothes

## 5. IMAGES AND LABS

- Point-of-care (POC) labs using a commercial portable/handheld blood analysis system:
  - Sodium, potassium, calcium, chloride, total $CO_2$ or bicarbonate, glucose, BUN, creatinine
  - Hemoglobin, hematocrit
- Tests: ECG, CXR, and/or US

## 6. ACTORS

- Patients: mannequins or SPs
- Nurse: should be knowledgeable and helpful
- Airway mannequin for intubation

## 7. CRITICAL ACTIONS

- Identify contaminated patients that require decontamination prior to treatment
- Appropriately decontaminate patients prior to treatment
- Recognize and treat hydrocarbon exposure and complications
- Recognize that the patient requires inpatient care and transfer after stabilization

## 8. TIMELINE AND TRANSITION POINTS

### Time: Two Minutes – Prebrief

You are physician member(s) of a Type 1 DMAT field hospital team. It is four days after a severe earthquake caused significant damage to local infrastructure. You are seeing patients when several trucks pull up with people in the back. They appeared to be covered in some sort of substance. (One patient should be designated as developing pulmonary complications. All others will be skin exposed only.)

### Time: 0–10 Minutes

Patient arrives at field hospital triage/emergency tent, initial evaluation and decon.

VS initial (all patients): BP 140/80, HR 95, RR 18, $O_2$ sat 97% RA, T 37°C (temporal scan), ECG sinus tachycardia

- Summary of initial presentation: desired number of patients brought by personal vehicle after exposure. (Note: Simulation lead should determine the number of involved patients based upon local capacity and the goals of the simulation and number of participants.) They were conducting an inspection of a damaged oil refinery when the structure collapsed. Everyone was able to evacuate but many were exposed to oil products. They were brought here rapidly by other uninjured personnel. All patients are endorsing being covered in oil but have no other complaints. No/minimal past medical history.
- Initial intervention: All patients should undergo decontamination and all clothing removed. Appropriate PPE should be worn for decontamination.
- Next intervention: head-to-toe physical exam
- Physical exam
  - General: prior to decon, covered in oil. Appears anxious. A&O ×3
  - HEENT: atraumatic, pupils 4 mm and reactive
  - Neck: supple, normal ROM
  - Chest: lungs clear to auscultation bilaterally, no chest wall trauma or bruising
  - Heart: sinus tachycardia
  - Abdomen: normal
  - Extremities: normal
  - Skin: similar prior to decon, covered in oily substance. After, mildly wet from decon
  - Neuro: normal
- Nurse
  - Obtains IV access and directs decontamination process.
    - If examined or interventions ordered prior to decontamination or without PPE, states "He's covered in oil; don't you think we should get that off first?"

**Critical Actions**

- Identify that patients are contaminated and require decontamination
- Successful decontaminate patients prior to interventions (soap and water)
- Obtain history and perform physical exam

## Time: 2–10 Minutes – Transition Point 1

**Evaluation and Disposition of Uninjured/Minorly Injured Patients**

VS: BP 120/55, HR 75, RR 18, $O_2$ sat 97% RA

- Oil is removed from all patients.
- No other injuries are found (or minor wounds/MSK complaints can be tended to if a more involved situation is desired)
- All patients can be discharged or observed.
- All patients should receive teaching regarding exposure to hydrocarbons

**Critical Actions**
- Treatment of any other injuries
- Appropriate disposition for discharge or observation

## Time: 2–10 Minutes – Transition Point 2

**Deterioration of Pulmonary Complication Patient**

VS: BP 140/75, HR 120, RR 26, $O_2$ sat 86% RA, temp not rechecked. (Repeat vitals should be made available only after order to obtain.)

- Nurse can prompt participants if treating/examining other patients and do not notice.
  - "One of the patients seems to be having trouble breathing. Can you come take a look at him again?"
- Patient begins to steadily develop increased work of breathing and coughing.
  - Can complain, "Hey, I'm having a lot of trouble breathing"
- Orders: XR, ECG, POC labs
- Interventions: Place patient on oxygen, start IV (if not previously).

**Critical Actions**
- Recognize pulmonary complication of hydrocarbon exposure.
- Begin initial management of respiratory distress including oxygen and IV access.
- Obtain testing as available.
- Discuss ultimate disposition and begin process of arranging transport.

## Time: 10+ Minutes – Transition Point 3

**Airway Management and Transfer**

VS: BP 145/75, HR 135, RR 32, $O_2$ sat 86% on 100 NRB (lower if NC)

- Verbalize the need for airway management
  - Acute respiratory distress syndrome (ARDS)-like picture developing, worsening despite oxygen
- Decision to manage airway
  - BiPAP if available can be an option. Otherwise, intubation with rapid-sequence intubation.
  - Nurse will assist with medications.

- Transport: Local hospitals have been damaged but have limited capacity for critical patients.
    - Transport to the nearest hospital is approximately 20–40 minutes due to road conditions. EMS can be made available but will need to have physician advocate for priority.
    - Air transport is available. When discussing with receiving hospital, they will ask if you would like air transport.
- Nurse verbal cues
    - "We'll probably need to get the patient to a hospital. Should I call to arrange transport?"
- Receiving hospital physician (facilitator via radio or phone) verbal cues
    - "Has the patient been decontaminated?"
    - "Are you sure he needs to come to us? Can't you manage him for a little while until a bed is ready?" (If discussed before intubation).
    - When rationale for transfer is appropriately addressed: "He sounds pretty sick. Do you think he needs air transport?"

**Critical Actions**
- Verbalize the need for advanced management
- Discuss transfer and transport
- Radio/phone discussion with receiving facility

## 9. STIMULI

- Initial ECG: NSR, sinus tachycardia with more respiratory distress
- CXR: diffuse bilateral hazy infiltrates (ARDS)
- BMP: Table 2.1

**Table 2.1** BMP

| Parameter | Value | Comment |
|---|---|---|
| Hemoglobin | 14.0 | |
| Hematocrit | 42.0 | |
| Chemistries | | |
| Sodium | 141 | BUN:Cr > 20 with normal Cr signifies dehydration |
| Potassium | 4.2 | |
| Bicarbonate | 16 | |
| Chloride | 98 | |
| BUN | 20 | |
| Creatinine | 1.1 | |
| Calcium | 9.3 | |
| Glucose | 75 | |

## BIBLIOGRAPHY

Aguilera F, Méndez J, Pásaro E, Laffon B. Review on the effects of exposure to spilled oils on human health. *J Appl Toxicol.* 2010;30(4):291–301. doi:10.1002/jat.1521.

Curtis J, Metheny E, Sergent SR. Hydrocarbon toxicity. [Updated 2022 Jun 27]. In: *StatPearls* [Internet]. Treasure Island, FL: StatPearls Publishing; 2022 Jan-. www.ncbi.nlm.nih.gov/books/NBK499883/. Accessed March 31, 2025.

D'Andrea MA, Reddy GK. Crude oil spill exposure and human health risks. *J Occup Environ Med.* 2014;56(10):1029-1041. doi:10.1097/JOM.0000000000000217.

Rusiecki J, Alexander M, Schwartz EG, et al. The Deepwater Horizon Oil Spill Coast Guard Cohort study. *Occup Environ Med.* 2018;75(3):165–175. doi:10.1136/oemed-2017-104343.

CASE 3

# Crisis in Indonesia

## Navigating Volcanic Eruptions, Ash Clouds, and Lightning Storm Injuries

Natalie Moore and Lauren Bacon

DISASTER PRINCIPLES

- Clinical diagnosis and treatment
- Timing of medical and surgical interventions
- Scene safety and security in the field
- Crisis standards of care
- Disaster triage concepts
- Scarce resource allocation protocols
- International systems
- Nongovernmental organizations (NGOs)
- Displaced populations
- Medical surge capacity
- Field operations and logistics
- Mass-casualty care in the field
- Field disaster triage
- Field stabilization, treatment, and transport
- Disaster operations
- Volcanic eruptions
- Medical care for refugee populations

### 1. SCENARIO OVERVIEW

You arrive in Indonesia as a medical volunteer through a nongovernmental organization one week after a series of volcanic eruptions resulted in significant destruction and population displacement. Since the start of the volcanic eruptions, ash clouds have been seen hundreds of miles downwind from the volcano and significant ash on the roads has made them slippery and traveling conditions treacherous. This has also triggered a series of thunderstorms around the area. Your organization has deployed a field hospital to help care for victims of this disaster. Your security team feels the area that the field hospital has been constructed on is safe for medical volunteers. However, on day 1 of your deployment, as you are orienting to the clinic, the storms become worse with the presence of thunder and lightning. All of a sudden, you hear a loud strike outside the clinic where there are approximately 30 patients waiting to be triaged. You look out and see a tree on fire and a group of people on the ground unconscious. You wait for confirmation from your security lead that you may exit the field hospital and you rush out to start triaging and assessing the patients who have been affected by the lightning strike. As you run out you ask anyone who can get up and walk to get themselves to cover into the field hospital, effectively triaging those patients as the "walking wounded," which according to the Simple Triage and Rapid Treatment (START) system classifies them as "minor." You then note approximately six other patients who were unable to move and who you quickly assess. You see that three patients are noted to be awake and talking with normal mentation but have lower extremity wounds from falling and you decide to address them after patients who are not moving. Of the remaining three patients, one patient appears to have an arterial bleed from his leg and is responding to pain, has respirations at 32 breaths/minute, as well as a radial pulse but a carotid pulse at 130 bpm so you classify him as "immediate" and quickly place a tourniquet on his leg. The next patient you come across is unresponsive with minor bleeding to the posterior occiput, snoring respirations, and a palpable radial pulse. You reposition their airway and note that the posterior aspect of the patient's right shoulder is unusually prominent with the anterior aspect appearing flattened. You classify them as "immediate." The last patient you come across is unresponsive, apneic, and pulseless. You label them as "expectant" and then recall when you learned about the START triage system that contrary to most mass causality incidents, these patients should be treated first in a lightening event. You immediately start doing chest compressions and call for help. While continuing to do chest compressions, your team places the patient on a backboard and in a cervical collar and evacuates the patient to the ED in the field hospital. There, the patient requires ACLS for approximately five minutes and then has return of spontaneous circulation. Ultimately, the patient is found to have head and neck injury from blunt trauma from the fall as well as rhabdomyolysis. The patient will require transfer to a higher level of care. The other three patients are categorized as "urgent" and transported after the "immediate" patients.

## 2. TEACHING OBJECTIVES AND DISCUSSION POINTS

### Clinical and Medical Management

- Resuscitation of lightening victim
- Post-return of spontaneous circulation care

### Communication and Teamwork

- Importance of scene safety
- Triage in a mass casualty incident
- Unique aspects of mass casualty incident triage in a lightning strike
- Evacuation

## 3. SUPPLIES

- Monitor with defibrillator
- IV supplies
- Medications
- IV fluids
- Intubation supplies: endotracheal tube, stylet, bougie, blade and handle, suction, BVM
- Ventilator

## 4. MOULAGE

- Hematoma to posterior occiput
- Lichtenberg burn to RLE
- Superficial first-degree burn to midline pelvis from belt buckle
- Arterial bleed from leg

## 5. IMAGES AND LABS

- Initial rhythm strip: asystole
- ECG: sinus tachycardia, peaked T waves
- Labs
  - CBC: WBC: 15, Hgb: 13, hematocrit: 37, platelets: 220
  - BMP: Na: 138 K: 5.8 Cl: 108 $HCO_3$: 21 Cr 1.7 BUN: 60 glucose: 130
  - CK: 11 000
  - Troponin: 1.24
  - Urinalysis: >50 RBCs
- Chest X-ray: ET tube in correct position, No signs of acute lung pathology
- Your facility does not have access to a CT scanner.

## 6. ACTORS

- Patient: can be actor or mannequin
- Nurse: assists provider and executes orders
- Technician: assists team

## 7. CRITICAL ACTIONS

- Scene safety
- Determine initial patient to care for (reverse triage)
- Initiate ACLS and intubate the patient
- Identify head and neck injury
- Identify patient has rhabdomyolysis
- Transfer patient to higher level of care

## 8. TIMELINE AND TRANSITION POINTS

### Time: Zero

- Physical exam
  - General: unresponsive
  - Head: hematoma to posterior occiput
  - Neck and back: crepitus to midline cervical spine. No midline step-offs or signs of trauma of thoracic or lumbar spine
  - Lungs: no spontaneous respirations
  - Cardiac: no heart sounds, Lichtenberg burn on right upper chest wall
  - Abdomen: soft, nondistended
  - Skin
    - Lichtenberg burn to RLE
    - Superficial first-degree burn to midline pelvis (from belt buckle)
- Initial intervention
  - Place IV and start IV fluid bolus
  - Place on cardiac monitor with pads: patient in asystole
  - Continue CPR and ACLS
- Monitor: reveals asystole

**Critical Actions**

- Continue ACLS
- Intubate patient
- Place in C-spine precautions

### Time: Five Minutes – Transition Point 1

- Patient has return of spontaneous circulation but still is not breathing spontaneously above the ventilator.
- Physical exam
  - Vital signs: T: 96.2°F BP: 90/50 HR: 120 RR: 12 $SpO_2$: 95%
  - General: unresponsive
  - Head: hematoma to posterior occiput
  - Neck: C-collar in place, crepitus to midline cervical spine
  - Lungs: Patient is intubated on ventilator, no spontaneous respirations above ventilator
  - Cardiac: tachycardic, no murmur. Lichtenberg burn on right upper chest wall
  - Abdomen: soft, nondistended
  - Skin
    - Lichtenberg burn to RLE
    - Superficial first-degree burn to midline pelvis
  - Vascular: palpable radial, dorsalis pedis, and popliteal pulses bilaterally

### Time: 10 Minutes – Transition Point 2

- Patient begins to breath over ventilator
- Physical exam
  - Vital signs: T: 98.2°F BP: 105/60 HR: 95 RR: 22 $SpO_2$: 95%
  - General: mild agitation, starting to breathe over ventilator
  - Head: hematoma to posterior occiput
  - Neck: C-collar in place, crepitus to midline cervical spine
  - Lungs: Patient is intubated breathing above the ventilator at 22 breaths/minute
  - Cardiac: normal S1 S2 RRR no murmur. Lichtenberg burn on right upper chest wall
  - Abdomen: soft, nondistended
  - Skin
    - Lichtenberg burn to RLE
    - Superficial first-degree burn to midline pelvis
  - Vascular: 2+ radial, dorsalis pedis and popliteal pulses bilaterally
- Labs return
  - CBC: WBC: 15, Hgb: 13, hematocrit: 37, platelets: 220
  - BMP: Na: 138 K: 7.0 Cl: 108 $HCO_3$: 21 Cr 1.7 BUN: 60 glucose: 130
  - CK: 11 000
  - Troponin: 1.24
  - Urinalysis: >50 RBCs
- Chest X-ray: ET tube in correct position, No signs of acute lung pathology
- ECG: sinus tachycardia with peaked T waves

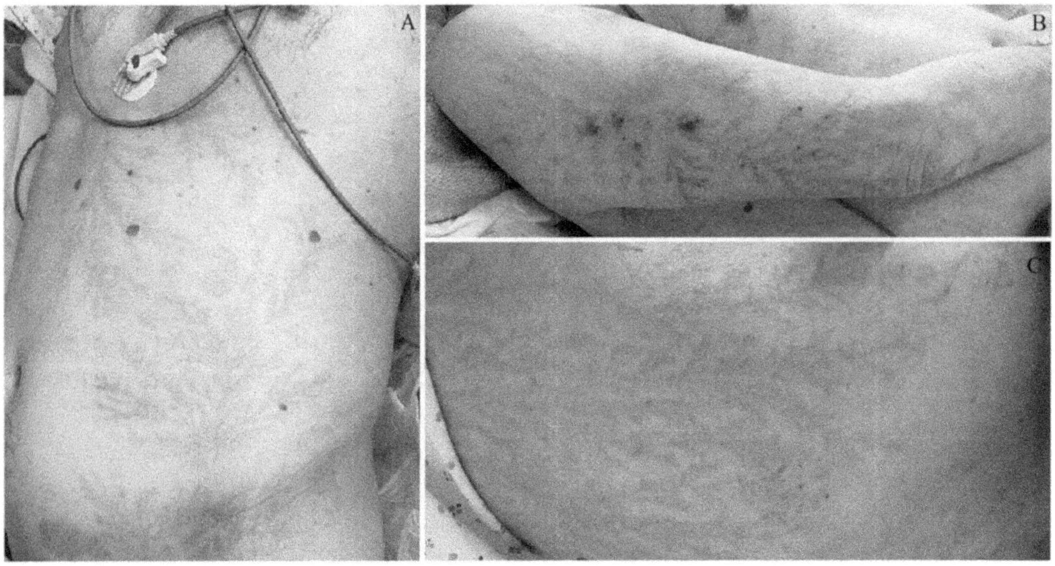


**Figure 3.1** Lichtenberg figures.
Reprinted from Legros, V., Floch, T., Leclercq-Rouget, M. et al. Lightning strike and Lichtenberg's figures. *Intensive Care Med* **49**, 1245–1246 (2023) with permission from Springer Nature.

## 9. STIMULI

When a human is struck by lightning, the electrical current can leave this common marking on the skin. It typically fades within 24–48 hours (Figure 3.1).

## BIBLIOGRAPHY

Ciottone GR, ed. *Ciottone's Disaster Medicine.* 2nd ed. Philadelphia: Elsevier; 2016.
Marx J, Hockberger R, Walls R, eds. *Rosen's Emergency Medicine.* 8th ed. Philadelphia: Elsevier; 2014.
Schmidhauser T, Azzola A. Lichtenberg figures. *N Engl J Med.* 2011 Dec 29;365(26):e49. doi:10.1056/NEJMicm1106008.

CASE 4

# Inhalational Injuries after Mount Kilauea Erupts

Natalie Moore, Lauren Bacon, and Andrew Milsten

DISASTER PRINCIPLES

- Scene safety and security in the field
- Clinical diagnosis and treatment
- Information management/communications
- Personal protective equipment
- Volcanic eruptions
- Personal preparedness
- EMS disaster operations
- Fireground safety
- Timing of medical and surgical interventions

## 1. SCENARIO OVERVIEW

You are working as an emergency physician at Hilo Medical Center, which is a level III trauma center in Hawaii. You receive a call that Mount Kilauea, one of the world's most active volcanoes located on the southeastern part of the island, has just erupted and there are at least 20 injured victims coming to the emergency department. The first patient to arrive is a 34-year-old male local volunteer firefighter who was one of the first responders on scene and, unfortunately, not in his PPE, including any respiratory protection. He managed to avoid the pyroclastic flow and any burns, but when rescuing civilians, he became trapped in a poorly ventilated house where he became overwhelmed by the volcanic ash clouds, which exacerbated his asthma. He also has a head injury likely from fragments of rocks and debris. His head CT is normal. He requires albuterol for an asthma exacerbation, but this quickly decompensates into him requiring intubation.

## 2. TEACHING OBJECTIVES AND DISCUSSION POINTS

### Clinical and Medical Management

- Discussion of inhalational injuries that can occur with volcanic eruptions
- Management of asthma exacerbation including when to proceed to invasive airway interventions and which pharmacological agents to use
- Management of a potentially difficult airway
- Management of head injuries

- Reassessment of airway in patients with inhalational injuries
- Postintubation care

**Communication and Teamwork**

- PPE for responders: N95 masks, eye wear, gloves, hard hats, boots, heat-resistant clothing for any first responders
- Discussion of how to activate your organization's disaster plan
- Discussion of local disaster resources that could be accessed and how to do that
- Deescalation of a worried family member

## 3. SUPPLIES

- IV supplies/fluids
- IV medications
- Nebulizer with albuterol

## 4. MOULAGE

- Hematoma and abrasion to posterior occiput
- Diaphoresis

## 5. IMAGES AND LABS

- Labs
  - CBC: WBC: 22, Hgb: 14, hematocrit: 41, platelets: 330
  - BMP: Na: 140 K: 5.6 Cl: 108 $HCO_3$: 23 Cr 1.4 BUN: 40 glucose: 140
- Head CT: no acute intracranial pathology
- CXR: no acute pathology
- ECG: sinus tachycardia at 150 bpm, no peaked T waves, no ST elevation, QTC normal

## 6. ACTORS

- Patient: can be actor or mannequin
- Nurse: assists provider and executes orders
- Respiratory therapist: can help with vent setting but is new on the job and unsure
- Mother: frantically asking if her son is okay

## 7. CRITICAL ACTIONS

- Identify and treat a potentially worsening respiratory situation due to a combination of inhalational injury and asthma exacerbation.
- Recognize and manage an asthma exacerbation with pharmacological interventions as there are escalating airway/oxygenation needs.
- CT head, primary and secondary surveys, and neurologic exam to assess extent of head injury.
- Continue to reassess posterior oropharynx for signs of swelling and edema (consider securing airway).
- Provide postintubation care and ventilator management.

## 8. TIMELINE AND TRANSITION POINTS

### Time: Zero

- Initial presentation
  - Physical exam
    - Vital signs: T: 98.1°F HR: 150 RR: 30 BP: 180/90 $SpO_2$: 92% on room air. Weight: 70 kg
    - General: 34-year-old male appears pale in moderate respiratory distress
    - HEENT: PEARRL, EOM intact, conjunctival injection, clear mucous discharge, sclera normal, posterior oropharynx has mild swelling, there is scattered evidence of soot to the airway, no burns noted to face.
    - Neck: supple
    - Lungs: diffuse expiratory wheezing. He speaks in broken sentences.
    - Cardiac: tachycardic, no murmur
    - Abdomen: soft, nontender abdomen, pelvis stable
    - Neuro: alert, oriented × 4, no cranial nerve deficits, 5/5 strength in all extremities
- Initial intervention
  - Place on cardiac monitor.
  - Place 18 G IVs, obtain labs and start IV fluids.
  - Acceptable supplemental oxygen interventions
    - Nasal cannula
    - Venti face mask
    - Nonrebreather
    - High-flow nasal cannula (HFNC)
    - Noninvasive positive pressure ventilation (NIPPV). Initial settings should aim for a tidal volume of 5–7 mL/kg with $FiO_2$ titrated to $SpO_2$ of >90%.
  - Pharmacological interventions that are acceptable
    - Albuterol nebulizer 2.5 mg q20 minutes × 3 or 5–20 mg run over 1 hour (continuous).
    - Ipratropium nebulizer 0.5–1.5 mg (with albuterol)
    - Magnesium sulfate 2 g IV once (over 20 minutes)
    - IV steroid.
  - Perform ECG (give to team)

#### Critical Actions

- Assess airway, breathing and circulation.
- Appropriate initial interventions for respiratory distress.
- Appropriate initial pharmacologic interventions for moderate asthma exacerbation, which includes bronchodilators and steroids, at a minimum.
- Appropriate initial oxygenation interventions for moderate asthma exacerbation.
- Discuss CT head imaging for a patient with a head injury but also tenuous respiratory status.

### Transition Point 1

- Vital signs: HR: 125 RR: 20 BP: 180/90 $SpO_2$: 85% on room air, 91% on supplemental oxygen.
  - Physical exam

- HEENT: PEARRL, EOM intact, conjunctival injection, clear mucous discharge, scleral normal, posterior oropharynx has mild swelling, there is scattered evidence of soot to the airway, no burns noted to face.
- Neck: supple
- Lungs: diffuse inspiratory and expiratory wheezing. His respiratory expiratory phase is prolonged. He speaks in broken phrases. He will not lie supine. He is sitting up with his hands on his thighs. He is using accessory muscles of respiration.
- Cardiac: tachycardic
- Abdomen: soft, nontender abdomen
- Neuro: He is not as responsive to questions. He seems confused and doesn't remember that he is in the hospital. He seems fatigued.

- Continued interventions
  - Acceptable supplemental oxygen interventions
    - Nonrebreather
    - HFNC
    - NIPPV. Initial settings should aim for a tidal volume of 5–7 mL/kg with $FiO_2$ titrated to $SpO_2$ of >90%.
    - Heliox. This agent has a lower density and may improve laminar flow when compared with plain oxygen. It is often used for respiratory support until other therapies take effect. Laminar flow decreases with increased oxygen content, so it is not appropriate for those requiring >30% $FiO_2$.
    - Intubation
  - Pharmacological interventions that are acceptable
    - Albuterol nebulizer 2.5 mg q20 minutes × 3 or 5–20 mg run over 1 hour (continuous)
    - Magnesium sulfate 2 g IV once (over 20 minutes), if not already given
    - IV steroid, if not already given
    - IM (Epi-Pen) or SQ epinephrine (1:1000 concentration, 0.01 mg/kg)
    - Consider IV terbutaline
- Patient will become progressively more confused and tired.
- If all appropriate medications and supplemental oxygenation interventions have been given, he will progress to Transition Point 2. If inadequate treatment has been provided, he will decompensate more quickly and go into cardiac arrest.
- Patient's mother comes in screaming frantically asking if son will be okay.

**Critical Actions**

- Update and try to deescalate his mother.
- Identify impending respiratory failure.
- Discuss how to approach a potentially difficult airway.

## Transition Point 2

- Vital signs: HR: 90 RR: 10 BP: 190/90 $SpO_2$: 75% on room air, 85% on supplemental oxygen.
  - Physical exam
    - Lungs: No breath sounds are audible. He will not lie supine. He is sitting up with his hands on his thighs. He is using accessory muscles of respiration.

- Cardiac: tachycardic
- Neuro: He is not responsive to questions. He is lethargic.

- Continued interventions
  - Acceptable supplemental oxygen interventions
    - NIPPV. Initial settings should aim for a tidal volume of 5–7 mL/kg with $FiO_2$ titrated to $SpO_2$ of >90%.
    - Intubation
  - Pharmacological interventions that are acceptable
    - Albuterol nebulizer 5–20 mg run over one hour (continuous).
    - Magnesium sulfate 2 g IV once (over 20 minutes), if not already given.
    - IV steroid, if not already given.
- Actions that will lead to a successful intubation by the team and stabilization of the patient. If these are not done, the patient rapidly decompensates and has a cardiac arrest.
  - Give an anxiolytic or ketamine prior to NIPPV.
  - Consider delayed sequence intubation with a dose of ketamine prior to intubating (if provider has experience with this procedure).
  - Use a large ETT.
  - **Avoid aggressive bag-mask ventilation.**
  - Plan for adequate sedation after intubation to ensure vent compliance and recognize that paralysis may be needed in some patients to ensure adequate ventilation.
- Intubation
  - Preoxygenate to >93% if possible. Asthmatic patients will have a rapid oxygen desaturation when performing rapid-sequence intubation (RSI), even with good preoxygenation.
  - Maintain the patient in an upright position during RSI and once they are unconscious, lay them supine for intubation.
  - Pretreat with albuterol.
  - Induction with ketamine (preferred) 1–1.5 mg/kg IV ketamine or 2 mg/kg IV propofol over two minutes.
  - Paralysis with 1.5–2 mg/kg succinylcholine given by IV push or rocuronium 1.2–1.5 mg/kg IV is used.
- Lactic acidosis. Prolonged beta agonist therapy may contribute to lactic acidosis, which can cause respiratory distress. Check repeated lactates.

**Critical Actions**

- Discuss RSI and pretreatment necessary for intubating an asthmatic patient.
- Discuss the correct medication choices for induction and paralysis.
- Discuss ventilator setting for the intubated asthmatic patient.

## Transition Point 3: Wrap-Up and Ventilator Management

- The goal of ventilator management in the intubated asthmatic patient is to maximize exhalation time (I:E of 1:3 or I:4), allow for lung deflation, minimize auto positive end-expiratory pressure (PEEP), and smaller tidal volumes.
- Initial tidal volume settings should be 6–8 mL/kg of predicted body weight; if plateau pressures are > 30 cm $H_2O$ tidal volume should be decreased to 4–5 mL/kg.

- Use lower PEEP settings 0–5 cm $H_2O$.
- Inspiratory flow rate: 80–120 L/minute
- Reduced respiratory rates will also allow longer exhalation times; initial recommended rates are 6–10 breaths per minute.
- The patient will need mechanical hypoventilation allowing "permissive" hypercapnia (pH around 7.2). One of the contraindications to this is CNS disease with increased intracranial pressure (in this scenario, the patient had head trauma. Faculty could allow the patient to have had a CT head or delete that part of the scenario).
- If the patient is fighting the ventilator, disconnect the ventilator, manually decompress the chest to facilitate exhalation and use a self-inflating bag with 100% oxygen.
- Hypotension could be from hypovolemia, air trapping (stop the positive-pressure ventilation, to permit exhalation of trapped air), or tension pneumothorax.

**Critical Actions**
- Proper ventilator management in the intubated asthmatic patient.
- Call to admit the patient to ICU.
- Consider transfer to a burn center because of the inhalational injury.

## 9. AUTHORS' NOTES

The inhalational effects of volcanic eruptions occur due to two separate phenomena, ash clouds and toxic gases.

**Ash Clouds**
- Ash clouds can travel hundreds of kilometers downwind from the active volcano and accumulate several meters in depth.
- There is very little research about the long-term respiratory effects of volcanic ash.
- Studies of eruptions at Soufriere Volcano in Montserrat and of the Mount St. Helens eruption, found a doubling of asthma and COPD exacerbations and bronchitis-related ED visits. There was no increase in the rate of pneumonia.
- If there is a high level of suspended particles in the ashfall, the number of ED visits for respiratory complaints was elevated for three weeks. This measurement (total suspended particles [TSP] is monitored and a level greater than 30 000 μg/m3, resulted in more ED visits).
- Rain dramatically decreases the TSP.
- Effective respiratory protection was achieved with an N95 or equivalent mask, but improvised cloth masks were ineffective.

**Volcanic Gases**
- The following gases are released: water vapor, carbon dioxide, sulfur dioxide (in large volumes). There are also smaller amounts of carbon monoxide, helium, hydrogen, hydrogen chloride, hydrogen fluoride and hydrogen sulfide.
- Hydrogen fluoride can cause an irritation of the respiratory tract.
- High concentrations of carbon dioxide (>20%–30%) can cause unconsciousness and death through asphyxiation. Since carbon dioxide is heavier than air, it collects in depressions or cellars in the affected area.

- Another dense gas that collects in low-lying areas is hydrogen sulfide. This gas smells like rotten eggs and causes eye and respiratory irritation, pulmonary edema, and death through cellular asphyxiation.
- Acid rain can occur after a volcano, when sulfur dioxide ($SO_2$) and nitrogen oxides ($NO_X$) react with water, oxygen, and other chemicals to form sulfuric and nitric acids.
- Inhaled toxic gases and acids can cause tracheobronchial burns, pulmonary edema, and acute respiratory distress syndrome.

## BIBLIOGRAPHY

Baxter PJ, Ing R, Falk H, et al. Mount St Helens eruptions, May 18 to June 12, 1980: an overview of the acute health impact. *JAMA.* 1981 Dec 4;246(22):2585–2589. PMID: 7029020.

Bergin CJ, Wilton S, Taylor MH, Locke M. Thoracic manifestations of inhalational injury caused by the Whakaari/White Island eruption. *J Med Imaging Radiat Oncol.* 2021 Jun;65(3):301–308. doi:10.1111/1754-9485.13159. Epub 2021 Feb 26. PMID: 33634571.

Bernstein RS, Baxter PJ, Falk H, et al. Immediate public health concerns and actions in volcanic eruptions: lessons from the Mount St. Helens eruptions, May 18–October 18, 1980. *Am J Public Health.* 1986 Mar;76(3 Suppl):25–37. doi:10.2105/ajph.76.suppl.25. PMID: 3946727; PMCID: PMC1651693.

Dianti J, Tisminetzky M, Ferreyro BL, et al. Association of PEEP and lung recruitment selection strategies with mortality in acute respiratory distress syndrome: a systematic review and network meta-analysis. *Am J Respir Crit Care Med.* 2022 Jun 1;205(11):1300–1310. doi:10.1164/rccm.202108-1972OC.

Gregory J. Chapter 102: volcanic eruption. In: Ciottone G, ed. *Ciottone's Disaster Medicine.* 3rd ed. Philadelphia: Elsevier; 2024:631–636.

Hodder R, Lougheed MD, FitzGerald JM, et al. Management of acute asthma in adults in the emergency department: assisted ventilation. *CMAJ.* 2010 Feb 23;182(3):265–272. doi:10.1503/cmaj.080073. Epub 2009 Nov 9.

Hurth KP, Jaworski A, Thomas KB, et al. The reemergence of ketamine for treatment in critically ill adults. *Crit Care Med.* 2020; 48:899–911.

Laher AE, Buchanan SK. Mechanically ventilating the severe asthmatic. *J Intensive Care Med.* 2018;33(9):491–501.

Lewis LM, Ferguson I, House SL, et al. Albuterol administration is commonly associated with increases in serum lactate in patients with asthma treated for acute exacerbation of asthma. *Chest.* 2014;145(1):53–59. doi:10.1378/chest.13-0930.

US Geological Survey. Respiratory effects. 2015. https://volcanoes.usgs.gov/volcanic_ash/respiratory_effects.html. Accessed March 31, 2025.

CASE 5

# Emergency Care in Volcanic Disasters

## A Case Study of Volcanic Burn Management after the Whakaari/White Island Eruption

Colleen M. Donovan, Emerson Franke, Paul Baker, and Michelle B. Locke

DISASTER PRINCIPLES

- Scene safety and security in the field
- Clinical diagnosis and treatment
- Information management/communications
- Field operations and logistics
- Disaster operations
- Crisis standards of care
- Disaster triage concepts
- Scarce resource allocation protocols
- Emergency operations plans for the healthcare environment
- Medical surge capacity
- Medical surge capability
- Mass-casualty incidents
- Mass-casualty care in the field
- Field disaster triage
- Decontamination
- Personal protective equipment (PPE)
- Burns
- Mass burn care
- Volcanic eruptions

### 1. SCENARIO OVERVIEW

The setting is a small community hospital in a Pacific Island tourist town. A nearby active strato-volcanic island is one of the biggest tourists draws and sources of income for the town. It is affectionately known as "the dramatic volcano" due to the near constant smoke plumes that can be seen from the town. The volcano is only 30 miles/48 kilometers from the port. It is a 90-minute boat ride or 20-minute helicopter ride from the port and there are multiple tours visiting the island daily. Volcanic activity had been rated at Alert Level 1 (minor volcanic unrest) for several years but was recently increased to Level 2 (moderate/heightened volcanic unrest, potential for eruption hazards) three weeks ago. The weather is mild, with partly cloudy skies, a high of 80°F/26°C, wind WSW 16 mph, 40% humidity, barometer 30 mmHg, visibility 12 miles.

The nearby community hospital is a 160-bed facility. The ED has 15 beds and two resuscitation bays. It is a weekday and the ED is staffed with two physicians and six nurses. The student learner teams are new to the ED, meaning that they are not totally familiar with hospital operations or polices yet. The student learners are not scheduled to work today, but just prior to the scenario and as part of the prebrief, they receive an emergency text message from the hospital. A mass casualty incident (MCI) has been declared by local authorities and the hospital disaster plan has been initiated. All off-duty healthcare professionals are ordered to report to the labor pool in the hospital cafeteria. Our participants are assigned to the ED to care for one of the incoming helicopter patients.

Participants are told that the nearby volcano erupted 60 minutes ago. On scene information provided to participants is at the faculty facilitator's discretion. The facilitator may use vague or inaccurate scene descriptions depending on the target audience. In reality, communications were confusing and unreliable, with initial reports of 0 to 100 incoming patients.

If the facilitator wishes to give more scene/rescue details, they may use the following:

- There were at least 50 tourists on the island.
- Initial communications from civilian boat and helicopter tourist companies who were on scene at the time of the eruption report that they are evacuating more than 30 people with severe burns and possible airway compromise.
- Rescue has been civilian only as conditions have been deemed too dangerous for new helicopters to fly (now Volcano Alert Level 4).
- Ten are dead on scene.
- At this time, one civilian helicopter has landed at the hospital helipad with five critically injured patients on board, who are currently being resuscitated in the ED.
- Two more civilian helicopters with a total of seven patients will be arriving imminently.
- Two tour boats are 10 minutes away from dock with a total of 28 passengers who have unknown injuries.
- Emergency medical services is staged at the dock to receive and triage patients.
- It is 10 minutes from the dock to the hospital.

John Doe Seven is male, appearing between 20–40 years old. He is initially able to answer minimal questions, including that he has no medical history. He can provide basic information but is in extreme pain. His tour guide reported that the sulfur odor was stronger than usual, and everyone donned their tour-issued gas masks (activated charcoal respirators) and helmets. While hiking away from the crater, the ground suddenly began to shake and the large white gas cloud turned black, shooting vertically into the air. In less than a minute, it became intensely hot, everything turned black, and the gas cloud rushed towards them as ash and rock rained down. He was able to seek shelter under a rocky outcropping. He was found by one of the helicopter pilots after shouting for help and was able to ambulate with some assistance to the helicopter. He was wearing a helmet, gas mask, torn short-sleeved T-shirt, and torn shorts with intact socks and boots.

John Doe Seven is the primary patient for the scenario. He should be considered for decontamination. The patient will have burns from the acidic pyroclastic density current (PDC) ash, requiring removal of clothes and copious irrigation. He will have multiple scattered abrasions and contusions from falling while running to seek cover. He will be slightly confused initially when he arrives at the ED; repetitive questions, delirium, memory loss, and will progress to unconsciousness. The team must treat his mental/airway status, his burns, and his hypovolemic shock.

## 2. TEACHING OBJECTIVES AND DISCUSSION POINTS

- Identify hazardous materials/contaminants that are part of a volcanic explosion
  - Ballistics (rocks, etc.)
  - PDC: Fast flowing, denser-than-air, superheated gas/ash cloud

- Lapilli (droplets of molten lava)
- Ash
- Magmatic asphyxiant gases
  - $H_2O$, $CO_2$, $SO_2$, $H_2S$, $NH_3$
- Acidic fluids
  - $H_2SO_4$, hydrohalic acids (HCl, HF, HBr, HI)

- Identify the possible injuries and medical complication of exposure
- Airway management for a severely burned trauma patient with altered mental status
  - Even patients without inhalation injury, but whose burn size is 40% or greater, should be intubated simply because progressive edema during the first 24–48 hours places the airway at risk (and makes intubation more difficult as time goes on). These patients may develop rapid airway obstruction soon after injury, or more insidiously during the first 24–48 hours post burn.
  - Anticipate a blood pressure drop during intubation induction in the catecholamine-depleted burn shock patient. Teams should be ready to pharmacologically support perfusion with push dose pressors.
  - ETT are difficult to secure as adhesives do not adhere to burned skin. Nonadhesive ET tube holders, including rudimentary umbilical ties, are recommended.
- Manage extensive burns
  - Fluid resuscitation
    - In prehospital and early hospital settings, it is appropriate to give 500 mL/hr for adults for a short period until an accurate weight and %TSBA can be calculated.
    - For adult patients with >20% TSBA burns, adjusted fluid calculations are recommended. The Modified Brooke formula (2 ml LR × kg × % TBSA second- and third-degree burns with half infused over the first 8 hours and the rest over the remaining 16 hours for a 24-hour total period) is preferred over the Parkland formula (4 ml LR × kg × % TBSA second- and third-degree burns with half infused over the first 8 hours and the rest over the remaining 16 hours), as the Parkland formula is known to result in excessive edema and over-resuscitation.
    - The modified Parkland formula now recommends 3 mL × kg × %TBSA due to risk of volume overload.
      - This said, volume resuscitation should be dictated by urine output and clinical response.
      - If initial resuscitation is delayed, the first half of the volume is given over the number of hours remaining in the first 8 hours post burn.
    - Close I/O measurements, foley. Urine output (UOP) is the most sensitive and reliable assessments of fluid resuscitation
      - Adults 0.5 mL/kg/hour (30–50 mL/hr, ideal body weight)
    - Upper extremities are preferred sites for IVs even if skin is burned due to risk of septic thrombophlebitis[9]
  - Burn wound care
    - Copious irrigation, consider warm water or saline
      - Dilute chlorhexidine gluconate or baby shampoo
      - Monitoring pH of effluent may provide quantitative measure for adequacy
    - Clean with surgical detergent if possible
    - Trim loose, nonviable skin, blisters >2 cm in size
    - Primary dressing: apply topical chemotherapeutic agent
      - Silver sulfadiazine (SSD 1%), bacitracin, triple antibiotic ointment, petroleum

            - HF acid burns (one of the rare exceptions of a direct neutralizing agent being used to acutely treat a chemical exposure): Topical calcium gluconate (1 amp in 100 gm of water-soluble lubricant or 2.5% calcium gluconate gel 3.5 gm mixed with 5 oz water-soluble lubricant).
        - Secondary dressing: loose mechanical dressing to hold primary dressing in place and absorb drainage.
        - In burn MCIs, teams need to think creatively about wound care as daily resources are consumed, such as using unconventional items like plastic wrap for dressings. The staff at Whakatane Hospital ran out of dressings and improvised by having team members get plastic wrap from local grocery stores.
        - Elevation of deep, circumferentially burned limbs
    - Pain control/analgesia
    - Close monitoring for hypothermia
    - Consider escharotomy, trunk or limbs
        - Indications
            - Full or deep partial thickness circumferential burn of limbs or trunk
            - Concern for compartment syndrome
            - Eschar present
            - On vent: Impaired ventilation with high vent pressures
            - Decreased pulse/$SpO_2$ in digits
        - Use electrocautery
- Anticipate an influx of additional patients
    - In a burn MCI, there is high risk for patient misidentification, as multiple patients will be unconscious due to injury or intubation and have similar injuries. Early history and identification are crucial, and this information should be physically attached to each patient.
- Prioritize staff self-care, including personal protective equipment (PPE) and debriefing

## 3. SUPPLIES

- Participant equipment (e.g. stethoscope, PPE including gloves, gowns, eye protection, N95 masks to prevent rescuer ash exposure)
- Mannequin clothing: short-sleeved T-shirt, shorts, boots (burned and charred), activated charcoal respirator (with patient, but not worn)
- Mannequin equipment (bedside monitor, etc.)
- 18 G IVs
- Oxygen delivery equipment: NRB mask, nasal cannula
- Medications: albuterol-ipratropium (nebulized), dexamethasone (IV), ketamine (IV/IM), lorazepam (IV/IM), SSD 1%, calcium gluconate (to be used topically), petroleum, rapid-sequence intubation (RSI) medications
- Wound care supplies including gauze, nonadherent dressings, tape, etc.
- Intubation equipment: Suction, bag-valve-mask, laryngoscope handles/blades, video laryngoscope with stylet, bougie, ETT size 6.5–8.0, 10 mL syringe, $EtCO_2$ monitor, adherent and non-adherent ETT holders

## 4. MOULAGE

- Several burns: Second-degree and third-degree burns to head and neck (5%; mouth and nose are spared due to gas mask), bilateral upper limbs including hands (right 9%, left 9%), abdomen

(5%), back (5%), buttocks (4%), bilateral lower limbs sparing bilateral thighs and feet (right 5%, left 5%): 47% TBSA
- Diffuse ash: Consider baby powder for ash on torso and clothing
- Scattered abrasions
- Hydrogen sulfide odor
  - Consider prank rotten egg spray, commercially available
- Noise pollution
  - Consider playing loud ED noises/screaming on a speaker. "Emergency response" sound effects may be found on various media streaming sites.

## 5. IMAGES AND LABS

- ECG: sinus tachycardia, but otherwise unremarkable
- CXR1: normal male (if ordered before intubation)
- CXR2: intubated male (if ordered after intubation)
- US: point of care testing (POCT) Extended Focused Assessment with Sonography for Trauma (EFAST), unremarkable
- Labs: POCT blood glucose, POCT ABG with lactate and whole blood chemistries/electrolytes, CBC-D, CMP, Mg, type and screen, coags, CPK, UA

## 6. ACTORS

- Mannequin: voice of the patient
- Nurse: at bedside, prompts for appropriate care
- Burn surgeon (optional: toxicologist/poison control/critical care physician): available via telephone, receives report, prompts for any missed critical actions

## 7. CRITICAL ACTIONS

- Perform H&P, including primary and secondary trauma surveys
- Identify need for exposure, decontamination, irrigation
- Initiate oxygen, IV fluids, and pain medications
- Prep for difficult airway and perform emergency intubation due to declining mental status
- Initiate pressor support for physiologic changes from intubation, burns, hypovolemic shock
- Calculate volume resuscitation for burns, modified Brooke formula preferred
- Consider causes of burns, including acid exposure like HF, and perform and/or describe appropriate burn wound care, including elevation of deep, circumferentially burned limbs
- Prevent hypothermia
- Obtain and interpret POCT, labs, imaging
- Give report to burn surgeon and disposition patient, transfer to burn center

## 8. TIMELINE

### Time: Two Minutes Before Simulation – Prebrief

The setting is a small community hospital in a Pacific Island tourist town. A nearby active stratovolcanic island is one of the biggest tourist draws and sources of income for the town.

The nearby community hospital is a 160-bed facility. The ED has 15 beds and two resuscitation bays. It is a weekday and the ED is staffed as usual with two physicians and six nurses.

You are a physician team that is new to the facility. You were not scheduled to work today but just received an emergency text message from the hospital. An MCI has been declared by local authorities and the hospital disaster plan has been initiated. All off-duty healthcare professionals are ordered to report to the labor pool in the hospital cafeteria.

We are now at the "labor pool."

The faculty facilitators should present either a vague or detailed scenario overview (see section 1).

You are assigned to the ED to care for one of the incoming helicopter patients. We have no additional patient information.

### Time: Zero to Four Minutes – Arrive at Bedside

VS: HR 120, BP 161/84, RR 24, $SPO_2$ 92% on room air, temp 98.4°F, wt: 70 kg

- Summary of initial presentation: male in T-shirt and shorts, crying/moaning in pain, in and out of consciousness but initially rousable to voice and able to give brief history. There is a strong sulfur odor.
- Initial interventions: Introduce the team, obtain history and physical exam
- Prehospital interventions: none. This was a civilian rescue.
    - History
        - As previously, given in short sentences
        - PMH: none, meds: none, allergies: none
    - Physical exam
        - Primary survey
            - Airway: phonating, mildly hoarse
            - Breathing: symmetric breath sounds bilaterally
            - Circulation: intact pulses, appropriate HR and BP
            - Disability: initial Glasgow Coma Scale (GCS) 14 (E3 V5 M6)
            - Exposure: diffuse severe burns with torn, singed clothing
        - Detailed relevant exam
            - General: semialert, burns 47% TSBA as in the skin exam findings (which follow), in severe painful
            - HEENT: normocephalic, facial burns (5%) with mouth/nose spared due to gas mask, no pooling of secretions, ash on face/hair, there is pharyngeal erythema, no pooling of secretions, trachea midline
            - Neck: supple
                - Team should apply C-collar for risk of traumatic injury
            - Chest: no burns, but ash on and under shirt (baby powder)
            - Cardiac: tachycardic, regular, no MGR
            - Respiratory: symmetric chest expansion, tachypnea, scattered wheeze/rales
            - Abdomen: soft, nondistended but with 5% burns as in the skin exam findings
            - Extremities: burns as in the skin exam findings, upper (9% bilaterally), lower (5% bilaterally)
            - Skin
                - Second-degree and third-degree burns to head and neck (5% – mouth and nose are spared due to gas mask), bilateral upper limbs including hands (right 9%, left 9%),

abdomen (5%), back (5%), buttocks (4%), bilateral lower limbs sparing bilateral thighs and feet (right 5%, left 5%): 47% TBSA

- Scattered abrasions

- Neuro: A&O ×3, strength and gross sensation intact and symmetric, anxious, agitated, in pain, repeating questions

- Nurse – verbal cues
  - "This is terrible! How do we even start helping him? Is he a trauma patient?"
    - Prompt for team organization, primary and secondary surveys
    - Prompt for C-spine protection
  - "What is all this white powder? Is it ash? It's getting all over my hands and scrubs."
    - Prompt for team PPE, decon/irrigation
  - "Looks at those burns! Is it his whole body? There's a lot of ash and debris stuck to him."
    - Prompt to start TBSA estimate, second prompt for decon/irrigation
  - "His arms are completely burned – can I put an IV here? What does the monitor show? Does he need oxygen?"
    - Prompt for large-bore IVs, upper extremities are preferred, even through burned skin
    - Prompt for interpretation of VS, supplemental $O_2$
  - "He's in extreme pain – do think we need to give him any medications? Or fluids?"
    - Prompt for pain control and fluid resuscitation, LR preferred
  - "What are your orders?"
    - Supplemental $O_2$
    - Initiate fluid resuscitation, LR preferred
    - Pain medications
    - POCT diagnostics (results available in next phase)
      - ➢ EFAST, ECG, CXR, blood glucose, ABG
    - Lab/imaging
      - ➢ Labs: CBC-D, CMP, Mg, type and screen, coags, CPK, UA
        - Labs pending, if requested
      - ➢ Imaging: trauma protocol CTs (pending)

**Critical Actions**

- Perform H&P, including primary trauma survey
- Identify need for exposure, decontamination, irrigation (vocalization is acceptable in this scenario)
- Initiate oxygen, IV fluids and pain medications
- Obtain POCT, including EFAST, ECG, CXR, blood glucose, ABG
- Order lab/imaging

## Time: Four to Six Minutes – Transition Point 1: Complete Secondary Survey, Clinically Worsening

VS: HR 135, BP 90/70, RR 30, $SPO_2$ 92% on room air, 98% on NRB

- No additional injuries found on secondary survey, other than minor abrasions
- Mental status worsening following secondary survey, moaning, not answering questions, GCS 6 (E1, V2, M3)

- Perform intubation with RSI
  - Team should anticipate inhalation injury and prepare for difficult intubation
  - Intubation is surprisingly uncomplicated, with only mild pharyngeal erythema and no laryngeal edema, likely due to the gas mask
  - Team will be unable to secure ET tube with tape, as it will not adhere to the burned facial skin. They will need to use or construct a nonadherent ETT holder (umbilical ties, etc.)
- Vent settings: low tidal volume (ARDSNet) settings are reasonable, given the following three conditions:
  - 100% $O_2$ until CO poising is ruled out
  - Escharotomy performed for chest eschar if indicated
  - If inhalation injury is a concern, consideration of high-frequency percussive ventilation.
- Initial fluid resuscitation and push dose pressors
  - If fluids and push dose pressors given prior to intubation with fluid resuscitation initiated, move to Transition Point 2.
    - ➢ Regardless of volume previously ordered, only ~200 mL have been administered
  - If hypotension NOT anticipated (e.g. fluids NOT bolused or push dose pressors NOT given prior to intubation), BP will drop to 70/40, due to increase intrathoracic pressure with positive pressure ventilation, decreased intravascular volume.
    - ➢ Team should address shock with additional IV fluids and pressor support.
    - ➢ Teams should optimize bolus infusion and consider pressor support.
    - ➢ Pressors often used to avoid fluid overload (preferred order: vasopressin > norepinephrine > epinephrine > phenylephrine).
- POCT results now available
  - EFAST, ECG, CXR, blood glucose, ABG
    - ➢ EFAST unremarkable
    - ➢ ECG sinus tachycardia
    - ➢ CXR currently normal
    - ➢ BG: 150 mg/dL
    - ➢ ABG: pH 7.17, $PO_2$ 96.7 mmHg, $PCO_2$ 31.5 mmHg, bicarb 9 mEq/L, sat 92%, carboxyhemoglobin 2%, lactate 9 mmol/L
    - ➢ Whole blood chemistries/electrolytes (if asked): Hgb 16mg/dL, hematocrit: 49%, Na138 mg/dL, K 5.2 mg/dL, Ca 3.3 mg/dL, glucose 150 mg/dL

- Nurse – verbal cues
  - "I'm wearing gloves, but I can still feel my skin tingling!" or "I'm wearing this surgical mask but I can still feel the ash at the back of my throat! Is there anything else to do?"
    - Second prompt for team PPE to minimize acidic ash exposure
    - Real-life teams initially used basic PPE: normal gloves and surgical masks. These precautions were then upgraded to double gloves and N95s when the teams were still symptomatic from the ash despite the basic PPE.
  - "He's a trauma patient, right? We did the ABCs, but should we check for other injuries?"
    - Prompt for secondary survey
  - "Doc – is he still responding? He's not really talking anymore . . . is he protecting his airway?"
    - Prompt for reeval, GCS, intubation
  - "Do we need to be careful with our RSI meds? I remember something about burns and paralytics . . ."
    - Prompt for RSI med consideration. Succinylcholine is probably acceptable for most burn patients prior to the 24-hour mark; however, this patient also has potential trauma and

unclear toxic gas exposures. It makes sense to avoid the nondepolarizing agent in case of hyperkalemia/rhabdomyolsis.

- "His BP is dropping . . . are we ok to push meds and intubate?"
    - Prompt to consider rapid bolus/pressure bags, pressor support just prior to intubating
- "What are your vent settings, doc? How about sedation/analgesia?"
    - Prompt for vent settings, ARDSNet recommendations are appropriate in early resuscitation
    - Prompt for post-RSI meds

**Critical Actions**

- Complete secondary trauma evaluation
- Recognize need for emergency intubation due to declining mental status
- Initiate pressor support for physiologic changes from intubation, burns, hypovolemic shock
- Interpret POCT

### Time: 6–10 Minutes – Transition Point 2 – Airway Established, Initiate Adjusted Fluid Resuscitation

VS: HR 125, BP 88/44 (without fluid, pressor support), HR: 110, 100/60 (with fluid, pressor support), on vent: RR 18, 98% on $FiO_2$ 100%, $EtCO_2$ 30 mmHg

- Calculate TBSA and use modified Brooke formula to calculate LR volume
    - 2 mL × kg × %TBSA, half in the first 8 hours, half over next 16 hours
        - 2 mL × 70 kg × 47% TBSA = 6580 mL over 24 hours, 3290 mL over first 8 hours, 3290 mL over next 16 hours
    - Team should subtract the volume already administered from the eight-hour total and divide over (eight hours – the time since the burn [two hours due to rescue/transport]), titrating to UOP 0.5–1 mL/kg/hr
        - If 1 L has already been given, 3290 mL–1000 mL = 2290 mL
        - Two hours have passed since the patient was burned: 8 hours – 2 hours = 6 hours
        - So resuscitative LR going forward should be
            - 2290 mL/6hr = 382 mL/hr for the next six hours
            - Then 3920 mL/16 hours = 205 mL/hr for 16 hours
    - If team uses Parkland formula, the total volume will result in twice the volume of the modified Brooke formula calculations: 4 mL × kg × %TBSA, half in the first 8 hours, half over next 16 hours
        - 4 mL × 70 kg × 47% TBSA = 13160 mL over 24 hours, 6580 mL over first 8 hours, 6580 mL over next 16 hours
    - Team should subtract the volume already administered from the eight-hour total and divide over (eight hours – the time since the burn [two hours due to rescue/transport]), titrating to UOP 0.5–1 mL/kg/hr
        - If 1 L has already been given, 6580 mL–1000 mL = 5580 mL
            - This is NOT double the modified Brooke calculation because the volume given in this resus is fixed at a given amount and not doubled
        - Two hours have passed since the patient was burned: eight hours – two hours = six hours
        - So resuscitative LR going forward would be:
            - 5580 mL/six hours = 930 mL/hr for the next six hours
            - Then 6 580 mL/16 hours = 411 mL/hr for 16 hours

    - There is no corrective action if the team decides to use the Parkland formula instead of the modified Brooke formula; however, this should be a focus point in the debrief, as many emergency physicians still default to the unmodified Parkland formula.
    - In burn MCIs, while awareness of fluid resuscitation formulae and output targets is an essential part of care, there is a role for limited/not overly aggressive immediate fluid resuscitation to preserve inventory. Over resuscitation can contribute to delayed onset limb ischemia and negative effects of burn swelling prior to transport to destination centers.
- Labs/imaging: not available yet
- Nurse – verbal cues
    - "This is awful – he's burned all over . . . it's not as bad as some of the others, but how bad is it?"
        - Prompt for best estimate of TSBA, may use Rule of Nines, Rule of Hands, or Lund–Browder diagram
    - "That's almost half his body – is there a way to figure out how to resuscitate this?"
        - Prompt for modified Brooke or Parkland formulas and initiation of fluid resuscitation
    - "That seems like a lot of fluid! How can we be sure we're not going to fluid overload him and make everything worse?"
        - Prompt to place urinary catheter and closely monitor UOP, aiming for 0.5–1 mL/kg/hr
    - If not already reviewed . . . "Doc – your POCT results are here"
        - Prompt to review EFAST, ECG, CXR, blood glucose, ABG
    - "Looks like K is up a little . . . why is the calcium so low?"
        - Prompt for recognition of hypocalcemia, concerning for HF burn/exposure

**Critical Actions**

- Calculate volume resuscitation, modified Brooke formula preferred
- Interpret POCT

### Time: 10+ Minutes – Transition Point 3 – Stabilization and Final Considerations

VS: HR 130, BP 88/44 (without appropriate resuscitation), HR: 100, 105/65 (with appropriate resuscitation), On vent: RR 18, 98% on $FiO_2$ 100%, $EtCO_2$ 30 mmHg

- Consider causes of burns
    - Ballistics (rocks, etc.)
    - PDC: fast flowing, denser-than-air, superheated gas/ash cloud
        - Lapilli (droplets of molten lava)
        - Ash
        - Magmatic asphyxiant gases
            - $H_2O$, $CO_2$, $SO_2$, $H_2S$, $NH_3$
        - Acidic fluids
            - $H_2SO_4$, HCl, HF, HBr, HI
        - Whakaari PDC: pH = 2
- Perform and/or describe appropriate burn wound care
    - Copious irrigation, consider warm water or saline
    - Clean with surgical detergent if possible
        - Cleaning agents include dilute chlorhexidine gluconate or baby shampoo
    - Trim loose, nonviable skin, blisters >2 cm in size
    - Primary dressing: Apply topical chemotherapeutic agent

        - SSD 1%, bacitracin, triple antibiotic ointment, petroleum
        - HF acid burns (one of the rare exceptions of a direct neutralizing agent being used to acutely treat a chemical exposure):
            - Topical calcium gluconate
                - 1 amp in 100 gm of water-soluble lubricant[1]
                - 2.5% calcium gluconate gel 3.5 gm mixed with 5 oz water-soluble lubricant.[9]
        - Secondary dressing: loose mechanical dressing to hold primary dressing in place and absorb drainage
            - If/when asked for, there are no more regular dressings, teams will have to improvise with what they have at hand
        - Elevation of burned limbs to limit impending swelling and subsequent effects
- Prevent hypothermia: warm fluids, blankets, patient warming systems
- Labs and imaging
    - Labs
        - CBC-D: WBC $18\times10^3$/dL, Hgb 16 mg/dL, hematocrit 49%, platelets 450, manual diff pending
        - CMP: Na 138 mg/dL, K 5.2 mg/dL, bicarb 9 mEq/L, chloride 108 mEq/L, BUN 22 mg/dL, creatinine 1.2 mg/dL, glucose 150 mg/dL, calcium 7.5 mg/dL, AST 44 units/L, ALT 50 units/L, AP 150 units/L, Tbili 1.5 mg/dL, protein 8.0 g/dL, albumin 3.0 g/dL
            - Concern for HF exposure
        - Mg: 1.5 mg/dL
        - Type and screen: pending
        - Coags: unremarkable
        - CPK: 550
        - UA: pending
    - Imaging: trauma protocol CTs
        - No traumatic injuries
        - CXR and CT images from Patient A and G from Bergin et al.[3] will be helpful in discussion, along with the comparison to Patient H.
- Call burn surgeon to discuss management and arrange for transfer.
    - In larger systems using formal Incident Command System/Structure, this information would be communicated with the medical unit/branch director, who would be in communication with consultant teams and assist in arranging the transfer. For this scenario, we will have a direct conversation between the care team and the burn surgeon.
    - Burn surgeon role can advise on management as described previously.
- Nurse – verbal cues
    - "This is awful – he's burned all over . . . what could have caused so much damage?"
        - Prompt for review of volcanic injury burn causes
    - "I've never had to do wound care like this – how can we dress these burns?"
        - Prompt for wound care
    - "Is the paralytic wearing off? It looks like he's shivering . . ."
        - Prompt to prevent hypothermia
        - Nondepolarizing agents like rocuronium have a duration of action of 30–90 minutes, so seeing shivering would be unlikely in this time frame, but we wanted a prompt to remind about hypothermia
    - "Doc – your labs and imaging are resulted."
        - Prompt to review labs and imaging
        - "Looks like K is up a little . . . why is the calcium so low?"
            - Additional clues for HF exposure

- "I'm not sure we have the resources to take care of him here . . . and I just got word that the two tour boats are pulling into port with 30 more patients, probably with similar injuries to this man. . . we're about to get hit, hard. Is there anyone we can hand this man off to?"
  - Prompt to discuss with higher level of care/burn surgeon
  - In a burn MCI, anticipate the need for patient distribution based on resources

**Critical Actions**

- Consider causes of burns
- Perform and/or describe appropriate burn wound care
- Prevent hypothermia
- Review diagnostic testing, concern for HF exposure
- Give report to burn surgeon and disposition patient, transfer to burn center

## 9. STIMULI

- Burn patient images. Consider referring to figures from Baker et al.[2] for examples.
- ECG: sinus tachycardia
- Normal male CXR
- Intubated male CXR. Consider referring to images from Bergin et al.[3] for examples.
- US: normal EFAST
- Optional: trauma CTs. Consider referring to images from Bergin et al.[3] for examples.
- Labs
  - CBC-D: WBC $18\times10^3$/dL, Hgb 16mg/dL, hematocrit 49%, platelets 450, manual diff pending
  - CMP: Na 138 mg/dL, K 5.2 mg/dL, bicarb 9 mEq/L, chloride 108 mEq/L, BUN 22 mg/dL, creatinine 1.2 mg/dL, glucose 15 0mg/dL, calcium 7. 5mg/dL, AST 44 units/L, ALT 50 units/L, AP 150 units/L, Tbili 1.5 mg/dL, protein 8.0 g/dL, albumin 3.0 g/dL
    - Concern for HF exposure
  - Mg: 1.5 mg/dL
  - Coags: unremarkable
  - CPK: 550
  - Type and screen, UA: pending
  - BG: 150 mg/dL
  - ABG: pH: 7.17, $PO_2$: 96.7 mmHg, $PCO_2$: 31.5 mmHg, bicarb: 9 mEq/L, sat 92%, carboxyhemoglobin 2%, lactate 9 mmol/L
  - Whole blood chemistries/electrolytes (if asked): Hgb 16 mg/dL, hematocrit 49%, Na 138 mg/dL, K 5.2 mg/dL, iCa 3.3 mg/dL, glucose 150 mg/dL[14]

## 10. CURVEBALLS: OPTIONS TO MAKE THE SCENARIO MORE COMPLEX

- Allergy to sulfa drugs: limits the sulfur containing topical medications that can be used, such as SSD (Silvadene)
- Third-degree burns with eschar on chest and/or arms, requiring emergent escharotomy
  - If adding escharotomy to the scenario, additional supplies will be needed, including electrocautery and an escharotomy task trainer.
- Delayed transfer to burn center: Discuss the plan for the next 24 hours for this patient.

  - Escharotomies will be required within next few hours, if patient not evacuated to tertiary center. Escharotomies are usually not performed during initial primary survey unless circumferential chest impairing ventilation.
- Pediatric patient: Due to extent of injuries, in can be differentiate adult versus teen pediatric patients. Implications for pediatric patients include the addition of maintenance fluid when caring for major pediatric burns (constant rate, not bolused and containing dextrose, etc.) and destination center may be different, depending upon local context.

## 11. AUTHORS' NOTE

This scenario is based on the Whakaari/White Island Disaster that occurred on December 9, 2019, in New Zealand, a Stage III burn disaster (local and regional systems overwhelmed, requiring national and international response).[1]

Although much has been documented about the scene rescue and medical care following transfer to tertiary centers, not much has been documented regarding the original receiving hospital and the experience of the on-shift medical staff. This scenario is dedicated to them, and to the victims, their families, the rescuers, and healthcare teams whose lives were forever changed on December 9, 2019.

The scenario is fictional, but it is constructed from documented first-hand accounts, media, and publications from the Whakaari eruption. We are awed by the efforts of local responders and hospital teams; and offer this scenario in the hopes that it may allow our colleagues in areas of volcanic activity to practice their skills before they need them.

This is a mannequin-based scenario. Please see the References section for more information on the Whakaari/White Island Disaster and potential reading/watching for participants.[2,3,4,7,10,12]

Special thanks to Tracey Perrett (Coordinator of the National Burn Service of New Zealand) and Colleen Bergin (Radiologist and Associate Professor, Anatomy with Medical Imaging, Department of Radiology Auckland Hospital, FMHS University of Auckland) for their first-person perspectives on this scenario.

## REFERENCES

1. Pham TN, Hollowed KA, Ahrenholz DH, Conlon KM, Carrougher GJ, eds. *Advanced Burn Life Support Course Provider Manual, 2018 Update*. Chicago: American Burn Association; 2018. http://ameriburn.org/wp-content/uploads/2019/08/2018-abls-providermanual.pdf. Accessed April 8, 2025.
2. Baker P, Locke M, Moazzam A, et al. Burn lessons learned from the Whakaari White Island volcanic eruption. *J Burn Care Res*. 2022;43(5):1105–1113. doi:10.1093/jbcr/irab246.
3. Bergin CJ, Wilton S, Taylor MH, Locke M. Thoracic manifestations of inhalational injury caused by the Whakaari/White Island eruption. *J Med Imaging Radiat Oncol*. 2021;65(3):301–308. doi:10.1111/1754-9485.13159.
4. Biddle D. Whakaari: bedlam at Whakatāne Hospital as worker describes eruption aftermath. Stuff. 2019, December 11. www.stuff.co.nz/national/118113442/whakaari-bedlam-at-whakatne-hospital-as-worker-describes-eruption-aftermath. Accessed April 8, 2025.
5. Cancio LC, Cancio JM. Initial management and resuscitation. In: Lee JO, ed. *Essential Burn Care for Non-Burn Specialists*. Cham: Springer International Publishing; 2023:113–143. doi:10.1007/978-3-031-28898-2_4.
6. Huson HB, Phelan HA. Chemical burns. In: Lee JO, ed. *Essential Burn Care for Non-Burn Specialists*. Cham: Springer International Publishing; 2023:285–300. doi:10.1007/978-3-031-28898-2_13.
7. Davisson J, DiCaprio L, Grazer B, et al. *The Volcano: Rescue from Whakaari*. [Motion Picture] Netflix. 2022. www.netflix.com/title/81410405. Accessed April 8, 2025.

8. Maj IR, Driscoll EA, Mann-Salinas NL, et al. *Burn Care (CPG ID: 12). Joint Trauma System Clinical Practice Guideline.* Fort Sam Houston, TX: Joint Trauma System, US Department of Defense; 2016. https://jts.health.mil/assets/docs/cpgs/Burn_Care_11_May_2016_ID12.pdf. Accessed April 7, 2025.
9. Mosier MJ, Sheridan RL, Heimbach DM. Emergency care of the burned patient. In: Auerbach PS, Cushing TA, Harris S, eds. *Auerbach's Wilderness Medicine.* 7th ed. Philadelphia: Elsevier; 2017:319–335.e2. doi:10.1016/B978–0-323-35942-9.00015-2.
10. Newton K. The day Whakaari/White Island erupted: a timeline of 9 December 2019. RNZ. 2019, December. https://shorthand.radionz.co.nz/White-Island-eruption-timeline/index.html. Accessed April 7, 2025.
11. South PJ, Ozhathil DK, El Ayadi A, Wolf SE. Burn wound management. In: Lee JO, ed. *Essential Burn Care for Non-Burn Specialists* Cham: Springer International Publishing; 2023:167–180. doi:10.1007/978-3-031-28898-2_6.
12. Sparkes L, Bernhardt A. *Survivors of White Island Disaster say they felt abandoned after eruption* [Video/DVD]. 60 Minutes Australia. 2020, November 1. www.youtube.com/watch?v = 5nGnXthjVgc. Accessed April 7, 2025.
13. Swan NA. Burn moulage made easy (and cheap). *J Burn Care Res.* 2013;34(4):e215–e220. doi:10.1097/BCR.0b013e3182721752.
14. Yeong E, Tung K, Chang C, Tsai S. The relationships between routine admission blood tests and burn size, and length of stay in intensive care unit. *J Formos Med Assoc.* 2022;121(12):2512–2519. doi:10.1016/j.jfma.2022.05.012.
15. Level 0: No volcanic unrest, Level 1: minor volcanic unrest, Level 2: moderate/heightened volcanic unrest, Level 3: minor volcanic eruption, Level 4: moderate volcanic eruption, Level 5: major volcanic eruption. NHC Toka Tū Ake; GNS Science.Volcanic alert levels. GeoNet. www.geonet.org.nz/about/volcano/val. Accessed April 7, 2025.

CASE 6

# Tsunami Survivor with Fever and Jaundice

## Pediatric Patient in a Refugee Clinic

Alexander Hart

DISASTER PRINCIPLES

- Crisis standards of care
- Scarce resource allocation protocols
- International systems
- Emergency medical teams and World Health Organization
- Nongovernmental organizations (NGO)
- Displaced populations
- Medical care for refugee populations
- Clinical diagnosis and treatment
- Climate change and disaster medicine
- Field operations and logistics
- Disaster operations
- Vulnerable populations

### 1. SCENARIO OVERVIEW

A 14-year-old boy with no past medical history presents to your refugee clinic three weeks after surviving a tsunami in Tanzania with daily fevers for the past week. His temperature is 104°F and he is restless. He also reports headaches, cough, myalgias, vomiting, diarrhea and over the past few days has begun to have jaundice. Brought to the clinic by his mother. No urinary symptoms, shortness of breath, rashes. Appears ill but not in distress. CXR shows no pneumonia, urinalysis shows no infection, basic metabolic panel and complete blood counts normal. Blood smear shows malarial parasites.

### 2. TEACHING OBJECTIVES AND DISCUSSION POINTS

a. Differential of fever in tropical endemic regions
b. Blood smear as the definitive diagnosis
c. Poor utility of other testing except to exclude alternative diagnoses
d. Natural course of malarial infection
e. Understand the importance of understanding local malaria species and resistance patterns
f. Understand that outbreaks of infectious diseases after disasters are typically due to endemic organisms and local disease knowledge is key to understanding likely infections.
g. Antimosquito interventions in endemic areas
h. Antimalarial drugs and the importance of completion of treatment course

## 3. SUPPLIES

a. IV start kit
b. IV fluids
c. Blood draw tubes
d. Syringes with medications

## 4. MOULAGE

a. Spray water on patient to simulate diaphoresis

## 5. IMAGES AND LABS

a. No imaging or ECGs
b. Labs
   i. CBC with hemoglobin of 8, hematocrit of 24, otherwise normal
   ii. Normal BMP
   iii. Liver function tests
      1. Total bilirubin 3.0
      2. ALT 190
      3. AST 160
      4. Alkaline phosphatase 100
   iv. Normal urinalysis
   v. Blood smear showing malarial parasites (*Plasmodium falciparum*)

## 6. ACTORS (CONFEDERATES) AND THEIR ROLES

a. Patient: actor, diaphoretic and ill appearing, but able to describe his symptoms
b. Mother: lacks medical knowledge, able only to describe symptoms, and asks repeatedly for antibiotics

## 7. CRITICAL ACTIONS

a. Obtain vital signs including temperature
b. Perform H&P
c. Draw blood smear
d. Prescribe appropriate antimalarial drug

## 8. TIMELINE WITH TRANSITION POINTS

### Time: Zero

a. VS: BP 120/80, HR 110, RR 18, T 104, $O_2$ 99% RA
b. If asks fingerstick glucose 90
c. If asks ECG sinus tachycardia without ischemia
d. Summary of initial presentation: A 14-year-old boy with no past medical history presents to the ED with his mother for intermittent daily fevers for the past week. He is a survivor of the recent tsunami three weeks ago and is living in the refugee camp by the lake. Patient is scratching

mosquito bites regularly. Mother mentions that a few other people in the camp are starting to develop fevers.

e. Physical exam
   i. General: He is nontoxic but looks fatigued and feverish.
   ii. HEENT: normal
   iii. Neck: supple, full ROM
   iv. Chest: clear to auscultation bilaterally
   v. Heart: mild tachycardia, regular rhythm, no extra heart sounds
   vi. Abdomen: soft, nontender, nondistended
   vii. Skin: diaphoresis, no cyanosis, no pallor, numerous mosquito bites
   viii. Neuro: cranial nerves, strength and sensation intact, A&O $\times 3$
f. Initial intervention:
   i. Blood drawn: sent to lab, but not immediately available
   ii. May ask for further testing: chest X-ray, urinalysis, other
   iii. IV placement
   iv. Further history from mother
   v. Antipyretics (acetaminophen or ibuprofen)
g. Patient: answers questions, not confused, but defers to mother on specifics (timing, focal symptoms)
h. Mother: concerned, states everything was fine until they moved to the refugee camp. Thinks he needs antibiotics. Able to answer questions directly.
i. Nurse: helpful and assists team with blood draw and IV placement. Tells participants that chest X-ray or urinalysis is "normal." Other tests not specified herein are "not available in this clinic."
   1. If team asks to consult infectious disease, nurse says "this is a post-tsunami refugee clinic, there are no consultants."

**Critical Actions**
- Obtain vital signs, obtain history from mother, perform physical exam

### Transition Point: Four Minutes – Labs Come Back

a. VS: BP 120/80, HR 95, RR 18, T 100°F, $O_2$ 100% RA
b. Patient says the fever and muscle aches feel better.
c. Physical exam
   i. General: Patient looks better and more energetic. Wipes off diaphoresis and does not return.
   ii. Able to tolerate PO
   iii. Rest of exam normal
   iv. Labs show mild anemia, moderate LFT abnormalities.
   v. If blood smear was asked for initially, it comes back showing two or more malarial parasites (*Plasmodium falciparum*).

**Critical Actions**
- Ask for blood smear if not asked for initially
- Diagnosis of malarial infection

### Transition Point: Six Minutes

a. VS: BP 120/80, HR 95, RR 18, T 100°F, $O_2$ 100% RA
b. Patient continues to feel better
c. Physical exam unchanged
d. Team must recognize malarial infection
e. Inform mother and patient of malarial infection
    i. Discuss ways to prevent mosquito bites. (Mother asks how to prevent from happening again if not prompted by team.)
        1. Mosquito nets
        2. Protective clothing
        3. Insect sprays (permethrin or DEET)
    ii. Prescribe antimalarial drug effective for treating *Plasmodium falciparum* malaria in a highly endemic area with known MDR malaria
        artemether + lumefantrine
        artesunate + amodiaquine
        artesunate + mefloquine
        dihydroartemisinin + piperaquine
        artesunate + sulfadoxine–pyrimethamine
f. Ensure that mother understands the importance of completing malaria treatment and reasons to return to the clinic

## 9. STIMULI

a. Lab results sheets
    i. CBC with hemoglobin of 10, hematocrit of 30, otherwise normal
    ii. Normal BMP
    iii. Liver function tests
        1. Total bilirubin 3.0
        2. ALT 190
        3. AST 160
        4. Alkaline phosphatase 100
    iv. Normal urinalysis
    v. Blood smear showing malarial parasites (*Plasmodium vivax*)

## BIBLIOGRAPHY

Cohee LM, Laufer MK. Malaria in children. *Pediatr Clin North Am.* 2017;64(4):851–866.

Fort GG. Malaria. In: Ferri FF, ed. *Ferri's Clinical Advisor.* 2023 ed. Elsevier; 2023:938–944.e1.

Severe Malaria Observatory. Tanzania malaria facts. www.severemalaria.org/countries/tanzania. Accessed March 31, 2025.

Woodford J, Shanks GD, Griffin P, Chalon S, McCarthy JS. The dynamics of liver function test abnormalities after malaria infection: a retrospective observational study. *Am J Trop Med Hyg.* 2018;98(4):1113–1119. doi:10.4269/AJTMH.17-0754.

World Health Organization. *Guidelines for Malaria.* Geneva: World Health Organization; 2024. www.who.int/publications/i/item/guidelines-for-malaria. Accessed March 31, 2025.

World Health Organization. Malaria. 2024. www.who.int/news-room/fact-sheets/detail/malaria. Accessed March 31, 2025.

CASE 7

# Severe Smoke Inhalation and Asthma Exacerbation after a Tsunami-Induced Fire

Alexander Hart

DISASTER PRINCIPLES

- Clinical diagnosis and treatment
- Climate change and disaster medicine
- Conventional standards of care
- Business continuity
- EMS disaster operations
- Fireground safety
- Asphyxiant agents
- Cyanide
- Timing of medical and surgical interventions
- Heat emergencies
- Technological disasters

## 1. SCENARIO OVERVIEW

A 45-year-old female with a history of asthma presents by EMS with cough, shortness of breath, headache, sore throat, and lightheadedness after a tsunami caused a fire at the local oil refinery. The patient works at the refinery and was exposed to smoke from the fire in a closed room. She is ill appearing and is wracked by paroxysms of cough and wheezing. She has soot in the mouth and nose. Chest X-ray has no obvious abnormalities. She has smoke inhalation injury with both upper and lower airway involvement. She decompensates and requires intubation for airway protection and ventilation.

## 2. TEACHING OBJECTIVES AND DISCUSSION POINTS

- Recognition of toxic smoke exposure/smoke inhalation injury
- Decision on need for intubation
- Check carboxyhemoglobin level
- Consider cyanide toxicity
- Ventilator management

## 3. SUPPLIES

- Mannequin
- Endotracheal tube

- Stylet
- Blade and handle for intubation
- Lubricant
- NC
- Ventimask
- Suction setup (tubing, yankour, +/- cannisters)
- Bag-valve-mask
- Backup airway (bougie, laryngeal mask airway, etc.)
- IV start kit
- IV fluids
- Syringes with medications
- Blood draw tubes
- Monitor/pulse oximetry
- Ventilator
- Optional: cricothyrotomy kit/mannequin

## 4. MOULAGE

- Black soot in nares and mouth of mannequin

## 5. IMAGES AND LABS

- Normal chest X-ray
- Repeat chest X-ray: normal with ETT or cricothyrotomy in place
- ECG: Sinus tachycardia
- Labs
    1. CBC (within normal limits)
    2. BMP (within normal limits)
    3. Carboxyhemoglobin level
    4. Hcg (negative)
    5. Lactate normal (may be measured as a surrogate for cyanide toxicity)

## 6. ACTORS (CONFEDERATES) AND THEIR ROLES

- Patient: intubation mannequin – soot on mouth and nares. Wheezing sounds. Initially able to speak in short sentences, but always interrupted by shortness of breath and/or coughing fits. Decompensates if not intubated.
- EMS: gives full history including enclosed space smoke inhalation. If asked, confirms that there was no visible plastic and no fire within the room. Patient does not have burn injuries.
- Nurse: draws blood, places IV, pushes medications, helpful to team.
- ICU consult (voice): discuss management with team, accept admission if all critical actions performed
- Respiratory therapist (optional): able to help with intubation by handing materials. Unable to set up equipment, needs help to manage ventilator settings. “I’m new.”

## 7. CRITICAL ACTIONS

- Recognize smoke inhalation injury
- Decision to control airway

- Rule out carboxyhemoglobinemia
- Low tidal volume ventilation (6–8 mL/kg)
- Admission to ICU

## 8. TIMELINE WITH TRANSITION POINTS

### Time: Zero

1. VS: BP 160/95, HR 115, RR 22, $O_2$ sat 92% on 2 L NC, T 98.6°F
2. Summary of initial presentation: A 45-year-old female with a history of asthma presents brought in by EMS with cough, shortness of breath, headache, sore throat, and lightheadedness after a tsunami caused a fire at the local oil refinery where she works. The patient was in a closed room where she was exposed to smoke. There was no fire in the room. Oxygen saturations were in the high 80s, so placed on NC by EMS.
3. Physical exam
   - General: anxious and in respiratory distress. Recurrent coughing fits interrupting sentences. Oriented ×3.
   - HEENT: soot in nares and oropharynx, no gross edema, no stridor. Pupils 3 mm equal/reactive
   - Neck: supple
   - Chest: wheezing, tachypnea
   - Heart: tachycardia, regular rhythm, no extra heart sounds
   - Abdomen: soft, nontender, nondistended
   - Skin: soot stains, NO burns, no cyanosis, no pallor
   - Neuro: cranial nerves, strength, sensation intact. Difficulty focusing due to focusing on breathing.
4. Initial intervention
   - IV placement
   - Draw bloodwork – especially carboxyhemoglobin
   - Place on cardiac monitor
   - Supplemental oxygen
   - Beta agonist nebulizer treatments
5. EMS: gives fuller story of the scene
6. Nurse: helpful and assists the team

**Critical Actions**
- Supplemental oxygen
- Cardiac monitor and $O_2$ saturations
- Recognize signs of smoke inhalation injury

### Time: Two Minutes – Transition Point 1

1. VS: BP 160/95, HR 125, RR 26, $O_2$ Sat 85% on 2 L NC (can increase to 90% if ventimask supplemental $O_2$ given), T 98.6°F
2. Chest X-ray if ordered: normal
3. Physical exam: increasing tachypnea, patient speaking in shorter and shorter sentences, increasing wheezing
4. Critical actions
   - Recognition of worsening respiratory status

- Decision to intubate
- Consent patient/explain intubation to patient
- Intubation setup (oxygen, call for appropriate medications, section, endotracheal tube, backup airway options)

5. Intubation
   - Nurse: pushes medications appropriately
   - Respiratory therapist: hands items to team and uses BVM appropriately, but then asks team their suggested ventilator settings
6. OPTIONAL: Team fails intubation and must proceed to cricothyrotomy
   - Patient becomes stridulous.
   - Respiratory therapist: I cannot ventilate the patient; the airway must be too tight.

**Critical Actions**

- Decision to proceed to cricothyrotomy
- Placement using cricothyrotomy kit

### Time: Eight Minutes – Transition Point 2 – Immediately after Intubation

1. VS: BP 120/80, HR 100, RR (per team's ventilator orders), $O_2$ sat 100% on ventilator, T 98.6°F
2. Postintubation chest X-ray: normal with ETT in good position
3. Physical exam: intubated, no distress, no movement if paralytic given, mild wheezing.

**Critical Actions**

- Ventilator management (6–8 mL/kg)
- Disposition to ICU

## 9. STIMULI

1. Chest X-ray 1: normal
2. Chest X-ray 2: normal with endotracheal tube or cricothyrotomy in place
3. Labs
   - CBC within normal limits
   - BMP: sodium 137, potassium 4.2, chloride 108, bicarbonate 20, BUN 15, creatinine 1.0, glucose 140, calcium 9.0
   - Carboxyhemoglobin level 7%

## BIBLIOGRAPHY

Campbell R. *Fires in Industrial and Manufacturing Properties.* Quincy, MA: National Fire Protection Association; 2016.

Hoek MR, Bracebridge S, Oliver I. Health impact of the Buncefield oil depot fire, December 2005: study of accident and emergency case records. *J Public Health (Oxf).* 2007;29(3):298–302. doi:10.1093/pubmed/fdm036.

Smollin C, Olson K. Carbon monoxide poisoning (acute). *BMJ Clin Evid.* 2010 Oct 12;2010:2103.

CASE 8

# Tsunami-Related Pulmonary Complications

## Respiratory Distress in an Internally Displaced Person

Jonathan Gammel

DISASTER PRINCIPLES

- Crisis standards of care
- Medical surge capacity
- Scarce resource allocation protocols
- International systems
- Emergency medical teams and World Health Organization
- Nongovernmental organizations (NGO)
- Displaced populations
- Medical care for refugee populations
- Clinical diagnosis and treatment
- Climate change and disaster medicine
- Field operations and logistics
- Disaster operations
- Vulnerable populations

### 1. SCENARIO OVERVIEW

A 66-year-old woman with a history of type 2 diabetes mellitus and hypertension is brought into the ED with shortness of breath, fever, and altered mental status. She is a survivor of a devastating tsunami that hit the coast of Indonesia 10 days ago. The team from a nearby internally displaced people (IDP) shelter bringing her in for evaluation tells you that she was swept up by the tsunami and nearly drowned. She survived and sought refuge at the shelter, which is crowded with limited resources and poor access to medical care. Since that time, she has developed progressive cough, fever, chills, and difficulty breathing. They have been unable to get her to the hospital until now due to destruction of roads and transportation systems, and she is now confused, febrile, and dyspneic. The patient is febrile to 102.2°F, hypotensive, tachycardic, hypoxic to 82% on room air, with increased work of breathing and decreased responsiveness. A chest X-ray reveals a significant pulmonary infiltrate in the right middle lobe with an air fluid level. Labs reveal significant leukocytosis and acute kidney injury. If chest CT is obtained it will reveal a pulmonary abscess in the right middle lobe. The patient is suffering from septic shock due to pneumonia and pulmonary abscess after aspirating tsunami water and ultimately will require intubation and admission to the ICU.

## 2. TEACHING OBJECTIVES AND DISCUSSION POINTS

1. Tsunami-associated aspiration pneumonia, or "tsunami lung," refers to severe pneumonia associated with aspiration of tsunami water contaminated with mud, bacteria, organic matter, and other potentially harmful material.
2. Tsunamis increase the incidence of acute respiratory infections and aspiration pneumonia.
3. Tsunami lung is often associated with multidrug resistant organisms, unusual pathogens, fungal infections, and abscess formation.
4. Devastated infrastructure including medical and transportation systems, lack of adequate nutrition, lack of access to home medications, and crowded shelters contribute to the spread and severity of disease after a tsunami disaster.
5. Management of aspiration pneumonia and septic shock includes timely initiation of broad-spectrum antibiotics with anaerobic coverage, fluid resuscitation, and vasoactive medications if needed.
6. This patient with altered mental status, profound respiratory failure, and septic shock must have adequate airway secured.
7. Appropriate disposition for this patient with unstable vital signs, septic shock, and acute hypoxic respiratory failure is to the ICU.

## 3. SUPPLIES

- IV fluids
- IV bags with medications (antibiotics, vasopressors)
- Syringes with medications (paralytics, sedatives)
- Noninvasive airway supplies (nasal cannula, NRB)
- Central line and arterial line set up if desired
- Intubation supplies (BVM, suction, ETT, stylet, laryngoscope, backup airway device)
- Intubation capable mannequin, placed out of view or covered with sheet (or the patient can be a high-fidelity intubatable mannequin from the start)

## 4. MOULAGE

- N/A

## 5. IMAGES AND LABS

- CXR: right middle lobe infiltrate with air fluid level (Figure 8.1)
- ECG: sinus tachycardia
- Point of care US (POCUS): hyperdynamic heart, collapsible IVC, focal B lines in right middle lobe
- Noncontrast head CT: unremarkable
- Chest CT (if requested): right middle lobe pneumonia with pulmonary abscess
- Labs: CBC, CMP, POC glucose, UA, lactate, blood cultures ×2

## 6. ACTORS AND ROLES

- Patient: standardized patient, in respiratory distress with increased work of breathing, lethargic and confused

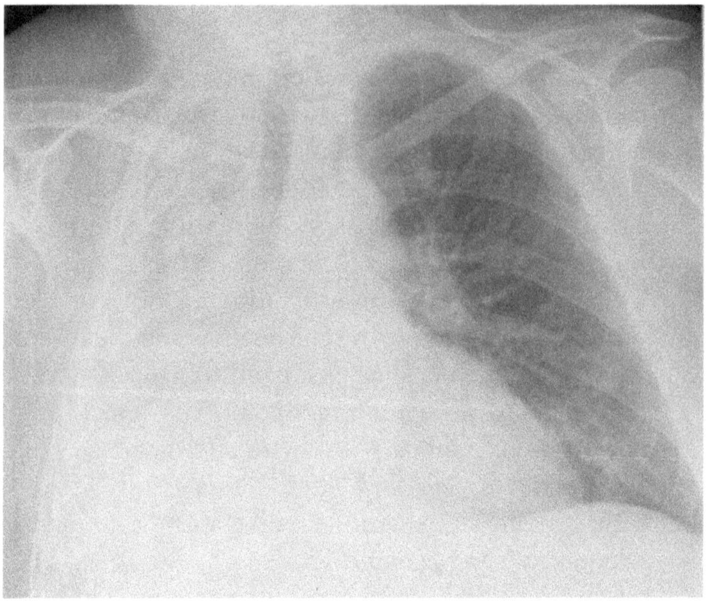

**Figure 8.1** CXR showing a right middle lobe infiltrate with air fluid level.
The original uploader was Pabloes at Spanish Wikipedia, CC BY-SA 3.0, http://creativecommons.org/licenses/by-sa/3.0/, via Wikimedia Commons.

- Staff from IDP shelter: limited medical training, resources completely overwhelmed at the shelter with no access to medications beyond basic first aid. Staff member knows the patient is very sick but was unable to secure transportation to your hospital earlier due to infrastructure devastation from the tsunami. They are helpful and provide the history, including patient being swept up in the tsunami wave, as well as their progressive respiratory illness and fevers.
- Nurse: assists team by executing orders.
- ICU doctor: accepts patient to medical ICU.

## 7. CRITICAL ACTIONS

- Assesses ABCs and places patient on cardiac monitor
- Obtains adequate IV access
- Provides fluid resuscitation
- Administers timely broad-spectrum antibiotics including anaerobic coverage for aspiration concerns
- Recognizes septic shock and initiates vasopressors
- Secures advanced airway
- Admits to medical ICU

## 8. TIMELINE WITH TRANSITION POINTS

### Time: Zero

- Initial ED VS: BP 78/54 HR 112 RR 30 oral temp 102.2°F (39°C) $SpO_2$ 82% on RA, FSBS 312
- Summary of initial presentation: A 66-year-old woman with a history of type 2 diabetes mellitus and hypertension is brought into the ED with shortness of breath, fever, and altered mental status. She is a survivor of a devastating tsunami that hit the coast of Indonesia 10 days ago. The team from a nearby IDP shelter bringing her in for evaluation tells you that she was swept up by the tsunami and nearly drowned. She survived and sought refuge at the shelter, which is

crowded with limited resources and poor access to medical care. Since that time, she has developed progressively worsening cough, fever, chills, and difficulty breathing. They have been unable to get her to the hospital until now due to destruction of roads and transportation systems, and she is now confused, febrile, and dyspneic. IDP shelter staff do not have prehospital vital signs but state her pulse is rapid and weak, and her breathing is rapid and shallow.

- Physical exam
  - General: altered, ill appearing
  - HEENT: pupils 3 mm bilaterally, PERRL. Dry mucous membranes.
  - Neck: supple
  - CV: rapid thready radial pulse, no MRG
  - Pulmonary: tachypneic, rhonchi noted to right middle lobe, coughing up thick yellow secretions, increased work of breathing with accessory muscle use
  - Abdomen: soft, nontender, nondistended
  - Skin: diaphoretic, pale
  - Neuro: moans and withdraws to pain ×4 extremities, no focal neuro deficits
- Initial intervention
  - Place on cardiac monitor and obtain initial set of vital signs
  - Obtain IV access
  - Begin fluid resuscitation
  - Begin broad spectrum antibiotics
  - Address hypoxia

**Critical Actions**

- Obtain history from IDP staff
- Recognize sepsis and acute respiratory failure with suspected aspiration
- Begin broad spectrum antibiotics and IV fluids
- Provide supplemental oxygen

## Time: Two Minutes – Transition Point 1

- VS: BP 82/56 HR 110 RR 26 $SpO_2$ 88% on NRB, ECG sinus tachycardia
- Physical exam: Patient remains hypotensive despite fluid resuscitation, obtunded, tachypneic with increased work of breathing, and rhonchi in right middle lobe.
- If POCUS obtained, reveals hyperdynamic heart with collapsable IVC and focal B-lines in right middle lobe
- If using a standardized patient, reveal intubatable mannequin when team indicates plans for intubation

**Critical Actions**

- Initiate vasopressors
- Secure advanced airway
- Send labs, imaging, and ECG

### Time: Six Minutes – Transition Point 2

- VS: BP 108/64 HR 105 RR 16 $SpO_2$ 97% on ventilator
- Physical exam: intubated, sedated, work of breathing improved
- Labs return to reveal leukocytosis, acute kidney injury, elevated lactate
- Portable chest X-ray reveals ETT in good position, consolidation in right middle lobe, and air fluid level
- Head CT: no acute abnormality
- CT chest (if obtained): right middle lobe pneumonia with pulmonary abscess in the right middle lobe
- If desired, can have ICU team request that learner place arterial line and/or central line prior to ICU acceptance
- Patient is accepted to ICU and scenario ends.

**Critical Actions**
- Place admission request to ICU
- Administer rectal or IV acetaminophen

## 9. STIMULI

- ECG: sinus tachycardia
- Cardiac and thoracic POCUS: hyperdynamic heart, collapsed
  - IVC, focal B-lines in right middle lobe
- Head CT: no acute intracranial abnormality
- Chest CT (if obtained): right middle lobe pneumonia with pulmonary abscess
- Labs
  - CBC: WBC 24, Hgb 14, hematocrit 42, platelets 310
  - POC glucose: 312
  - BMP: sodium: 136, potassium 4.0, chloride 96, bicarbonate 18, BUN 38, creatinine 1.6, glucose 312 calcium 9.5
  - LFTs: ALT 32, AST 28, alkaline phosphatase 84, Tbili 0.9
  - Troponin: <0.01 ng/mL
  - Lactate: 4.2
  - TSH/T4: 3.5/1.8 (WNL)
  - UA: color yellow, specific gravity 1.021, glucose 2+, protein 2+, ketones 1+, nitrite neg, leukocyte esterase neg, urine WBC 0–3, urine RBC 0–2, bacteria none

## BIBLIOGRAPHY


Garzoni C, Emonet S, Legout L, et al. Atypical infections in tsunami survivors. *Emerg Infect Dis.* 2005;11(10):1591–1593. doi:10.3201/eid1110.050715.

Mavrouli M, Mavroulis S, Lekkas E, Tsakris A. Respiratory infections following earthquake-induced tsunamis: transmission risk factors and lessons learned for disaster risk management. *Int J Environ Res Public Health.* 2021;18(9):4952. doi:10.3390/ijerph18094952.

Nakadate T, Nakamura Y, Yamauchii K, Endo S. Two cases of severe pneumonia after the 2011 Great East Japan Earthquake. *Western Pac Surveill Response J*. 2012 Oct 30;3(4):67–70. doi:10.5365/WPSAR.2012.3.2.002. PMID: 23908944; PMCID: PMC3729095.

Potera C. In disaster's wake: tsunami lung. *Environ Health Perspect*. 2005;113(11):A734. doi:10.1289/ehp.113-a734.

Shibata Y, Ojima T, Tomata Y, et al. Characteristics of pneumonia deaths after an earthquake and tsunami: an ecological study of 5.7 million participants in 131 municipalities, Japan. *BMJ Open*. 2016;6(2):e009190. doi:10.1136/bmjopen-2015-009190.

SECTION 3

# METEOROLOGICAL NATURAL DISASTERS

CASE 9

# Delayed Blunt Trauma Sustained during Debris Removal after Hurricane

Morgan Ritz and Romeo Fairley

DISASTER PRINCIPLES

- Conventional standards of care
- Personal preparedness
- Hurricanes/cyclones/typhoons
- Climate change and disaster medicine
- Care of animals
- Clinical diagnosis and treatment
- Communication systems and informatics

## 1. SCENARIO OVERVIEW

Patient brought in by neighbors via private vehicle is a 63-year-old female with left arm, right flank, and right leg pain. She says they have been hurting for several days now. The patient states she was out initially in the storm trying to bring in her outdoor furniture when something flew through the air and struck her. She thinks she blocked it with her left arm, but it knocked her down and she fell on her right side. She denies hitting her head or loss of consciousness. The patient was able to stand afterwards and bear weight without difficulty. She notes she would have presented earlier but the roads were flooded, and she had to care for her pets. She endorses limited left arm use secondary to pain.

## 2. TEACHING OBJECTIVES

i. Discuss initial and delayed presentation of blunt trauma after hurricanes.
ii. Discuss common traumatic injuries from a hurricane: Almost half are lacerations or abrasions. A large percentage are from falls, trips, and slipping. About 15% occur from being hit by or against an object.
iii. Understand the importance of obtaining an emergent trauma consult.
iv. Obtain initial and repeat vital signs.
v. Understand when to complete an Extended Focused Assessment with Sonography for Trauma (EFAST) exam.
vi. Discuss which patient population requires a CT head.

vii. Review how to diagnose and treat Morel-Lavallée lesions.
viii. Discuss clinical findings indicating a need for blood transfusions.

## 3. SUPPLIES

i. Cardiac monitoring
ii. Pulse oximetry
iii. Bedside ultrasound
iv. IV supplies
v. Standard ED medications

## 4. MOULAGE

i. Abrasion left upper arm
ii. Right lateral thigh contusion
iii. Right upper quadrant/flank ecchymosis

## 5. IMAGES AND LABS

i. X-rays of the chest, left shoulder, left humerus, left elbow, pelvis, right hip, and right knee
ii. CT chest, abdomen, and pelvis with IV contrast
iii. CBC, chemistry panel, coagulation studies, type and screen, troponin, and lactate
iv. ECG
v. Optional: having EFAST images for the students to view
vi. Optional: having right thigh US images for the students to view

## 6. ACTORS AND THEIR ROLES

i. Nurse who can obtain IV access, place on monitor, and obtain labs
ii. Trauma consultant

## 7. CRITICAL ACTIONS

i. Perform a thorough history of present illness.
ii. Determine whether the patient is on anticoagulating medications.
iii. Assess for additional symptoms prior to the fall such as chest pain, dizziness, or weakness.
iv. Obtain initial and repeat vital signs.
v. Fully undress patient and complete physical exam to find additional injuries.
vi. Have labs drawn including coagulation studies, type and screen, and lactic acid.
vii. Obtain an ECG (which shows sinus tachycardia).
viii. Obtain a CXR.
ix. Obtain a CT chest, abdomen, and pelvis with IV contrast to include runoffs of lower extremities through the knees.
x. Blood transfusion of packed RBCs
xi. Compression dressing for Morel-Lavallée lesion
xii. Trauma consult and admission

## 8. TIMELINE WITH TRANSITION POINTS

### Time: Zero

Vital signs: BP 117/86, HR 101, RR 16, temp 37.1°C oral, sat 96% RA, point of care glucose 92 (if requested).

i. Summary of initial presentation: A 63-year-old female with history of hypertension and hyperlipidemia presents with several days of left arm, right flank, and right leg pain after a fall secondary to blocking an object being flown through the air during the hurricane. Patient denies loss of consciousness. When asked she denies anticoagulation. Patient notes she delayed presentation secondary to road closures, flooded routes, caring for her pets, and lack of transport.
ii. Initial physical exam
   a. General: sitting upright, alert, and oriented, mild acute distress
   b. Head: atraumatic, normocephalic
   c. Neck: supple, trachea midline, no midline spinal tenderness
   d. Chest: right anterior and lateral lower rib pain on palpation, no crepitus. The lungs are clear to auscultation bilaterally.
   e. Cardiac: tachycardia, regular rhythm
   f. Abdomen: right upper quadrant and flank ecchymosis, which is tender to palpation with no crepitus or peritoneal signs
   g. Back: no midline spinal tenderness
   h. Extremities: no deformities. Stable pelvis. Left upper arm is without tenderness to palpation and has soft compartments. The right lateral thigh has a contusion with slight tenderness to palpation, there is edema present, no crepitus and the compartments are soft. The patient is able to flex and extend the left elbow and shoulder as well as the right hip and knee without difficulty.
   i. Skin: abrasion to the left upper humerus, healing contusion to the right lateral thigh but there is moderate edema present. Ecchymosis to the right upper abdominal quadrant and flank. The skin is warm, dry.
   j. Vascular: capillary refill is less than three seconds.
   k. Neuro: Glasgow Coma Scale 15 with no focal deficits
iii. Initial intervention
   a. IV placement, large bore (18 G or larger), bilateral upon request
   b. Labs drawn including coagulation studies, type and screen, and lactic acid
   c. Placed on cardiac monitor and pulse oximetry
   d. ECG obtained

### Time: Two Minutes – Transition Point 1

Vital signs: BP 115/84, HR 102, RR 16, sat 96% RA

i. EFAST at bedside is negative.
ii. Bedside point of care ultrasound musculoskeletal ultrasound of right thigh shows Morel-Lavallée lesion (upon request).
iii. CXR is negative for pneumothorax.
iv. X-rays left shoulder, left humerus, left elbow, pelvis, right hip, and right knee are negative for fractures or dislocations.

v. The nurse has sent the labs.
vi. The patient is taken to CT.

### Time: Five Minutes – Transition Point 2

Vital signs: BP 105/72, HR 109, RR 16, sat 96% RA

i. Patient comes back from CT.
ii. CT shows nondisplaced fractures of right 7–8 ribs as well as a grade 2 subcapsular liver hematoma, and a right lateral thigh Morel-Lavallée lesion.
iii. Students have the option to confirm the Morel-Lavallée lesion on bedside US.
iv. Labs reveal Hgb 6.8 (from a baseline 12.4).
v. Students should order a transfusion of packed RBCs.
vi. Students should apply a compression dressing to right thigh.

### Transition Point 3: Final Disposition

Vital signs: BP 110/75, HR 101, RR 16, sat 96% RA.

i. Consult trauma surgery.
ii. Admit to a monitored trauma surgery bed for serial abdominal exams, right thigh compression dressing, BP monitoring, and serial labs (as indicated).
iii. May need further inpatient transfusion and/or operative management of liver hematoma or Morel-Lavallée lesion.

## 9. STIMULI

i. CBC: WBC 12, Hgb 6.8, hematocrit 23, platelets 250
ii. CMP: AST 40, ALT 60
iii. PT 12, PTT 40, INR 1.0
iv. Type and screen O+
v. Lactate 2.5
vi. EFAST: negative
vii. Right thigh US positive for Morel-Lavallée lesion
viii. CXR: negative for pneumothorax
ix. CT chest, abdomen, and pelvis: nondisplaced fractures of right 7–8 ribs as well as a grade 2 subcapsular liver hematoma and right lateral thigh Morel-Lavallée lesion.

## BIBLIOGRAPHY

Frasqueri-Quintana VM, Oliveras García CA, Adams LE, et al. Injury-related emergency department visits after Hurricane Maria in a southern Puerto Rico hospital. *Disaster Med Public Health Prep.* 2020;14(1):63–70. doi:10.1017/dmp.2019.75.

Kaplan U, Hatoum OA, Chulsky A, et al. Two weeks delayed bleeding in blunt liver injury: case report and review of the literature. *World J Emerg Surg.* 2011;6:article 14. doi:10.1186/1749-7922-6-14.

Scolaro JA, Chao T, Zamorano DP. The Morel-Lavallée lesion. *J Am Acad Orthop Surg.* 2016;24(10):667–672. doi:10.5435/jaaos-d-15-00181.

CASE 10

# Sheltering in the Storm

## Delayed Extrication of an Elderly Man after a Southern US Hurricane

Michael Weiner

DISASTER PRINCIPLES

- National disaster response
- Disaster Medical Assistance Teams (DMAT)
- Incident Command System (ICS) basics
- Field operations and logistics
- Mass-casualty care in the field
- Field stabilization, treatment, and transport
- EMS disaster operations
- Search and rescue
- Hurricanes
- Scene safety and security in the field
- Clinical diagnosis and treatment
- Communication systems and informatics

### 1. SCENARIO OVERVIEW

a. This is a standardized patient (SP) scenario, with options for wound care/hemorrhage task trainer or mannequin, based on desired complexity. It takes place at the scene. The geographic region is a hurricane-prone region inland from the coast.

b. Karl Barning is a 72-year-old male smoker with a diagnosed history of hyperlipidemia. It is seven days after a category 3 hurricane swept through a small town in the southern United States. There has been extensive damage to housing and road infrastructure. Mr. Barning had sheltered in his basement throughout the storm instead of evacuating. His house had a partial collapse which barricaded the basement door and the bulkhead doors shut and he has been trapped. A neighbor who had evacuated and was coming back to survey the damage noticed that his car was in the driveway and found that he was trapped in the basement. She went to retrieve help.

c. Learner(s) is/are physician and/or nurse member(s) of a six-person Federal Emergency Management Agency (FEMA) Search and Rescue task force. They are deployed in the area for search and rescue (SAR) operations. The learner arrives soon after the search and rescue team has gained access to the basement. They find the patient seated in a leather armchair, feeling too weak to stand. They are partnered with emergency medical technician–paramedic providers and firefighters. Learners should focus on medical care and transportation. The learner should demonstrate situational awareness and inquire about scene safety. They may request additional resources, although they may not be necessary. They may assume the rest of the SAR team is standing by at a safe scene within earshot of the patient scene. They may assume that once extricated and transport is initiated, that appropriate safe transport of the patient will occur.

## 2. TEACHING OBJECTIVES AND DISCUSSION POINTS

### Clinical and Medical Management

a. Situational awareness, PPE, and scene safety
b. Evaluation of the patient's initial clinical stability in the context of anticipated extrication
c. Management of a dehydrated, hypoglycemic, individual with moisture damage

### Communication and Teamwork

a. Discussion of plan with patient
b. Interprofessional communication with on-scene team member(s)
c. Communication with receiving facility, such as a casualty collection point, Disaster Medical Assistance Team field hospital, ED

## 3. SUPPLIES

a. Standardized patient
    i. Clothing: dirty, wet clothing
b. Personal equipment
    i. Stethoscope, PPE, wristwatch
    ii. Optional
        1. Helmets, high-visibility vests for added fidelity
        2. Two-way radios for communications with team
    iii. Sphygmomanometer, stethoscope
    iv. Pulse oximeter
    v. Glucometer
    vi. Standard care kit
        1. PPE, gloves, facemask with shield
        2. Syringes and various needles/cannulas. IV normal saline
        3. Saline, distilled water in bottles, dextrose-containing fluids
        4. Povidone-iodine, alcohol wipes
        5. Bandaging, gauze, elastic rolls, tape
        6. Oxygen tank, NRBs, NCs, BVM
            a. Option for laryngoscopes, endotracheal tubes, rapid-sequence intubation medications if potential airway requirement
        7. Option for antibiotics, insulin, and full complement of additional medications available with additional staff or by request from command
    vii. Additional search and rescue stability tools and staff per scenario (engineer and shoring equipment)

## 4. MOULAGE

a. Dirty clothing
b. Dark makeup for sunken eyes and bitemporal wasting

## 5. IMAGES AND LABS

a. Fingerstick blood sugar

## 6. ACTORS AND THEIR ROLES

a. Patient: SP
b. Paramedic: partner assist with initial stabilizing and prompt for appropriate care.
c. Receiving physician at ED: receives report, prompts any missed critical actions.

## 7. CRITICAL ACTIONS

a. Demonstrate situational awareness, inquire about scene safety.
b. Make contact and introduce self/team to SP.
c. Obtain history.
d. Perform physical exam.
e. Communications
   i. Discuss need for higher level of care and next steps with SP.
   ii. Discuss transport with the team.
   iii. Radio discussion with receiving facility

## 8. TIMELINE WITH TRANSITION POINTS

### Time: Two Minutes – Prebrief

You are a physician member of a six-person FEMA search and rescue task force. It is one week after a category 3 hurricane hit a small community in the southern United States. You are deployed in the area for search and rescue operations but believe most victims have been found. As you are searching, a well-appearing woman comes to you and tells you of her neighbor who is trapped in his basement. She states she came to see if her home was still standing after evacuating and saw her neighbor's car in the driveway. She looked into the basement window and saw him sitting in an armchair and called out to him. He weakly raised his arm in response but seemed to be unable to say much in response. There is ankle-level water due to a leaking pipe from structure damage.

*If asked:*

1. There are other teams in the area with various resources, one of which includes a technical specialist for structural support and to assist in extrication.

### Time: Zero – Arrival on Scene

a. Summary of initial presentation: Elderly-appearing man in an armchair, mouth agape, pale, and dirty. Breathing, raises his arm in response to verbal stimulating before initial contact.
b. Initial interventions
   i. Situational awareness: evaluate structural stability (partner may prompt to suggest instability, technical specialist assistance can be requested, which will state structurally stable and safe for extrication)
   ii. Ensure proper PPE before approaching patient.

c. Partner prompts
   i. Comment about personal safety concerns if scene safety not discussed or considered.
d. Audio of structural creaking, leaking, or spraying pipes may be played loudly.
e. Facilitator may confirm structural stability depending on situation chosen.

**Critical Actions**
- Ensuring scene safety
- Considering structural stability, calling for technical specialist if not stable
- Recognizing need for PPE

### Time: Two Minutes – Transition Point 1 – Patient Contact and History

VS: BP 70/30, HR 115, RR 18, sat 92%, temp not available, warm to touch. If asked, FSBS 50 mg/dL.

a. Once structure is deemed stable (if necessary, make contact, introduce self and team.
b. SP: groans, moans, grumbles
c. Obtain history
   i. When attempted, patient unable to participate in interview
d. Partner "obtains" VS during attempted history and reports them as they are obtained.

**Critical Actions**
- Attempt to obtain history

### Time: Two to Four Minutes – Transition Point 2 – Physical Exam

a. Physical exam
   i. Learner should perform head-to-toe exam if able to access entirety of patient's body. If not able to access lower aspect of right lower extremity, performs exam on all else.
      1. Exposure can be performed after extrication to dry land
   ii. General/constitutional: fatigued appearing. (optional: vomited material around the mouth)
   iii. HEENT: dry mucus membranes, otherwise unremarkable
   iv. Heart: fast rate and regular rhythm, unremarkable sounds.
   v. Lungs: coarse, reduced lung sounds in right lower lobe
   vi. Abdomen: soft, nontender, nondistended.
   vii. Skin: pale, poor skin turgor
   viii. Extremities: weak radial and posterior tibial pulses. (if socks and shoes removed: severe boggy edema to bilateral feet)

**Critical Actions**
- VS obtained before next transition point, can be obtained as early as with history.
- Exam of all possible aspects of patient.

### Time: 4–10 Minutes – Transition Point 3 – Field Management and Extrication

a. Extricate patient from the home to dry land/ambulance.
b. Consider field management options
    i. Given hypoglycemia, hypotension and tachycardia, patient should be given IV NS/LR or dextrose-containing IV fluids.
        1. If dextrose containing IV fluids only are given, FSBS should be rechecked, and patient will have moderate improvement in vital signs but unchanged or slightly worsened mental status. FSBS is brought to the 200s, BP becomes 80s/40s, HR becomes 110s, and oxygen saturation becomes 92%.
            a. For the purpose of brevity, the paramedic partner can state "the dextrose infusion has completed" and report the change in patient status and vital signs.
            b. If IV NS/LR is given after that, VS show FSBS 180s, BP 100/50, HR becomes 95, oxygen saturation remains 92%.
        2. If both dextrose containing IV fluids and IV NS/LR are given, patient can improve to baseline mental status and speak clearly.
            a. VS show FSBS 180s, BP 100/50, HR becomes 95, oxygen saturation remains 92%.
        3. If IV NS/LR is given first, FSBS becomes 35, BP becomes 95/40, HR becomes 100, and oxygen saturation remains 92%
            a. Once dextrose containing fluids are given, VS show FSBS 180s, BP 100/50, HR becomes 95, oxygen saturation remains 92%.
    ii. May begin community-acquired pneumonia treatment with antibiotics given reduction in right lower lobe breath sounds.
c. Consider transport and destination.
    i. Call for ambulance or other transportation.
        1. Transport to field hospital will take 30 minutes.
            a. Has same supply of medications as SAR team but has days-worth of supplies.
            b. Has a simple X-ray machine, portable ultrasound, and point of care labs.
        2. Transport to local ED will take about 90 minutes.
            a. Has more expanded capability for medications, specialists, and basic and advanced imaging.
        3. Prompt learner on call for transport on destination, "team member" or partner can provide capabilities of destinations if requested by learner.

**Critical Actions**
- Extricated when safe to do so.
- Both dextrose-containing IV fluids and IV NS/LR given.

### Time: 10+ Minutes – Transition Point 4 – Transport and Final Considerations

a. Transport: Local hospitals are damaged but are able to take some patients if resources are present, requires discussion with the receiving facility.
    i. The nearest facility is one to two hours away and has a staffed and functioning emergency department and has X-ray capability but very limited surgical and advanced imaging capabilities.

  ii. Surgery-capable and undamaged facility is three to four hours away.
  iii. Partner can prompt learner if incorrect facility chosen.

b. Communication
  i. SP may help prompt verbalization of a more detailed and advanced plan by asking for what he is being sent to the hospital.
    1. Imaging (chest X-ray)
    2. Antibiotics
    3. Monitoring of renal function and electrolytes and giving IV fluids.

**Critical Actions**

- Decide on appropriate facility depending.
- Discuss patient's care with receiving facility and with transporting team.

## BIBLIOGRAPHY

1. Schultz CH, Schlesinger SA. Earthquakes. In: Koenig KL, Schultz CH, eds. *Koenig and Schultz's Disaster Medicine: Comprehensive Principles and Practices.* New York: Cambridge University Press; 2016:642–660.
2. US Department of Health and Human Services. *Response Teams Description Manual.* 1999, May. www.odmt.org/docs/DMAT_OPS_NDMS.pdf. Accessed April 8, 2025.

CASE 11

# "I Lost My Medications"

## Primary Care Interruption after a Hurricane

Liam Porter

DISASTER PRINCIPLES

- Disaster Medical Assistance Teams (DMAT)
- Field operations and logistics
- Mass-casualty care in the field
- Hurricanes
- Medical surge capacity
- Information management/communications
- Hospital preparedness
- Disaster triage concepts
- Scarce resource allocation protocols
- Climate change and disaster medicine
- Hospital preparedness
- Clinical diagnosis and treatment
- Communication systems and informatics

### 1. SCENARIO OVERVIEW

Ten days ago, a category 4 hurricane caused moderate to severe damage to a town's infrastructure. Your Disaster Medical Assistance Team (DMAT) was deployed and set up the medical tents two days ago. You and the team have been treating patients and assisting with local Urban Search and Rescue operations when available. Most search and rescue operations have ceased, and work is beginning on clearing rubble and restoring infrastructure. Local hospitals have been overwhelmed and are not yet operating at 100%. After treating initial injuries, your tent has started to see an uptick in chronic medical conditions.

In this scenario, patients will be presenting with exacerbations of chronic disease due to inability to access medications or primary care. There will be two patients, who can be incorporated into a larger simulation or as a standalone. Patient 1 will be hyperglycemic from type 2 diabetes due to inability to refrigerate insulin or obtain refills. Patient 2 will have type 1 diabetes and hyperglycemia and DKA due to loss of insulin as well.

Learner(s) is/are a physician or team at the triage/emergency tent of a DMAT field hospital.

## 2. TEACHING OBJECTIVES AND DISCUSSION POINTS

**Clinical and Medical Management**

- Recognize exacerbations of chronic medical diseases
- Provide initial stabilization and treatment of two patients with hyperglycemia, one with and one without DKA
- Discuss options for long-term management of chronic illness in the setting of infrastructure damage

**Communication and Teamwork**

- Work as a team to appropriately manage several patients at once
- Have appropriate and timely discussion with receiving hospital for transfer of patient needing dialysis

## 3. SUPPLIES

- IV fluids
- Standardized patient or mannequin
- Oxygen mask, nebulizing equipment and medication
- ECG, point of care (POC) labs (BMP, glucose, blood gas), urine dipstick

## 4. IMAGES AND LABS

- POC labs using a commercial portable/handheld blood analysis system
  - Sodium, potassium, calcium, chloride, total $CO_2$ or bicarbonate, glucose, BUN, creatinine
  - Hemoglobin, hematocrit
- Tests: ECG, CXR

## 5. ACTORS

- Patients: mannequin or standardized patients
- Nurse: should be knowledgeable and helpful

## 6. CRITICAL ACTIONS

- Identify symptoms of uncontrolled chronic medical problems
- Perform initial diagnostic steps for exacerbations of chronic diseases
- Provide initial stabilization of chronic diseases
- Arrange appropriate disposition and follow-up for patients

## 7. TIMELINE

### Time: Two Minutes – Prebrief

You are physician member(s) of a Type 1 DMAT field hospital team. It is 10 days after a severe hurricane caused significant damage to local infrastructure. You are seeing patients in the medical tent. There are several people waiting in chairs to be seen.

## Patient 1

### Time: Zero–Five Minutes – Patient Arrives at Field Hospital Triage/Emergency Tent, Initial Evaluation

VS initial: BP 140/80, HR 95, RR 18, $O_2$ Sat 97% RA, T 37°C (temporal scan). 90 kg

- Summary of initial presentation: A 64-year-old male with history of HTN, hyperlipidemia, DM2, presents for fatigue. He has been without his medication for the last week. He was not able to use his usual insulin because he lost power and had to get rid of it. In the last few days, he has been more fatigued. He has been urinating a lot and trying to stay hydrated. Denies fevers, cough, abdominal pain, n/v/d. Patient takes metformin 1000 mg BID and insulin glargine 20 units with insulin lispro 4 units with meals.
- Initial intervention: fingerstick glucose, urine dip (if available), POC BMP
- Next interventions: head-to-toe physical exam
- Physical exam
  - General: A&O ×3, NAD
  - HEENT: atraumatic, pupils 4 mm and reactive
  - Neck: supple, normal ROM
  - Chest: lungs clear to auscultation bilaterally, no chest wall trauma or bruising
  - Heart: RRR. Normal S1, S2.
  - Abdomen: normal
  - Extremities: normal
  - Skin: mucous membranes dry. Otherwise normal.
  - Neuro: normal
- Nurse
  - Obtains IV access (if directed). Checks POC labs as directed.
  - If no interventions ordered, can prompt by "He's diabetic. Would you like to check a blood sugar?"
- Labs: initial FSBG 540

#### Critical Actions

- Obtain history of diabetes and lack of access to medication
- Order and interpret elevated blood glucose

### Time: 5–10 Minutes – Transition Point 1 – Evaluation and Disposition of Diabetic Hyperglycemia

VS: BP 120/55, HR 75, RR 18, $O_2$ sat 97% RA

- POC BMP and urine dipstick ordered. Urine shows 3+ glucose, low specific gravity, otherwise normal. BMP in Table 11.1.
- Nurse will start IV and give IV fluid bolus as directed.
  - If not ordered, can prompt. "He looks pretty dehydrated. Should we give fluids to bring down the sugar?"
- If available, insulin or other diabetic medications can be given.
- Repeat vitals will be the same.
- After 1 L of fluid, recheck will be 340. Patient states he is feeling better.
- After 2 L of fluid (or 1 liter and insulin), fingerstick will be 210.

**Table 11.1** Patient 1 lab values

| Parameter | Value |
|---|---|
| Hemoglobin | 14.0 |
| Hematocrit | 42.0 |
| Chemistries | |
| Sodium | 132 |
| Potassium | 4.2 |
| Bicarbonate | 24 |
| Chloride | 92 |
| BUN | 23 |
| Creatinine | 1.3 |
| Calcium | 9.3 |
| Glucose | 521 |

**Critical Actions**

- Administration of IVF
- Diagnose that patient is not in DKA
- Reevaluation and disposition of patient with prescriptions for home medications.

#### Time: 10–15 Minutes – Transition Point 2 – Discharge Planning and Other Issues

VS: BP 120/55, HR 75, RR 18, $O_2$ sat 97% RA

- Patient is feeling better. He would like to go home.
- Discussion of medication options
  - If asked, patient will state that power is restored but he doesn't have his insulin anymore.
  - If asked if he has other adequate supplies, he will say yes.
  - Other acceptable options would be discharge with oral meds such as a sulfonylurea with plans to resume insulin when able.
- Before discharge, patient mentions that he is almost out of his oxycodone. He takes 10 mg every 6 hours due to chronic back pain. He wants to know if he can get some until the pharmacy is available again.

### Patient 2

#### Time: Zero–Five Minutes – Patient Arrives at Field Hospital Triage/Emergency Tent, Initial Evaluation

VS initial: BP 100/50, HR 135, RR 30, $O_2$ sat 97% RA, T 37°C (temporal scan), 70 kg

- Summary of initial presentation: A 41-year-old male with history of DM1, presents for shortness of breath, abdominal pain, nausea and vomiting. He was brought by personal vehicle. He was traveling to the area and only had a couple days' supply of his insulin before it ran out. He has not used it in the last four days. In the last few days, he has been more fatigued. He has been urinating a lot and trying to stay hydrated. Today he started to get very short of breath, and he has abdominal pain, nausea, and vomiting. Patient takes 15 units of long-acting insulin nightly, and a carbohydrate-dosed meal-time insulin (usually around six to eight units of short-acting insulin).

- Initial intervention: fingerstick glucose, urine dip (if available), POC BMP, blood gas
- Next interventions: head-to-toe physical exam
- Physical exam
  - General: A&O ×3, NAD
  - HEENT: atraumatic, pupils 4 mm and reactive
  - Neck: supple, normal ROM
  - Chest: tachypneic with deep breathing. Lungs clear to auscultation bilaterally, no chest wall trauma or bruising
  - Heart: tachycardic, regular rhythm. Normal S1, S2.
  - Abdomen: mildly tender. No guarding or rebound. Nondistended
  - Extremities: increased skin turgor.
  - Skin: mucous membranes dry. Otherwise normal.
  - Neuro: normal
- Nurse
  - Obtains IV access (if directed). Checks POC labs as directed.
    - If no interventions ordered, can prompt by "He's diabetic. Would you like to check a blood sugar?"
- Labs: initial FSBG 475

**Critical Actions**

- Obtain history of type 1 diabetes and lack of access to medication
- Order and interpret elevated blood glucose
- Suspect DKA

**Time: 5–10 Minutes – Transition Point 1 – Evaluation and Disposition of Diabetic Hyperglycemia**

VS: BP 100/50, HR 135, RR 30, $O_2$ sat 97% RA

- POC BMP and urine dipstick ordered. Urine shows 3+ glucose, 3+ ketones, low specific gravity, otherwise normal. BMP follows.
- Nurse will start IV and give IV fluid bolus as directed.
  - If not ordered, can prompt. "He looks pretty dehydrated. Should we give fluids to bring down the sugar?"
- IV insulin will need to be given.
  - Initial bolus of 0.1 units per kg IV regular insulin
  - Insulin drip can be given if available. 0.1 units/kg/hr IV regular insulin. Typical concentration is 100 units/100mL NS.
- Repeat vitals in Table 11.2

**Critical Actions**

- Administration of IVF and IV insulin
- Diagnose that patient is in DKA
- Reevaluation and disposition of patient to hospital for admission

**Table 11.2** Patient 2 lab values

| Parameter | Value |
|---|---|
| Hemoglobin | 14.0 |
| Hematocrit | 42.0 |
| Chemistries | |
| Sodium | 128 |
| Potassium | 5.5 |
| Bicarbonate | 4 |
| Chloride | 90 |
| BUN | 27 |
| Creatinine | 1.5 |
| Calcium | 9.3 |
| Glucose | 475 |

**Time: 10–15 Minutes – Transition Point 2 – Disposition Planning**

VS: BP 110/55, HR 105, RR 24, $O_2$ sat 97% RA

- Patient is feeling a little better.
- Repeat glucose is 400 after one hour (if patient still at field hospital)
- Discussion of disposition
  - Patient requires admission, preferrable to ICU
- Transport: Local hospitals have been damaged but have limited capacity for critical patients.
  - Transport to the nearest hospital is approximately 20–40 minutes due to road conditions. EMS can be made available but will need to have physician advocate for priority.
  - Air transport is available. When discussing with receiving hospital, they will ask if you would like air transport.
- Nurse verbal cues
  - "We'll probably need to get the patient to a hospital. Should I call to arrange transport?"
- Receiving hospital physician (facilitator via radio or phone) verbal cues:
  - "His blood glucose is high. Are you sure he is in DKA?"
  - When rationale for transfer is appropriately addressed: "He sounds pretty sick. Do you think he needs air transport?"

## BIBLIOGRAPHY

Munoz C, Villanueva G, Fogg L, et al. Impact of a subcutaneous insulin protocol in the emergency department: Rush Emergency Department Hyperglycemia Intervention (REDHI). *J Emerg Med.* 2011;40(5):493–498. doi:10.1016/j.jemermed.2008.03.017.

Sharma AJ, Weiss EC, Young SL, et al. Chronic disease and related conditions at emergency treatment facilities in the New Orleans area after Hurricane Katrina. *Disaster Med Public Health Prep.* 2008;2(1):27–32. doi:10.1097/DMP.0b013e31816452f0.

CASE 12

# Tornado Bloodbath

## Addressing Major Trauma from a Chainsaw Complicated by Anticoagulation in a Rural Emergency Setting

Ameer F. Ibrahim

DISASTER PRINCIPLES

- Conventional standards of care
- Community preparedness and resiliency
- Rehabilitation and reconstruction
- Field stabilization, treatment, and transport
- Timing of medical and surgical interventions
- Tornadoes
- Scene safety and security in the field
- Clinical diagnosis and treatment
- Communication systems and informatics

### 1. SCENARIO OVERVIEW

A 35-year-old-man with a history of recurrent deep vein thromboses on Eliquis for prevention is working on scene clearing up debris from a recent tornado. He is using a chain saw to cut through fallen trees. Suddenly he loses footing and one of his legs slip. This causes him to lose control of the chain saw and it swings downward and inward towards him. He attempts to readjust; however, it happens too quickly and the chain saw strikes him in the midthigh on the left side. He falls to the ground in pain. He is bleeding profusely and becomes weak and diaphoretic. His colleagues called 911. The EMS crew placed a tourniquet proximal to the wound, established large-bore IV, and start IV NS bolus. They also place a dressing on the wound and immediately transport patient to the ED. The injury happens in a rural town, with the nearest ED 1 hour away. The weather is not amenable to activate helicopter transport. The patient arrives in the ED hypotensive, tachycardic, pale, diaphoretic, and in extreme pain. His tourniquet has been on for 70 minutes. The ED physicians and trauma team work diligently to resuscitate him, stabilize him, and get him to the OR for definitive care to save his limb.

### 2. TEACHING OBJECTIVES AND DISCUSSION POINTS

- Activating trauma team
- Assigning individual roles to team members
- Performing the primary survey (ABCs)
- Performing the secondary survey
- Recognizing time sensitivity of removing tourniquets

- Reversing anticoagulation
- Giving uncrossed matched blood
- Getting patient to OR as soon as possible

## 3. SUPPLIES

- Large-bore IV
- Oxygen
- Uncrossmatched blood
- IV crystalloids
- Morphine
- KCentra
- TXA
- Laryngoscope
- Epinephrine
- Endotracheal tube
- Bag-valve mask

## 4. MOULAGE

- SimMan or actor with laceration to left midthigh with tourniquet proximal to wound. Color of limb distally should be mottled compared to the right leg due to lack of blood supply.

## 5. IMAGES AND LABS

- X-ray: Left femur shows no fracture.
- Labs: CBC, BMP, INR, PTT, lactate
- CBC: WBC 14.3, H/H 12/36, platelets 150
- BMP: Na+ 134, potassium 4, chloride 98, HCO3 14, BUN 25, creatinine 1.2, glucose 88
- INR: 1.3
- PTT: 40
- Lactic acid: 4.2

## 6. ACTORS

- EMS medic
- Emergency physician
- Trauma surgeon
- RN

## 7. CRITICAL ACTIONS

- Activate trauma team
- Do primary survey
- Place large-bore IV catheter – $O_2$ – monitor
- Team leader assigns roles
- Provide analgesia
- Perform secondary survey

- Order uncrossmatched blood
- Reverse anticoagulation
- Keep tourniquet on until arrival at OR
- Go straight to OR

## 8. TIMELINE

### Time: Zero

a. VS: T 35.5°C HR 150 RR 40 BP 75/35 $O_2$ sat 95% RA
b. Summary: Patient (Pt) arrives by ambulance with tourniquet on left leg above large wound wrapped. Pt hypothermic, hypotensive, diaphoretic, and with a thready pulse. Pt is moaning in pain.
c. Physical exam
   i. General: Pt in acute distress, pale, and diaphoretic
   ii. HEENT: PERRA, EOMI
   iii. Neuro: A&O ×3, no focal deficits
   iv. Vascular: thready pulse, tachycardic, regular rhythm, no murmurs
   v. Pulmonary: Pt with equal breath bilaterally
   vi. Abdomen: soft, nontender, nonddistended, with no peritoneal signs
   vii. Skin: Left thigh tourniquet is proximal to wound. Large wound wrapped in gauze. Leg is dusky and pale in appearance. No pulses palpable to extremity distal to tourniquet.

**Critical Actions**

- Activate trauma team
- Do primary survey
- Place large-bore IV catheter
- Place on oxygen
- Place on monitor
- Start uncrossmatched blood
- Provide analgesia

### Time: Five Minutes – Transition Point 1

a. VS: T 36°C HR 130 RR 35 BP 80/40 $O_2$ sat 95%
b. Summary: Pt improves with resuscitation and pain control. Nurse yells, "Should we remove the tourniquet?"
c. Physical exam
   i. General: Pt remains in distress but improved
   ii. HEENT: PERRA, EOMI
   iii. Neuro: A&O ×3, no focal deficits
   iv. Vascular: tachycardic, regular rhythm, no MRG
   v. Pulmonary: clear lungs bilaterally
   vi. Abdomen: soft, nontender, nondistended
   vii. Skin: large deep laceration to left midthigh with vessels and muscles exposed. Leg remains dusky and pale in appearance. No pulses palpable to extremity distal to tourniquet.

**Critical Actions**
- Perform secondary survey including removing bandage to expose wound.
- Reverse anticoagulation with KCentra and TXA.
- If <2 hours and OR readily available, consider removing tourniquet in OR.
- Update tetanus status

### Time: 10 Minutes – Transition Point 2A – If Any of the Following Happens

Tourniquet removed in the emergency room or uncrossed match blood not given

a. VS: T 37°C HR 95 RR 0 BP undetectable $O_2$ sat undetectable
b. Summary: Pt goes into PEA arrest
c. Physical exam
   i. General: unresponsive
   ii. HEENT: PERRA
   iii. Neuro: unresponsive
   iv. CVS: no pulse
   v. Pulmonary: apneic
   vi. Abdomen: soft, nontender, nondistended
   vii. Skin: active bleeding from the left thigh wound if tourniquet removed (arterial bleeding) or can consider oozing through dressing if anticoagulation not reversed and torniquet may need to be readjusted as well

**Critical Actions**
- Secure airway with intubation
- Initiate chest compressions
- Give epinephrine
- Give uncrossmatched blood
- Reverse anticoagulation with KCentra and TXA if not already given
- Take to OR once ROSC achieved
- Reapply tourniquet

### Time: 10–15 Minutes – Transition Point 2B – If All Critical Actions Happen after Transition Point 2A

a. VS: T 37°C HR 115 RR 25 BP 90/50 $O_2$ 100% ETT
b. Summary: ROSC achieved
c. Physical exam
   i. General: unresponsive, intubated
   ii. HEENT: PERRA, eyes closed
   iii. Neuro: unresponsive
   iv. CVS: tachy, regular, no MRG
   v. Pulmonary: clear to auscultation bilaterally
   vi. Abdomen: soft, nondistended
   vii. Skin: left thigh tourniquet is proximal to wound. Large wound wrapped in gauze.

**Critical Actions**

- CXR to confirm ETT placement
- Take to OR immediately

### Time: 10–20 Minutes – Transition Point 3 – Final Actions

If everything done correctly from Time Zero and Transition Point 1, skip 2A and 2B.

a. VS: T 37°C HR 115 RR 25 BP 90/50 $O_2$ 100%
b. Summary: Pt stabilized to go to OR
c. Physical exam
   i. General: Pt pain improved
   ii. HEENT: PERRA, EOMI
   iii. Neuro: A&O ×3, no focal deficits
   iv. CVS: tachy, regular rhythm, no MRG
   v. Pulmonary: BS clear to auscultation bilaterally and equal
   vi. Abdomen: soft, nontender, nondistended
   vii. Skin: Left thigh tourniquet is proximal to wound. Large wound wrapped in gauze.

**Critical Actions**

- Goes straight to OR

## 9. STIMULI

- Pulseless leg with wound and tourniquet
- Nurse pushing to remove tourniquet
- Delayed management leads to PEA arrest

## BIBLIOGRAPHY

Levy MJ, Pasley J, Remick KN, et al. Removal of the prehospital tourniquet in the emergency department. *J Emerg Med.* 2021 Jan;60(1):98–102. doi:10.1016/j.jemermed.2020.10.018. Epub 2020 Dec 7. PMID: 33303278.

CASE 13

# Tornado Chasing Gone Wrong

## Managing Patients with Impaled Objects in the Emergency Department

Ameer F. Ibrahim

**DISASTER PRINCIPLES**

- Field stabilization, treatment, and transport
- EMS disaster operations
- Tornadoes
- Conventional standards of care
- Personal preparedness
- Hospital preparedness
- Timing of medical and surgical interventions
- Scene safety and security in the field
- Clinical diagnosis and treatment
- Communication systems and informatics

## 1. SCENARIO OVERVIEW

A 50-year-old male storm chaser is videotaping a tornado when it takes a sudden turn in an unexpected direction and begins heading towards his vehicle. He stops recording, places his seatbelt on and begins driving as fast as possible. However, the vehicle is propelled a few feet off the ground and is thrown backwards several hundred feet by the tornado. The vehicle luckily lands in the correct position with its tires contacting the ground first. However, there is flying debris everywhere and a piece of large metal pierces the windshield and hits the driver in the LUQ of his abdomen in a caudocranial direction (cranial orientation of leading edge). The patient is transported to the ED by rescue crews and arrives in the ED with an impaled object in his abdomen heading upwards into his chest. Patient presents awake and in acute distress. He becomes tachycardic, hypoxic, and hypotensive from a tension pneumothorax. He requires needle decompression followed by chest tube insertion which reveals a hemopneumothorax. His exam is notable for abdominal tenderness and diffuse guarding. His Focused Assessment with Sonography for Trauma (FAST) exam is positive for free fluid in the peritoneal cavity. Patient is stabilized and receives uncrossmatched blood and is taken to the OR for definitive management.

## 2. TEACHING OBJECTIVES AND DISCUSSION POINTS

- Activating trauma team
- Assigning individual roles to team members
- Performing primary survey (ABCs)

- Performing secondary survey
- Avoiding distracting injury (impaled object)
- Performing FAST exam
- Recognizing penetrating injury to the abdomen that pierces the diaphragm and causes hemopneumothorax.
- Recognizing tension pneumothorax and acting quickly to needle decompress
- Placing chest tube after needle decompression
- Giving uncrossmatched blood
- Leaving impaled object in place if possible until patient gets to OR. Removal only with surgical colleague consultation.
- Getting patient to the OR ASAP

## 3. SUPPLIES

- Large-bore IV
- Oxygen
- Uncrossmatched blood
- IV crystalloids
- Morphine
- Bedside ultrasound
- Large-bore needle for needle decompression
- Chest tube
- Scalpel
- Kelly clamps
- Pleurovac

## 4. MOULAGE

- SimMan with ecchymosis to LUQ of abdomen and left flank.
- Large impaled metal object piercing upper abdomen of SimMan

## 5. IMAGES AND LABS

- US: extended FAST (EFAST) positive for free fluid and no-sliding left lung
- CXR: left-sided hemopneumothorax or reexpanded lung with left-sided chest tube
- Labs: CBC, BMP, INR, PTT, lactate
- CBC 13, H/H 12.3/36.9, platelets 235
- BMP: sodium 135, potassium 3.3, chloride 95, $HCO_3$ 16, BUN 29, creatinine 1.0, glucose 92
- INR 1.0, PTT 25, lactic acid 2.5

## 6. ACTORS

- EMS medic
- Emergency physician
- Trauma surgeon
- RN

## 7. CRITICAL ACTIONS

- Activate trauma team
- Do primary survey
- Place large-bore IV catheter – $O_2$ – monitor
- Team leader assigns roles
- Identify tension pneumothorax on exam
- Needle decompression on left side
- Provide analgesia
- Perform secondary survey
- Complete FAST exam
- Order uncrossmatched blood
- Place left-sided chest tube
- Order CXR
- Goes straight to OR

## 8. TIMELINE

### Time: Zero

a. VS: T 37°C HR 110 RR 25 BP 100/50 $O_2$ sat 94% RA
b. Summary: Patient (Pt) arrives by ambulance after prolonged extrication with impaled object in the abdominothoracic region. Pt is moaning in pain. Is awake but in acute distress.
c. Physical exam
   i. General: Pt in acute distress
   ii. HEENT: PERRA, EOMI
   iii. Neuro: A&O ×3, no focal deficits
   iv. CVS: tachycardic, regular rhythm, no MRG
   v. Pulmonary: Pt with diminished breath sounds on left side
   vi. Abdomen: impaled object in LUQ, tending and guarding in all four quadrants
   vii. Skin: ecchymosis to LUQ, entrance wound LUQ of abdomen, no exit wound

**Critical Actions**

- Activate trauma team
- Do primary survey
- Place large-bore IV catheter
- Place on oxygen
- Place on monitor

### Time: Two Minutes – Transition Point 1

a. VS: T 37°C HR 150 RR 35 BP 75/35 $O_2$ sat 88% on $O_2$ NC
b. Summary: Pt develops tension pneumothorax on left side
c. Physical exam
   i. General: Pt in acute distress
   ii. HEENT: PERRA, EOMI

iii. Neuro: A&O ×3, no focal deficits
iv. CVS: tachycardic, regular rhythm, no MRG, JVD (distended neck veins present)
v. Pulmonary: absent breath sounds on left side
vi. Abdomen: impaled object in LUQ, tending and guarding in all four quadrants
vii. Skin: ecchymosis to LUQ, entrance wound LUQ of abdomen, no exit wound

**Critical Actions**

- Identify tension pneumothorax on exam
- OK to rapidly confirm no lung sliding on bedside US
- Needle decompression on left side

### Time: Five Minutes – Transition Point 2A – If Needle Decompression or Simple (Finger) Thoracostomy DONE IMMEDIATELY

a. VS: T 37°C HR 95 RR 25 BP 100/50 $O_2$ sat 97% on $O_2$ NC
b. Summary: Pt improves after $O_2$ and needle decompression
c. Physical exam
 i. General: Pt in acute distress
 ii. HEENT: PERRA, EOMI
 iii. Neuro: A&O ×3, no focal deficits
 iv. CVS: RRR, no MRG
 v. Pulmonary: absent breath sounds on left side
 vi. Abdomen: impaled object in LUQ, tender and guarding in all four quadrants
 vii. Skin: ecchymosis to LUQ, entrance wound LUQ of abdomen, no exit wound

**Critical Actions**

- Provide analgesia
- Perform secondary survey
- Complete FAST exam
- Order uncrossmatched blood
- Place left-sided chest tube

### Time: Five Minutes – Transition Point 2B – If Chest Decompression Delayed

a. VS: T 37°C HR 150 RR 0 BP undetectable $O_2$ 95% on NRB
b. Summary: Pt goes into PEA cardiac arrest
c. Physical exam
 i. General: unresponsive
 ii. HEENT: PERRA, eyes closed
 iii. Neuro: unresponsive
 iv. CVS: no pulse
 v. Pulmonary: absent breath sounds on left side
 vi. Abdomen: impaled object in LUQ
 vii. Skin: ecchymosis to LUQ, entrance wound LUQ of abdomen, no exit wound

**Critical Actions**
- CPR
- Needle decompression

### Time: 10 Minutes – Transition Point 3 – Final Actions

a. VS: T 37°C HR 95 RR 25 BP 100/50 $O_2$ sat 97% on $O_2$ NC
b. Summary: If needle decompression done, patient improves. If was in PEA arrest has ROSC and is neuro intact without need for intubation. Chest tube should be placed. Blood products should be administered and patient should go directly to OR.
c. Physical exam
   i. General: Pt pain improved
   ii. HEENT: PERRA, EOMI
   iii. Neuro: A&O ×3, no focal deficits
   iv. CVS: RRR, no MRG
   v. Pulmonary: BS clear to auscultation bilaterally and equal
   vi. Abdomen: impaled object in LUQ, tender and guarding in all four quadrants
   vii. Skin: ecchymosis to LUQ, entrance wound LUQ of abdomen, no exit wound

**Critical Actions**
- CXR ordered
- Goes straight to OR

## 9. STIMULI

- Impaled object in abdomen
- Tension pneumothroax
- Free fluid in abdomen
- Delayed management leads to PEA arrest

## BIBLIOGRAPHY

Barlotta KS, Stack LB, Knoop KJ. Impaled foreign body. In: Knoop KJ, Stack LB, Storrow AB, Thurman R. eds. *The Atlas of Emergency Medicine*. 5th ed. New York: McGraw Hill; 2021. https://accessmedicine.mhmedical.com/content.aspx?bookid = 2969&sectionid = 250456692. Accessed June 29, 2022.

Muhammad Afzal R, Armughan M, Javed MW, Rizvi UA, Naseem S. Thoracic impalement injury: a survivor with large metallic object in-situ. *Chin J Traumatol*. 2018 Dec;21(6):369–372. doi: 10.1016/j.cjtee.2018.08.002. Epub 2018 Sep 20. PMID: 30348473; PMCID: PMC6354130.

CASE 14

# Tornado in the Farmland

## Multisystem Trauma Response in Rural Alabama

Guy Carmelli

DISASTER PRINCIPLES

- Field stabilization, treatment, and transport
- EMS disaster operations
- Tornadoes
- Conventional standards of care
- Personal preparedness
- Hospital preparedness
- Timing of medical and surgical interventions
- Scene safety and security in the field
- Clinical diagnosis and treatment
- Communication systems and informatics

### 1. SCENARIO OVERVIEW

A 61-year-old female with history of DM, HTN, and obesity presents to a tertiary care center in Birmingham, Alabama by EMS ground transportation after she was a victim of an EF4 tornado disaster in the farmland outside of the city. She was helmeted and riding her bike at the time when the tornado started and was subsequently blown off her bike into a field of crops, where she was found awake and alert by EMS personnel. Patient's injuries include a closed fracture to her right femur and multiple soft tissue injuries to her hands including abrasions, lacerations, and impaled foreign bodies, all of which appear to be covered in soil and debris. She also has a lot of pain and swelling to her left eye with evidence of globe rupture on exam. Her care involves stabilization, pain control, consultation with ophthalmology and orthopedics/hand surgery, systemic antibiotics/anti-fungal therapy, and admission for surgical debridement of contaminated tissue.

### 2. TEACHING OBJECTIVES AND DISCUSSION POINTS

**Tornado Basics**

- Tornado disasters are high risk for traumatic injuries, related to high-velocity projectile injuries, falls, and injuries related to impact.
- Survivors of tornado disasters typically present with multiple (on average four or more) injuries, including long bone fractures, amputations, and crush injuries.
- Soft tissue injuries such as punctures, abrasions, lacerations, and sometimes even degloving injuries may occur.

- Subsequent soft tissue infections are common, especially if wounds are contaminated with dirt, soil, mud, water, or debris.
- Prompt broad-spectrum antibiotics to cover gram positive and gram-negative species (including *Pseudomonas*) is important. A good option might include vancomycin and Zosyn.
- Furthermore, data from tornado disasters in Joplin, Missouri and multiple tornados from the Jiangsu Province, China, show a high rate of mucormycosis secondary fungal infections.
  - As a result, heavily soiled wounds would benefit from surgical debridement and addition of an antifungal agent such as amphotericin B.

**Globe Rupture**

- Thoroughly examine traumatic eye injuries to identify signs of traumatic globe rupture.
- Initiation of IV antibiotics to cover gram-positive and gram-negative species (including *Pseudomonas*) to prevent secondary endophthalmitis infections.
- Prompt ophthalmology consultation for closure of open globe injuries.

**Femur Fracture**

- Musculoskeletal injuries, while often alarming, should not distract providers from more urgent resuscitation priorities. Upon arrival at the ED, physicians must assess for life-threatening injuries in the primary survey before addressing extremity injuries during the secondary survey.
- The initial management of closed femur fractures is traction immobilization of the affected extremity in order to realign the fractured bones into anatomical proximity.
- After splinting, be sure to reassess the neurologic and vascular status of the extremity and closely monitor the patient for signs of compartment syndrome.
- Finally, adequate pain control and orthopedic consultation are necessary for definitive management.

**Communication and Teamwork**

- Structured approach to the evaluation of a polytrauma patient is important, utilizing both the primary and secondary surveys, to identify and manage all traumatic injuries.
- Clear and concise consultation is necessary to encourage consultants to aid in preventing long-term morbidity.
- Frequent reassessment of the patient to identify additional injuries and complications is important.

## 3. SUPPLIES

- Gurney
- Patient (standardized or mannequin)
- Stethoscope
- Monitor
- Ability to provide oxygen and/or suction
- IV supplies, blood draw supplies, syringes labeled with medications, IV fluids, and IVPB for medications
- External traction immobilization device (such as Hare or Sager traction splint).
- Wound care supplies: gauze, iodine povidone, saline, tape
- Ophthalmoscope, fluoresceine strip, Wood's lamp

## 4. MOULAGE

- Patient or mannequin should have left eye closed and covered with gauze/tape.
- Patient or mannequin should have makeup indicating swelling in the right middle thigh.

- Patient or mannequin should have both hands contaminated with black soil and other makeup to signify abrasions, lacerations, and punctures with impaled pieces of wood.
- If possible, patient or mannequin should have clothes dirty and soiled.

## 5. IMAGES AND LABS

- Black eye (Figure 14.1)
- Seidel test positive after corneal perforation (Figure 14.2)
- Femur X-ray (Figure 14.3)
- Chest X-ray: lungs clear. No pneumothorax. No acute pathology.
- Pelvis X-ray: bones in alignment. No fracture or dislocation.
- CT head (if ordered): no intracranial bleed. Evidence of globe rupture in the left eye with linear foreign body material impaled in cornea.

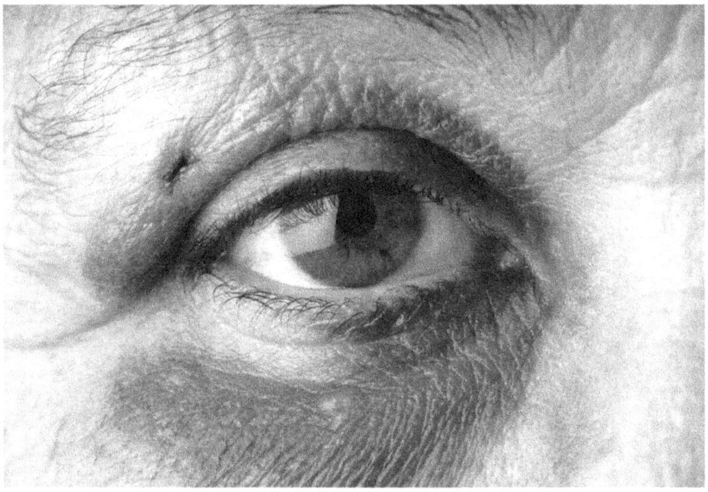

**Figure 14.1** Black eye.
Image credit Roc Canals/Moment/Getty Images.

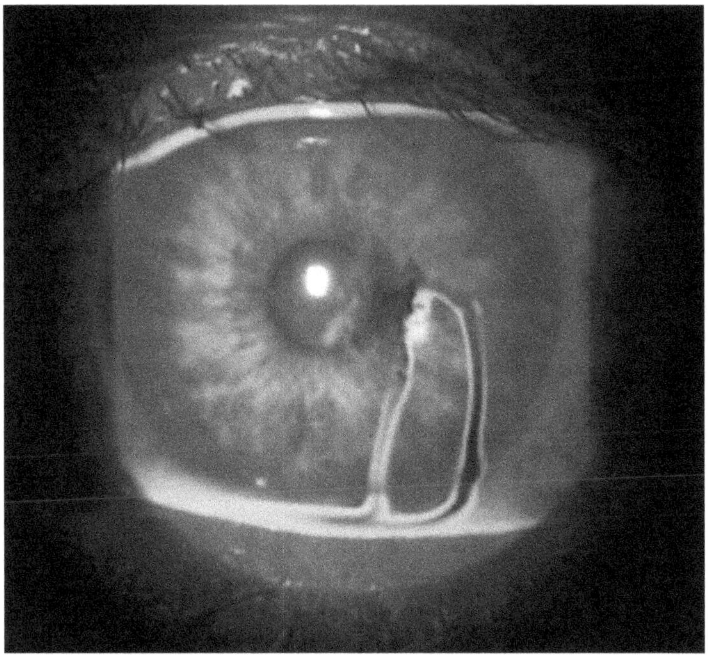

**Figure 14.2** Seidel test positive after corneal perforation.
Reproduced from Mahoney H. Ocular trauma, in *Trauma: A Comprehensive Emergency Medicine Approach*. Ed. Legome E, Shockley LW. Cambridge University Press; 2011:105–125.

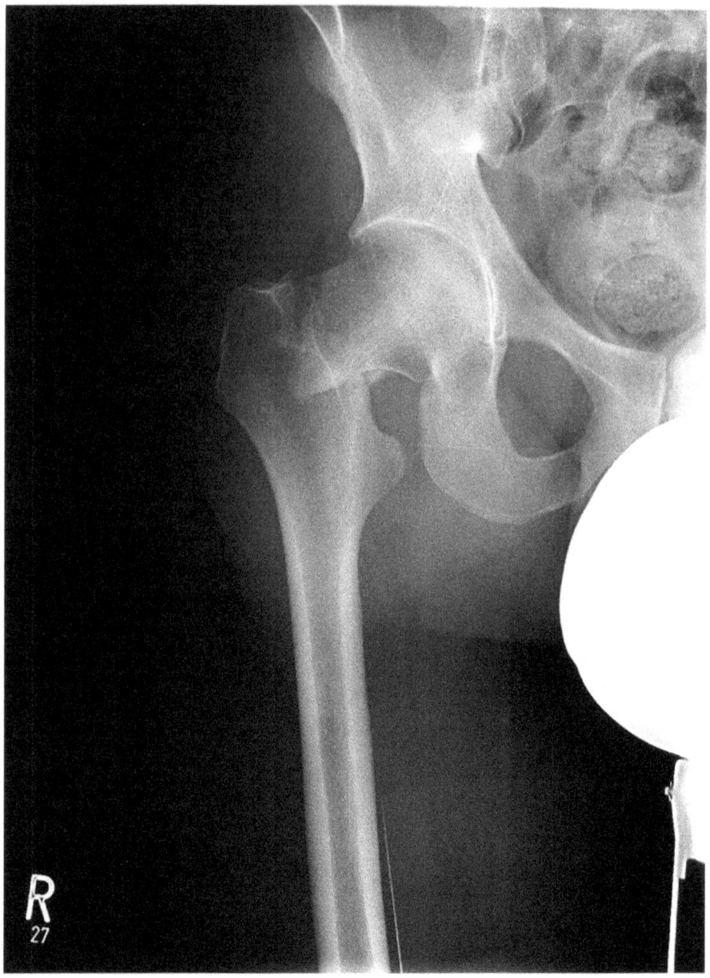


**Figure 14.3** Femur X-ray.
Image credit Prof. Dr. med. Ralf Puls, CC BY 3.0 de.

- Extended Focused Assessment with Sonography for Trauma (EFAST) ultrasound: negative
- Labs (if ordered): all normal.

## 6. ACTORS (CONFEDERATES) AND THEIR ROLES

- Patient or mannequin: scared and in pain (initially to her right leg, then her left eye). Won't let manipulate legs, examine eye, or clean hands without pain medicine.
- Nurse: assists team with administration and execution of orders.
- Ophthalmology consult: initially won't listen to consult until the providers examine the eye and provide basic information (such as visual acuity, gross examination, possibly fluoresceine staining of cornea).
- Orthopedics/hand surgery: will recommend external traction splint and operating room planning for tomorrow if only the femur fracture is discussed. If contaminated complex hand wounds are discussed, will be willing to come do a surgical debridement for infection control.

## 7. CRITICAL ACTIONS

- Perform primary and secondary surveys in a polytrauma patient
- Give adequate pain control to assist with examination and management

- Identify femur fracture and place in external traction immobilization
- Verbalize assessment of neurovascular status after immobilization
- Examine the patient's eye for injury and identify globe rupture
- Initiate broad spectrum antibiotics with coverage for *Pseudomonas* and fungal infections
- Consultation with ophthalmology for operative management of globe rupture and orthopedics/hand surgery for the femur fracture and surgical debridement of contaminated wounds.

## 8. TIMELINE WITH TRANSITION POINTS

Initial stimulus: You are working in a large emergency department at a tertiary care trauma center in Birmingham, Alabama. You are alerted to an EF4 tornado with wind speeds of up to 200 mph coming through a high-risk area of "tornado alley" in the farmland 30 minutes outside the city. You receive EMS notification that they are bringing in a patient who survived this tornado disaster.

EMS prehospital report upon arrival:

A 61-year-old female with history of DM, HTN and obesity was helmeted and riding her bike at the time when the tornado started and was subsequently blown off her bike into a field of crops, where she was found awake and alert by EMS personnel. EMS removed her helmet for transport. Patient is complaining of pain to her left eye, right thigh and has grossly contaminated soft-tissue wounds to both her hands. No treatment was initiated.

### Time: Zero

V/S: BP 130/80, HR 80, RR 14, O2 sat 99% on RA, temp 99°F

General appearance: Patient is awake, alert, conversive with EMS, complaining of pain. Her clothes are grossly contaminated with soil and debride. Her left eye is covered in gauze. She is holding her right leg.

#### Primary Survey

- Airway: intact, patient conversive, phonating well, tolerating secretions
- Breathing: breathing comfortably, good air movement, and equal breath sounds bilateral. Good chest excursion, no splinting
- Circulation: normal cardiac sounds, pulses 4+ in all four extremities, no obvious external hemorrhage
- Disability: Glasgow Coma Scale 15, Right pupil 3 mm, reactive to light. Left pupil distorted and minimally reactive to light, patient moving all extremities (limited movement to right leg secondary to pain)
- Exposure: contaminated clothing removed. Patient fully exposed. Has obvious deformity to right thigh. No additional obvious injuries identified.

#### Initial Interventions

- IV(s) placed (labs may be sent at this time), preferably two large bores.
- Patient refuses further examination without pain control
- Patient should be placed on cardiac monitor
- Patient should be kept warm after exposed with warm blanket.
- EFAST exam, chest X-ray and pelvis X-ray may be ordered (if so, can get results immediately after)
- IV fluids may be given (although not required)

## Time: Five Minutes – Transition Point 1

VS: unchanged

### Secondary Survey

- HEENT: Patient has swollen left eyelid (see Figure 14.1) and refuses to open her eye (she is in too much pain). Right eye normal exam and normal visual acuity. No facial bone tenderness, no nasal septal hematoma, no oral injury
- Neck: supple, no midline cervical tenderness
- CV/chest: no signs of trauma, no tenderness, normal s1/s2, no MRG
- Pulmonary: clear and equal bilaterally
- Abdomen: soft, nontender, nondistended. No signs of trauma
- GU/pelvis: stable, no signs of trauma
- MSK: right thigh swollen and deformed with tenderness. Compartments are soft, good distal pulses, motor, and sensation. Closed skin overlying deformity. Bilateral hands are grossly contaminated with debride and soil. Several impaled wood splinters in digits of both hands. Many small superficial lacerations on both palms (not deep, not actively bleeding) covered in soil. Deep contaminated abrasions down both forearms. Hands are neurovascularly intact with no obvious deformities, amputations or bony tenderness.

### Further Actions

- Providers should identify concern for right femur fracture.
- If femur X-ray is ordered, they will be provided with image (Figure 14.3).
- Providers should place patient into an external traction immobilization splint (such as a Hare or Sager traction) or attempt to call orthopedics for traction pinning.
- Providers should reassess neurovascular status after immobilization splint.
- Providers should also consult ophthalmology.
  - Ophthalmology will call back and refuse to hear about the patient without an examination of the eye and provide basic information (such as visual acuity, gross examination, possibly fluoresceine staining of cornea).

## Time: 15 Minutes – Transition Point 2

VS: unchanged

Patient should be encouraged to allow further examination of the eye now that their femur fracture is immobilized, and their pain has subsided.

- Eye exam: VA to left eye is 20/40. Patient has conjunctival injection. Slight distortion of the pupil is noted. Small subconjunctival hemorrhage on the superior aspect of eye. EOMI. Eye pressure (deferred or not available). If fluorescein staining is performed, provide image of Seidel sign (Figure 14.2).

### Further Actions

- Ophthalmology is called back with update for concern of globe rupture. Consultation question regarding surgical management of globe rupture.
  - If the eye is not examined, providers may ask for CT head. If so, the CT head identifies globe rupture, which should prompt ophthalmology to be called.
- Providers should initiate prophylactic antibiotics for both gram-positive and gram-negative (*Pseudomonas*) bacteria and fungal infections (for both the globe rupture and the contaminated soft-tissue wounds).

- Tetanus should also be updated.
- Minor wound care management of bilateral hands may be initiated (although not required if hand surgery is doing surgical debridement).
- Orthopedics/hand surgery should not only be consulted about the femur fracture but also be informed of the grossly contaminated wounds and encouraged to come to the ED for surgical debridement.
  - If orthopedics only is consulted on the femur fracture, they will not want to come down, but rather will say the patient can have surgical planning for the fracture once admitted. If hand wounds are discussed and concern for contaminated wound are mentioned, they will come down.
  - If trauma or other surgery is consulted for surgical debridement, they will refer to ortho/hand surgery.
- Labs, if ordered, are all normal.
- Patient will need to be admitted for pain control and wound care management.

## 9. STIMULI

See 5. Images and Labs.

## BIBLIOGRAPHY

Ahmed Y, Schimel AM, Pathengay A, Colyer MH, Flynn HW. Endophthalmitis following open-globe injuries. *Eye*. 2012;26(2):212–217.

American College of Surgeons Committee on Trauma. *Advanced Trauma Life Support: Student Course Manual*. 10th ed. Chicago, IL: American College of Surgeons; 2018.

Barrett TW, Moran GJ. Update on emerging infections: news from the Centers for Disease Control and Prevention. *Ann Emerg Med*. 2004;43(1):43–45.

Federal Emergency Management Agency. *Taking Shelter from the Storm: Building a Safe Room for Your Home or Small Business*. 3rd ed. Washington, DC: FEMA; 2008.

Hua Mu G, Li X, Shan Hou S, Qian Lu Z, Jun Deng Y. Injury patterns and outcomes of victims after the 2016 Jiangsu tornado in China: a retrospective analysis of injuries treated at a teaching hospital. *Disaster Med Public Health Prep*. 2020;14(2):208–213.

Neblett Fanfair R, Benedict K, Bos J, et al. Necrotizing cutaneous mucormycosis after a tornado in Joplin, Missouri, in 2011. *New Engl J Med*. 2012;367(23):2214–2225.

Williams DF, Mieler WF, Abrams GW, Lewis H. Results and prognostic factors in penetrating ocular injuries with retained intraocular foreign bodies. *Ophthalmology*. 1988;95(7):911–916.

CASE 15

# Stranded in the Heat

## Severe Hyperthermia and Multisystem Organ Failure

Jonathan Gammel

DISASTER PRINCIPLES

- Clinical diagnosis and treatment
- Conventional standards of care
- Timing of medical and surgical interventions
- Heat emergencies
- Role of public health agencies in disaster medicine

## 1. SCENARIO OVERVIEW

You are called to the resuscitation bay to see a 71-year-old man who is confused and febrile. He was found slumped over in his wheelchair outside your hospital. There has been a heat wave in the area for the last three days, and today it is 112°F. EMS reports that he was discharged from the ED several hours ago after being seen for an ingrown toenail and was outside waiting for transportation home. When valet services realized he was confused and not responding appropriately, he was rushed back to the ED resuscitation bay. On arrival, he is tachycardic, tachypneic, hypotensive, moaning, and unable to answer questions. Rectal temperature is 42°C (107.6°F). Learner initiates aggressive cooling measures and labs reveal an acute kidney injury, hyperkalemia, significantly elevated creatinine kinase, and transaminitis. Despite cooling measures and IV fluid resuscitation, the patient has a seizure. He remains tachypneic with noncardiogenic pulmonary edema, hypoxia, and tachypnea ultimately requiring intubation. Patient will be admitted to the ICU.

## 2. TEACHING OBJECTIVES AND DISCUSSION POINTS

### Educational Goal

1. To expose learners to environmental heat stroke and understand evaluation and management priorities.

### Teaching Objectives

1. Preparation of team for patient with altered mental status and concern for instability
2. Broad differential of altered and hyperthermic patient
3. How to recognize environmental heat stroke
4. Appropriate management of heat stroke including core temperature measurement, resuscitation with IV fluids, aggressive cooling measures

5. Complications of heat stroke including vital sign instability, organ failure, rhabdomyolysis, neurologic symptoms such as seizure and altered mental status, pulmonary edema, hypoglycemia, and electrolyte abnormalities

**Discussion Points**

1. Epidemiology of heat stroke
2. Core temperature monitoring
3. Cooling techniques for heat stroke patients
4. Temperature target during cooling and avoiding hypothermic overshoot
5. Fluid management in heat stroke
6. Complications of heat stroke, including vital sign instability, organ failure, rhabdomyolysis, neurologic symptoms such as seizure and altered mental status, pulmonary edema, hypoglycemia, and electrolyte abnormalities
7. Airway management including securing advanced airway
8. Appropriate disposition

## 3. SUPPLIES

- Wheelchair
- Ultrasound
- IV fluids
- Temperature measurement devices (rectal thermometer, oral thermometer, rectal temperature probe, temperature sensing foley)
- Cooling supplies (cold packs, ice/ice water, spray bottles, fans, arctic sun if available)
- Gauze wrap for right great toe s/p ingrown toenail treatment
- Syringes with medications (paralytics, sedatives, benzodiazepines)
- Noninvasive airway supplies (NC, NRB)
- Intubation supplies (BVM, suction, ETT, stylet, laryngoscope, backup airway device)
- Intubation-capable mannequin, placed out of view or covered with sheet (or the patient can be a high-fidelity intubatable mannequin from the start)

## 4. MOULAGE

- N/A

## 5. IMAGES AND LABS

- CXR: pulmonary edema
- ECG: sinus tachycardia
- Point of care ultrasound (POCUS): hyperdynamic heart, collapsible IVC, bilateral B-lines
- Noncontrast head CT: unremarkable
- Labs: CBC, CMP, CK, lactate, troponin, coags, POC glucose, TSH/free T4, UA

## 6. ACTORS AND ROLES

- Patient: standardized patient, acts confused with decreased responsiveness, Glasgow Coma Scale (GCS) 9, becomes progressively more somnolent throughout the scenario and ultimately has a seizure. Also develops increasing respiratory distress due to pulmonary edema. When team moves to intubate, can reveal the mannequin for intubation.

- Nurse: assists team by executing orders. Provides prompts to keep scenario moving as needed. Questions team if acetaminophen should be administered.
- ICU doctor: accepts patient to medical ICU (MICU). If team did not consider broad differential, can prompt by asking about alternative possibilities such as sepsis, thyroid storm, toxicologic etiologies.

## 7. CRITICAL ACTIONS

- Assesses ABCs and places patient on cardiac monitor
- Obtains adequate IV access
- Obtains core temperature measurement and set up continuous core temperature monitoring (or frequent reassessments)
- Rapidly cools patient utilizing evaporative and/or immersion cooling techniques
- Provides fluid resuscitation
- Identifies rhabdomyolysis, hyperkalemia, and pulmonary edema
- Conducts appropriate seizure management (gives benzodiazepines, aggressive cooling)
- Recognizes need for intubation
- Admits to MICU

## 8. TIMELINE WITH TRANSITION POINTS

### Time: Zero

- Initial VS: BP 88/62 HR 124 RR 22 oral temp 102.2°F (39°C) $SpO_2$ 94%, FSBS 52
  With core temperature (must specifically request), temperature is revealed to be 107.6°F (42°C)
- Summary of initial presentation: A 71-year-old man rushed in from outside the ED, confused and febrile. He was found slumped over in his wheelchair outside your hospital in the southwest United States. There has been a heat wave in the area for the last three days, and today it is 112°F. EMS reports that he was discharged from the ED several hours ago and had been waiting outside since that time.
- Physical exam
  - General: altered, moaning, GCS 9 (E2, V2, M5)
  - HEENT: pupils 3 mm bilaterally, PERRL
  - Neck: supple
  - Cardiovascular: tachycardic rate, regular rhythm, no MRG
  - Pulmonary: tachypneic, lungs clear to auscultation bilaterally
  - Abdomen: soft, nontender, nondistended
  - Skin: hot, dry, right great toe wrapped in a bandage, s/p ingrown toenail excision without evidence for infection
  - Neuro: confused, GCS 9 (E2, V2, M5), moves all extremities, no focal neuro deficits
- Initial intervention
  - Place on cardiac monitor, obtain IV access
  - Obtain core temperature, begin cooling
  - Begin fluid resuscitation
  - Address hypoglycemia
- If team is not considering heat emergency and has not obtained core temperature, RN notes the ongoing heat wave and wonders if this could be related to the patient's presentation.

**Critical Actions**
- Establish IV access and cardiac monitoring
- Obtain core temperature
- Recognize heat stroke and immediately begin aggressive cooling measures
- Obtain FSBS in altered patient
- Address hypoglycemia
- Begin IV fluids

### Time: Three Minutes – Transition Point 1

- VS: BP 98/64 HR 118 RR 24 core temp 106.5°F (41.4°C) (if aggressive cooling has begun) $SpO_2$ 91%, ECG sinus tachycardia, FSBS recheck 68
- Physical exam: patient with increasing work of breathing, crackles noted to lung bases bilaterally, becoming more hypoxic, otherwise unchanged.
- Once heat stroke is recognized, if team has not begun aggressive cooling RN will ask if they can give acetaminophen "or do something else" to cool the patient.

**Critical Actions**
- Establish continuous core temperature monitoring
- Continue aggressive cooling measures
- Address hypoxia
- Send labs and obtain imaging and ECG

### Time: Six Minutes – Transition Point 2

- VS: BP 96/64 HR 118 RR 26 core temp 105°F (40.6°C) $SpO_2$ 88% despite supplemental $O_2$
- Labs return to reveal rhabdomyolysis, acute kidney injury with hyperkalemia, and mild transaminitis
- Chest X-ray reveals pulmonary edema, no cardiomegaly
- If POCUS obtained, reveals hyper-dynamic heart with collapsible IVC and bilateral B-lines
- Despite appropriate management, patient will have a generalized tonic-clonic seizure
- If team moves to intubate, reveal airway mannequin for intubation

**Critical Actions**
- Continue aggressive cooling measures
- Address hyperkalemia
- Once patient has seizure, initiate benzodiazepines and anticonvulsive therapy
- Obtain definitive airway (succinycholine should not be used during rapid sequence intubationdue to concern for hyperkalemia)

### Time: Nine Minutes – Transition Point 3

- VS: BP 96/64 HR 118 RR 26 or vent settings core temp 104°F (40.0°C) $SpO_2$ 97% if intubated
- If benzos are given, seizure stops.

- If patient is not intubated, $SpO_2$ will continue to drop and patient will continue to have increased work of breathing.
- After intubation, patient should be admitted to MICU.
- Learners will discuss patient with MICU. MICU team can ask about alternative etiologies if learner did not consider a differential beyond heat emergency (thyroid storm, toxic ingestion, neuroleptic malignant syndrome, etc.).
- Patient is accepted by MICU team and scenario ends.

**Critical Actions**
- Continue aggressive cooling measures
- Call MICU for admission

## 9. STIMULI

- ECG: sinus tachycardia
- CXR: pulmonary edema, no cardiomegaly
- Cardiac and thoracic POCUS: hyperdynamic heart, collapsed IVC, bilateral B-lines
- Head CT (if obtained): no acute intracranial abnormality
- Labs
  - CBC: WBC 14, Hgb 13.5, hematocrit 40.5, platelets 110
  - POC glucose: 52
  - Repeat POC glucose: 68
  - BMP: sodium: 146, potassium 6.5, chloride 112, bicarbonate 20, BUN 42, creatinine 1.8, glucose 70 (if requested after glucose repletion, otherwise 52), calcium 9.5
  - LFTs: ALT 80, AST 75, alkaline phosphatase 110, Tbili 0.9
  - CK: 4000
  - Troponin T: <0.01 ng/mL
  - Lactate: 3.6
  - TSH/T4: 3.5/1.8 (WNL)
  - UA: color reddish brown, pH 6.0, glucose neg, bilirubin neg, ketones neg, blood 3+, protein neg, nitrite neg, Leukocyte esterase neg, urine WBC 0–3, urine RBC 0–2

## BIBLIOGRAPHY

Epstein Y, Yanovich R. Heatstroke. *N Engl J Med.* 2019;380:2449–2459. doi: 10.1056/NEJMra1810762.

Kraska E. Heat emergencies. In: Cydulka RK, Fitch MT, Joing SA, et al., eds. *Tintinalli's Emergency Medicine Manual.* 8th ed. New York: McGraw-Hill Education; 2017:1368–1371. https://accessemergencymedicine.mhmedical.com/content.aspx?bookid=2158&sectionid=162272869. Accessed March 23, 2025.

Lipman G, Gaudio FG, Eifling KP, et al. Wilderness Medical Society practice guidelines for the prevention and treatment of heat-related illness: 2019 update. *Wilderness Environ Med.* 2019;30(4S):S33–S46. doi:10.1016/j.wem.2018.10.004.

Pratt M, LoVecchio F. Nonexertional (classic) heat stroke in adults. In: Danzl D ed. *UpToDate.* Waltham, MA: UpToDate; updated February 10, 2025. www.uptodate.com/contents/nonexertional-classic-heat-stroke-in-adults. Accessed April 7, 2025.

CASE 16

# Out Cold

## Hypothermia from Environmental Exposure in a Winter Storm

Daniel Saltzman

DISASTER PRINCIPLES

- Clinical diagnosis and treatment
- Conventional standards of care
- Timing of medical and surgical interventions
- Healthcare coalitions and community integration
- Personal preparedness

## 1. SCENARIO OVERVIEW

In this scenario a 50-year-old male is brought in from the bus station where he was found sleeping on a covered park bench during a severe winter storm. Several other homeless patients have arrived in the ED due to cold related injuries because shelters are overwhelmed. He arrives obtunded with limited history, severely hypothermic (core temperature of 26°C or 78.8°F) and bradycardic in slow atrial fibrillation. The patient decompensates and suffers a v-fib arrest, requires volume resuscitation, active rewarming in addition to typical ACLS measures. If such measures are taken, then the patient will have return of spontaneous circulation, at which point the team will have the opportunity to contact either their institution's cardiopulmonary bypass personnel or contact the nearest center with this capability.

## 2. TEACHING OBJECTIVES AND DISCUSSION POINTS

a. Definition: Hypothermia is defined as a core temperature below 35°C (95.0°F).
b. Clinical presentation: The signs and symptoms of mild hypothermia include tachycardia, increases in muscle tone, and shivering, which serve to increase basal metabolic rate and thermogenesis. As body temperature falls, patients might have apathy, confusion, or dysarthria. Diuresis occurs independent of hydration status which leads to volume depletion. Peripheral vasoconstriction occurs with shunting of blood from the periphery to the core, a phenomenon that can result in worsening hypotension during treatment when external warming leads to peripheral vasodilation and a reduction on peripheral vascular resistance. At lower core temperatures, bradycardia becomes common and Osborn waves (J waves) can be seen as a positive deflection at the junction between the QRS complex and ST segment, but these are neither sensitive nor specific for hypothermia (Figure 16.1). Below 32°C (89.6°F), consciousness is impaired and shivering ceases. Cardiac arrhythmias such as atrial fibrillation are more common at this point but tend to resolve with rewarming. At 28°C (82.4°F) and lower there is greater risk of

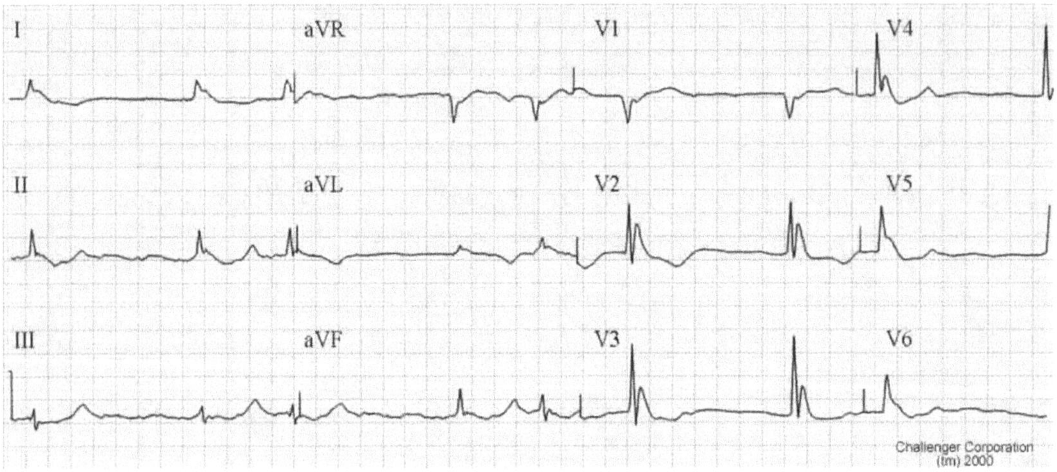


**Figure 16.1** ECG showing hypothermia with J waves.
WikiSysop, CC BY 3.0 https://creativecommons.org/licenses/by/3.0, via Wikimedia Commons.

ventricular fibrillation, and this may be refractory to usual measures such as defibrillation and antiarrhythmics until the body temperature increases. Asystolic arrest can also occur at these temperatures.

c. Management: In addition to usual stabilization, hypothermic patients require rewarming. In the most stable patients with mild hypothermia (32–35°C or 89.6–95.0°F), this might only consist of removal from the cold environment, removal of wet clothing, and application of warm blankets in a warm room. In patients with a lower temperature (<32°C or 89.6°F) but still conscious, active warming with warming blankets and warm IV fluids is a good strategy. IV fluids can be warmed in a microwave or rapid infuser with the goal IV fluid temperature being 40–42°C (104–107.6°F). In patients who are obtunded or with more severe hypothermia (<28°C or <82.4°F), in addition to these measures, transfer to a center capable of cardiopulmonary bypass should be considered. Cardiopulmonary bypass is the most effective warming technique, able to increase body temperature at a rate of 9°C/hour of 16.2°F). Other invasive approaches such as thoracic lavage, peritoneal or hemodialysis have been tried and can increase body temperature (1–3°C/hour or 1.8–5.4°F/hour) and could be an option if bypass is completely unavailable, but there is less evidence to support them. In cases of severe hypothermia that requires invasive rewarming, it might be best to focus efforts on transfer to a center with bypass capability if that is possible.

d. Electrolyte shifts are common in hypothermia. Potassium levels in particular can fluctuate. Potassium levels are likely to be low in early or mild hypothermia but can become elevated in prolonged or severe cases. If rapid-sequence intubation needed, avoid succinycholine because this drug could worsen hyperkalemia, and hyperkalemia is common in patients who have been hypothermic for prolonged periods.

e. Cardiac arrest: In patients who present in cardiac arrest, prognosis depends greatly on whether cooling occurred before or after the arrest and it can be challenging to determine who could survive. Patients who had an arrest (from trauma or submersion/drowning) are very unlikely to survive. However, patients who have been immersed in cold water (but did not drown) and arrested primarily due to hypothermia rather than hypoxia are more likely to survive. In the hypothermic arrest population, the amount of time undergoing CPR has not been found to be the key determinant of survival. Serum markers such as potassium are of limited utility in predicting mortality in this population as well: One pediatric patient survived a hypothermic arrest despite a serum potassium level of 11.8 mmol/L. Some authors have advocated a cutoff of 12 mmol/L when considering futility. It is also important to know that patients have survived profound hypothermia: one patient survived accidental hypothermia with a body temperature of 14°C (57°F).

## 3. SUPPLIES

a. Simulation mannequin
b. Towels
c. Blankets
d. External warming blanket (i.e. Bair hugger)
e. IV set-ups and warm IV fluids (IV fluids can be put in a microwave)
f. ACLS medications, sedative and induction agents
g. Airway management supplies: nasal cannula, non-rebreather mask, bag-valve mask, oxygen, oropharyngeal airway, nasopharyngeal airway, endotracheal tubes and stylets, 10 cc syringe, laryngoscope (direct or video), laryngeal mask airways, suction set up, end-tidal $CO_2$ monitoring or colorimetric $CO_2$ detector

## 4. MOULAGE

a. Worn and soiled winter clothing and footwear
b. Hard liquor to apply to the clothing

## 5. IMAGES AND LABS

a. ECG shows atrial fibrillation with slow ventricular response, Osborn waves.
b. Chest X-ray is grossly negative.
c. CBC shows hemoconcentration, leukopenia, thrombocytopenia.
d. Chemistry shows mild hypokalemia, low magnesium, normal kidney function.
e. Ethanol level is elevated.
f. CT scan of the head without contrast is negative for intracranial hemorrhage.

## 6. ACTORS (CONFEDERATES) AND THEIR ROLES

a. EMS provider (BLS) will give limited initial history and rush to another call.
b. Bedside nurse: will assist with care, will offer prompts to check temperature ("Wow, he is ice cold") and to initiate warming if not already being done ("Do you want me to get some blankets? He feels really cold"). If the learners do not recognize cardiac arrest/VF then the nurse will call it out ("That looks like v-fib").

## 7. CRITICAL ACTIONS

a. Removal of cold and wet clothing and application of blankets
b. Check a fingerstick blood glucose
c. Obtain IV access
d. Place patient on telemetry and pulse oximetry
e. Obtain and interpret a 12-lead ECG
f. Recognize VF arrest
g. Secure an advanced airway (LMA or ETT) during arrest if not done earlier

h. Obtain laboratory studies including basic chemistry profile
i. Measure a core temperature to identify and determine degree of hypothermia
j. Initiate passive external warming while active rewarming is considered
k. Give volume resuscitation with warmed IV fluids and apply a warming blanket while more invasive measures are considered
l. Consider consultation or transfer for cardiopulmonary bypass

## 8. TIMELINE WITH TRANSITION POINTS

### Time: Zero

a. A severe winter storm has caused widespread power outages in the area. Shelters are overwhelmed. Temperatures are in the 20s Fahrenheit. EMS brings in a gentleman who appears to be in his 50s who was found at the bus station sleeping on a bench. When security at the bus terminal tried to wake him, they were unable to do so and called 911. EMS reports that the patient was wet, cold to touch, and bradycardic.
b. Past medical history: unknown
c. Past surgical history: unknown
d. Allergies: unknown
e. Medications: unknown
f. Examination
g. Vital signs: temperature 26°C (78.8°F), pulse 40 bpm, BP 80/40 mmHg, RR 10, unable to obtain pulse oximetry reading (poor waveform)
h. Head: normocephalic, atraumatic
i. Neck: no JVD, trachea midline
j. Chest and respiratory: normal excursion, bilateral rhonchi throughout
k. Cardiovascular: bradycardic, irregularly irregular rhythm, thready distal pulses, normal carotid and femoral pulses
l. Abdomen: soft, nontender, nondistended
m. Skin: cool to touch
n. Neurologic: obtunded, no eye opening, moans, withdraws from pain in all extremities, cranial nerve reflexes intact, depressed deep tendon reflexes

### Time: Five Minutes

Patient has a VF arrest.

### Time: 10 Minutes

If active warming measures (warm IV fluids, warming blanket) have been started then a repeat attempt at defibrillation will yield return of spontaneous circulation. If warming has not been initiated despite prompts from simulation actors, then the case will end here.

## 9. STIMULI

a. 12-lead ECG showing atrial fibrillation with bradycardia, with Osborn waves
b. Clear chest X-ray
c. CT head without contrast: no intracranial hemorrhage, no acute findings

d. Labs
   i. CBC: WBC 5.0, Hgb 17, hematocrit 51, platelets 125;
   ii. CMP: sodium 135, potassium 3.0, chloride 108, bicarbonate 20, BUN 20, creatinine 1.1, glucose 90, calcium 9.0, magnesium 1.4, albumin 4.0, AST 250, ALT 150, alkaline phosphatase 75, bilirubin 1.0
   iii. INR: 1.0
   iv. Troponin 0.01 ng/dL
   v. Ethanol 250 mg/dL
   vi. Drug screen: negative for THC, cocaine, opioids, benzodiazepines

## BIBLIOGRAPHY

Bickle I. Normal chest radiograph – male. Case study. Radiopaedia.org; 2016. doi:10.53347/rID-46452.

Brown DJ, Brugger H, Boyd J, Paal P. Accidental hypothermia. *N Engl J Med.* 2012 Nov 15;367(20):1930–1938. doi:10.1056/NEJMra1114208. Erratum in: *N Engl J Med.* 2013 Jan 24;368(4):394. PMID: 23150960.

Dobson JAR, Burgess JJ. Resuscitation of severe hypothermia by extracorporeal rewarming in a while. *J Trauma.* 1996;40:483–485.

Gilbert M, Busund R, Skagseth A, Nilsen PÅ, Solbø JP. Resuscitation from accidental hypothermia of 13.7 degrees C with circulatory arrest. *Lancet.* 2000;355:375–376.

Plaisier BR. Thoracic lavage in accidental hypothermia with cardiac arrest - report of a case and review of the literature. *Resuscitation.* 2005;66:99–104.

Strohmer B, Pichler M. Atrial fibrillation and prominent J (Osborn) waves in critical hypothermia. *Int J Cardiol.* 2004 Aug;96(2):291–293. doi:10.1016/j.ijcard.2003.04.065. PMID: 15262049.

Zafren K, Danzl D. Accidental hypothermia. In: Walls R, Hockberger RS, Gausche-Hill M, Bakes KM, eds. *Rosen's Emergency Medicine: Concepts and Clinical Practice.* 9th ed. Philadelphia: Elsevier; 2018:1743–1754.

CASE 17

# An Invisible Killer

## Carbon Monoxide Toxicity from Gasoline Generator Use during a Winter Storm

Daniel Saltzman

DISASTER PRINCIPLES

- Clinical diagnosis and treatment
- Conventional standards of care
- Timing of medical and surgical interventions
- Community preparedness and resiliency
- Scene safety and security in the field

## 1. SCENARIO OVERVIEW

A severe winter storm has caused widespread power outages in the area. Temperatures are in the 20s Fahrenheit. To power their multifamily home, a group of families has set up a gasoline-powered generator in the basement, which has been running overnight. This has caused elevated carbon monoxide (CO) levels in the home as the CO has permeated the drywall and reached every part of the home. Multiple members of the families have begun feeling ill, complaining of headaches, nausea, and fatigue. They have arrived by private vehicles primarily due to concern that one of them, the 75-year-old grandfather with multiple medical problems, is confused, lethargic, and cannot walk. He has a carboxyhemoglobin level of 30%, ischemic changes on his ECG and an elevated troponin. If asked, he will admit to chest pain. If high-flow oxygen is not applied the patient will have unstable ventricular tachycardia requiring synchronized cardioversion. He will stabilize with appropriate therapy. Family members will complain of symptoms, and this should prompt their evaluation or referral to be evaluated. If this does not happen, one of them will collapse on the floor.

## 2. TEACHING OBJECTIVES AND DISCUSSION POINTS

a. Carbon monoxide accounts for more toxicity than any other substance due to its ubiquity. Most often toxicity occurs from inhalation in gaseous form. Carbon monoxide is produced by the incomplete combustion of carbon containing compounds such as wood, gasoline and other fuels. It is hard to detect because it is odorless, colorless, and tasteless.
b. During severe weather events with power outages, the indoor use of gasoline powered generators can lead to epidemic carbon monoxide poisoning outbreaks.
c. The symptoms of carbon monoxide toxicity are wide ranging and can be vague, so a high index of suspicion is important. Common symptoms and signs include ataxia, cardiac dysrhythmias, chest pain, coma, confusion, dizziness, dyspnea, headache, metabolic acidosis, myocardial ischemia, nausea, seizures, syncope, tachypnea, blurry vision, vomiting, and weakness.

d. In addition to usual stabilization, patients with carbon monoxide toxicity should be treated with high-flow oxygen. Carbon monoxide binds deoxyhemoglobin with 200–250 times greater affinity than oxygen and causes the formation of carboxyhemoglobin. In addition to its hemoglobin binding, CO inhibits the final cytochrome complex in mitochondrial oxidative phosphorylation, resulting in a shift from aerobic to anaerobic metabolism. This results in metabolic acidosis and cell death. Finally, CO activates sodium channels and increases nitric oxide levels and injures brain tissue due to an inflammatory cascade. This is especially problematic for high oxygen-consuming areas such as the basal ganglia and occiput.
e. The diagnosis of CO toxicity is confirmed using co-oximetry testing. A venous sample can be used; an arterial sample is not required to Measure the carboxyhemoglobin level. A level of >3% is considered abnormal in nonsmokers and a level >10% is considered abnormal in smokers. Standard pulse oximetry is not helpful and will give spuriously elevated values because the devices cannot differentiate the different wavelengths produced by carboxyhemoglobin and oxyhemoglobin. Co-oximeters that can differentiate between carboxyhemoglobin and oxyhemoglobin do exist but can be less reliable than serum studies.
f. Oxygen therapy is the mainstay of CO toxicity treatment. The half-life of the carboxyhemoglobin complex while breathing room air is about five or six hours but can be reduced to one hour while breathing 100% oxygen. Hyperbaric oxygenation at 2.8 atmospheres can reduce the half-life further to just 20–30 minutes. Hyperbaric oxygenation can improve outcomes, in particular reducing long-term neurologic sequelae. Evidence does not support hyperbaric treatment for all patients with CO toxicity, so discussion with a toxicologist can helpful. Hyperbaric treatment should be considered in the following cases:
    i. CO level of >25%
    ii. CO level of >15% in pregnancy
    iii. Syncope
    iv. Coma
    v. Seizure
    vi. Altered mental status
    vii. Abnormal cerebellar function
    viii. Prolonged CO exposure (long "soak" time)

## 3. SUPPLIES

a. Simulation mannequin or actor (If using an actor, certain procedures would need to be verbalized such as IV placement)
b. Cardiac monitor with telemetry and pulse oximetry
c. non-rebreather mask and oxygen
d. Defibrillator set up
e. ACLS medications
f. IV sedatives and analgesics

## 4. MOULAGE

a. Cherry red lips (lipstick or mannequin feature), oxygen saturation set at 100%

## 5. IMAGES AND LABS

a. ECG showing ischemic changes, diffuse ST depressions but no ST elevations
b. CO level of 30%

c. Elevated troponin at 0.50 ng/mL (reference range 0.01–0.04 ng/mL)
d. Mild metabolic acidosis
e. CT scan of the head without contrast that is negative for intracranial hemorrhage

## 6. ACTORS (CONFEDERATES) AND THEIR ROLES

a. Multiple family members (if simulation resources allow) should report more mild symptoms prompting the care team to consider epidemic carbon monoxide toxicity. In more advanced learners, these family members can distract the care team from the critical patient. In novice learners they can provide clues to the care team that there is concern for "bad air" in the house.
b. Bedside nurse: will assist with care delivery to varying degrees depending on the level of learner

## 7. CRITICAL ACTIONS

a. Check a fingerstick blood glucose
b. Obtain a CT scan of the head to rule out intracranial hemorrhage
c. Obtain and interpret a 12-lead ECG
d. Obtain serum studies including a basic metabolic profile, blood gas, and troponin
e. Include carbon monoxide toxicity on the differential diagnosis based upon exposure history and order appropriate testing to determine carbon monoxide levels: co-oximetry laboratory studies or bedside finger probe with co-oximetry capability
f. Apply high-flow oxygen to the patient
g. Identify potential need for hyperbaric oxygenation and contact either a dive center, toxicologist, or poison control center
h. Recognize that the family members have carbon monoxide toxicity and activate resources to care for them such as activating protocols for mass casualty or disaster events
i. Alert the local fire department and/or department of public health

## 8. TIMELINE WITH TRANSITION POINTS

### Time: Zero

a. The patient presents in a wheelchair as his family drove him in by private vehicle. He is lethargic but able to answer questions. Multiple members of the families with whom he lives accompany him. He will admit to chest pain if asked and family will report that he took 324 mg aspirin prior to arrival.
b. Past medical history: diabetes mellitus, hypertension, hyperlipidemia
c. Past surgical history: none
d. Allergies: none
e. Medications: Lantus 20 U nightly, metformin 1000 mg twice daily, lisinopril 20 mg daily, metoprolol tartrate 50 mg twice daily, aspirin 81 mg daily
f. Examination
    i. Vital signs: temperature 37.2°C, pulse 80 bpm, BP 160/85 mmHg, RR 20, $O_2$ saturation 100% on room air
    ii. Head: normocephalic, atraumatic
    iii. Neck: no JVD, trachea midline
    iv. Chest and respiratory: normal excursion, lungs clear bilaterally
    v. Cardiovascular: normal rate, regular rhythm, no murmurs; strong distal pulses throughout

vi. Abdomen: soft, nontender, nondistended
vii. Skin: warm, dry, flushed
viii. Neurologic: sleepy but arousable to voice, mostly moans but able to tell his name and answer some yes or no questions; oriented to self only, CNs 2–12 intact, 5 of 5 strength in all extremities, sensation grossly intact to light touch, unable to stand up to test gait

### Time: Five Minutes

If oxygen therapy is not initiated, the patient will have worsening chest pain and a run of ventricular tachycardia with hypotension requiring electrical cardioversion.

### Time: 10 Minutes

If the family members have not been evaluated or referred to be evaluated for CO toxicity, then one of them will collapse on the floor.

## 9. STIMULI

- ECG showing ischemic changes (but not ST elevations)
- Clear chest X-ray
- VBG: pH 7.30, $pCO_2$ 45, $pO_2$ 40, $HCO_3$ 17
- Co-oximetry: carboxyhemoglobin 30%, methemoglobin 1%, oxyhemoglobin 65%
- CBC: WBC 9.0, Hgb 15, hematocrit 45, platelets 250
- Chemistry (CMP): Na 135, potassium 4.0, chloride 105, bicarbonate 16, BUN 25, creatinine 1.4, glucose 250, calcium 9.0, magnesium 1.8, albumin 4.0, AST 40, ALT 35, alkaline phosphatase 45, bilirubin 1.0
- CPK 4000 U/L
- Lactic acid 3.5 mmol/L
- Troponin 0.50 ng/dL
- CT head without contrast: no intracranial hemorrhage, no acute findings

## BIBLIOGRAPHY

Buckley NA, Juurlink DN, Isbister G, Bennett MH, Lavonas EJ. Hyperbaric oxygen for carbon monoxide poisoning. *Cochrane Database Syst Rev.* 2011;(4):CD002041.

Nelson L, Hoffman R. Inhaled toxins. In: Walls R, Hockberger RS, Gausche-Hill M, Bakes KM, eds. *Rosen's Emergency Medicine: Concepts and Clinical Practice.* 9th ed. Philadelphia: Elsevier; 2018;1926–1933.

Tomaszewski C. Carbon monoxide. In: Nelson LS, Howland M, Lewin NA, et al. eds. *Goldfrank's Toxicologic Emergencies.* 11th ed. New York: McGraw Hill; 2019. https://accessemergencymedicine.mhmedical.com/content.aspx?bookid = 2569&sectionid = 210264419. Accessed July 14, 2022.

Touger M, Gallagher EJ, Tyrell J. Relationship between venous and arterial carboxyhemoglobin levels in patients with suspected carbon monoxide poisoning. *Ann Emerg Med.* 1995;25(4):481–483. doi:10.1016/s0196-0644(95)70262-8. PMID: 7710152.

Weaver L, Hopkins RO, Chan KJ, et al. Hyperbaric oxygen for acute carbon monoxide poisoning. *N Engl J Med.* 2002;347(14):1057–1067.

SECTION 4

# HYDROLOGICAL NATURAL DISASTERS

CASE 18

# Helping Turns Hazardous

## Blunt Trauma and Respiratory Distress during Flash Flood Rescue

Morgan Ritz and Romeo Fairley

DISASTER PRINCIPLES

- Conventional standards of care
- Local disaster response
- Community preparedness and resiliency
- EMS disaster operations
- Hurricanes/cyclones/typhoons
- Climate change and disaster medicine
- Flooding
- Scene safety and security in the field
- Clinical diagnosis and treatment
- Communication systems and informatics

### 1. SCENARIO OVERVIEW

EMS brings in a 31-year-old male with hypoxia and cough. The patient attempted to help his older neighbor after the flash flood warning was announced. EMS notes the water in the area got up to 5 feet deep. The patient is sitting up and talking. EMS notes an oxygen saturation of 86% prehospital on room air with improvement to 96% on 4 L NC. Patient thinks he got hit by something in the water and remembers waking up in the water several houses down from where he started. He called EMS after feeling short of breath when assisting his neighbor. The patient is actively coughing and shivering upon arrival.

### 2. TEACHING OBJECTIVES AND DISCUSSION POINTS

1. Complete primary assessment with ABCs.
2. Obtain initial vitals and temperature.
3. Discuss management of drowning in both prehospital and hospital environments.
4. Discuss when passive versus active rewarming is necessary.
5. Discuss treatment for mild, moderate, and severe hypothermia.
6. Evaluate for blunt trauma and other injuries.
7. Complete workup, imaging, and labs needed for drowning victims.
8. Discuss drowning without morbidity, drowning with morbidity, and drowning with death and mortality.
9. Discuss risk factors for drowning in pediatrics, adults, and special populations during disasters.
10. Discuss the role of antibiotics for drowning patients.

11. Discuss which drowning victims can be discharged and which should be admitted, including which require ICU admission.

## 3. SUPPLIES

1. Cardiac monitor, $SpO_2$
2. Noninvasive respiratory therapies such as NRB, HFNC, or BiPAP
3. Intubation supplies in the room for backup airway in case of decompensation: BVM, ETT, stylet, blade, suction
4. Warm blankets and Bair hugger, warmed IVF if necessary

## 4. MOULAGE

1. Forehead abrasion on the patient (mannequin or actor).
2. Skin pallor and patient should be shivering.

## 5. IMAGING AND LABS

1. Diagnostic testing will vary based on the patient's severity of illness. Vital signs with cardiac monitoring, core temperature, end-tidal $CO_2$, and $SpO_2$ are required.
2. CXR should be obtained to evaluate for aspiration and pneumonitis.
3. ECG.
4. CT head (as indicated, at discretion of simulation proctor).
5. Basic labs including CBC, CMP, troponin, lactate.

## 6. ACTORS AND THEIR ROLES

1. Nurse who is able to obtain IV access, give medications, etc.
2. Respiratory therapist: set up HFNC, BiPAP, etc. as indicated.
3. Confederate (optional role): neighbor (whom the patient was helping) barge in and distract the team midway through the case.

## 7. CRITICAL ACTIONS

1. Complete primary survey with ABCs.
2. Obtain initial vital signs.
3. Request core temperature.
4. Continue oxygen supplementation and escalate as needed to HFNC or BiPAP.
5. Passive and active rewarming are necessary. Make sure the patient is undressed and dried off. Warm blankets and a Bair hugger should be applied.
6. CXR obtained.
7. Patient can be admitted to ICU as he requires advanced non-invasive ventilatory support.

## 8. TIMELINE WITH TRANSITION POINTS

### Time: Zero

1. VS: BP 142/89, HR 58, RR 18, sat 96% 4 L NC, temp 32.1°C axillary, point of care glucose 84.
2. ECG shows sinus bradycardia and Osborn waves.

3. Core temperature is 32.4°C core.
4. Summary of initial presentation: A 31-year-old-male with no significant past medical history who presents via EMS for shortness of breath. Patient with unknown water submersion, endorsing blunt injury with loss of consciousness while being in the water. He is awake without respiratory distress while on 4 L NC.
5. Primary assessment: Airway intact, lungs with mild rales bilaterally, 2+ bilateral radial and DP pulses.

**Initial Intervention**

1. Continue supplemental oxygen on NC.
2. Placed on cardiac monitor and end-tidal $CO_2$.
3. Undress the patient to remove wet clothes and expose any underlying injuries. Cover with warm blankets.
4. IV placement of bilateral large-bore IVs.
5. Have labs drawn.
6. Obtain an ECG.

## Time: Two Minutes – Transition Point 1

1. Confederate (optional role): Confederate actor enters case as patient's neighbor. Actor demands the medical team help the patient immediately, that he is dying, etc. Team must effectively deal with the neighbor to not block medical care.
2. Full physical exam: VS: BP 140/82, HR 57, RR 24, sat 93% 4 L NC, core temperature 32.9°C.
3. General: sitting upright, alert and oriented, no acute distress but shivering.
   a. HEENT: forehead abrasion, normal voice.
   b. Neck: supple, trachea midline.
   c. Chest: mild bibasilar rales, mild respiratory distress on oxygen.
   d. Cardiac: bradycardic, regular rhythm.
   e. Abdomen: soft, nontender, nondistended.
   f. Skin: some areas are wet, cool, with minimal peripheral cyanosis, capillary refill four to five seconds.
   g. Neuro: Glasgow Coma Scale 15, no focal deficits.
4. Nurse sends off blood work.
5. CXR obtained showing small pneumonitis versus aspiration right greater than left lower bases.
6. Antibiotic not needed at this time.
7. Respiratory therapist obtains ABG if requested by team to evaluate oxygenation.

## Time: Four Minutes – Transition Point 2

1. VS: BP 135/82, HR 61, RR 25, sat 92% 6 L NC, core temperature 34.1°C core.
2. Patient still shivering and the Bair hugger placed on the patient.
3. Patient now has tachypnea with slowly declining oxygenation, moderate respiratory distress, minimal CXR findings, escalate to HFNC or BiPAP.

## Transition Point 3: Final Disposition

1. VS: BP 136/78, HR 67, RR 19, sat 98% HFNC or BiPAP, core temperature 35.9°C.
2. Admit to the ICU.

## 9. STIMULI

1. ECG showing sinus bradycardia.
2. CXR showing small bilateral, pneumonitis versus aspiration right greater than left lower bases.
3. CT head negative.
4. CBC: WBC 14, Hgb 13
5. CMP: sodium 136, potassium, 4.8, chloride 100, bicarbonate 20, creatinine 1.3.
6. Troponin: 0.03.
7. Lactic acid: 2.4.
8. ABG w/ $O_2$ sat: pH 7.32, $PaO_2$ 84, $PaCO_2$ 39, $HCO_3$ 17, $O_2$ sat 93% on 6 L NC.

## BIBLIOGRAPHY

Centers for Disease Control and Prevention. *About Hurricanes and Other Tropical Storms.* Atlanta: Centers for Disease Control and Prevention. 2024, October 15. www.cdc.gov/disasters/hurricanes/index.html. Accessed April 8, 2025.

Szpilman D, Bierens JJLM, Handley AJ, Orlowski JP. Drowning. *New Engl J Med.* 2012;366(22):2102–2110. doi:10.1056/nejmra1013317.

CASE 19

# Trapped by the Flood

## Rescue of an Elderly Man after 24 Hours

Guy Carmelli

DISASTER PRINCIPLES

- Field stabilization, treatment, and transport
- EMS disaster operations
- Conventional standards of care
- Personal preparedness
- Hospital preparedness
- Flooding
- Scene safety and security in the field
- Clinical diagnosis and treatment
- Communication systems and informatics

## 1. SCENARIO OVERVIEW

A 70-year-old male with history of peripheral vascular disease, diabetes, and bipolar disorder presenting found trapped in a flooded one-story house. The initial bystander call to EMS was concerning for a near drowning; however, upon EMS arrival to the patient's residence, they found him trapped inside his bedroom by an overturned dresser, wading through 3 feet of freshwater. Patient reports he had been trapped for over 24 hours, without access to food, water, warmth, or dry clothes. EMS did not note any immediate airway issues but found the patient shivering in the cold, shoeless, with concerns of trench foot and possibly an overlying skin and soft tissue infection. His care involved rewarming of hypothermia, initiation of treatment for trench foot, diagnosis of soft tissue infection with abscess, and antibiotic management. The patient will ultimately need to be admitted for his injuries.

## 2. TEACHING OBJECTIVES AND DISCUSSION POINTS

### Water Immersion and Hypothermia

- Most often occurring in low- and middle-income areas. More common overall in young but higher mortality in elderly.
- Drowning refers to a submersion injury into a medium of liquid that often involves a primary respiratory impairment and may lead to cardiac irregularities.
- Prolonged water immersion is a high-risk factor for hypothermia (defined as a core temperature below 35°C/95°F) as a result of convective heat loss to cold air and conductive heat loss to water.

- Older patients are at increased risk of injury from hypothermia, secondary to underlying chronic diseases, medications, social isolation, and difficulty in localizing exam findings.
- While managing hypothermia, patients are very sensitive to sudden movement (which could precipitate arrhythmias) and care should be taken to avoid jostling the patient.
- Rewarming includes removing wet clothing and providing slow rewarming at a rate of 0.5 and 2°C/hour, while being careful not to burn the skin.

**Nonfreezing Cold Injuries and Soft Tissue Infections**

- Nonfreezing cold injuries (NFCI), formally trench foot or immersion foot, are injuries of the soft tissue, nerves, and vasculature exposed to a nonfreezing cold and wet environment.
- NFCI is often seen after days of exposure, but during extreme situations (such as fatigue, malnutrition, stress), may develop after only 14–22 hours of exposure to temps 0–15°C.
- Risk factors including older age, smoking, diabetes, peripheral vascular disease, mental illness, and substance/alcohol usage.
- Treatment includes drying, wound management, and slow rewarming of the extremity.
- While prophylactic antibiotics are not always needed, signs of secondary infections or abscesses may prompt early antimicrobial management.
  - Treatment for freshwater, nonsoil, or sewage contaminated injuries should cover staphylococci, streptococci, and *Pseudomonas* species (e.g. Ancef and Levaquin)
- Rewarming is often a painful process and providers should consider management with NSAIDs, opioids, and possibly amitriptyline.

**Communication and Teamwork**

- Clear communication with EMS staff is necessary to get an adequate understanding about the conditions that a patient was exposed to prehospital.
- When history is limited, careful examination and understanding of local environment conditions can help aid in emergency management.
- Closed loop communication with team members can avoid miscommunication errors.

## 3. SUPPLIES

- Gurney
- Patient (standardized or mannequin)
- Stethoscope
- Monitor, including continuous temperature monitoring (such as rectal probe)
- Ability to provide oxygen and/or suction
- IV supplies, blood draw supplies, syringes to signify medication, IV fluids, and IVPB for medications
- IV fluid warmer, hot packs, and warm blankets
- Wound care supplies: gauze, scissors, tissue forceps
- Intradermal lidocaine and scalpel for bedside incision and drainage (I&D)

## 4. MOULAGE

- Patient or mannequin can have makeup to look a little blue in the face and hands.
- Patient or mannequin can have makeup on both feet that make them look white, with some linear lacerations on the bottom of the feet with overlying redness.
- If possible, patient or mannequin should have clothes dirty and soiled.

## 5. IMAGES AND LABS

- Fingerstick 160, lactate 1.2, CPK 40
- CBC: WBC 8, Hgb 12.5, hematocrit 37, platelets 180
- Chemistry: Na 132, K 3.5, creatinine 2.0, BUN 40
- ECG: sinus bradycardia (Figure 19.1)
- Trench foot (Figure 19.2)

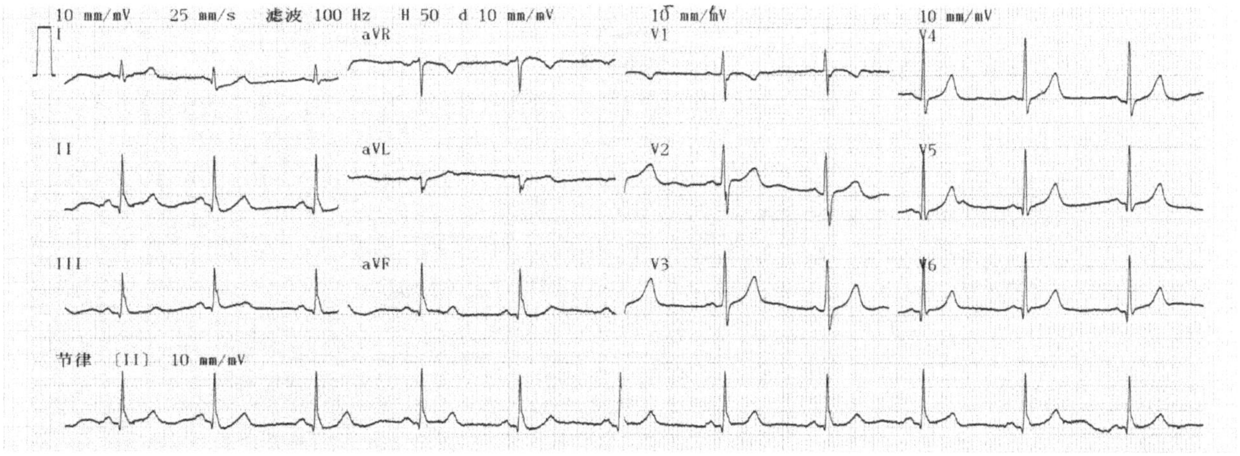


**Figure 19.1** ECG: Sinus bradycardia.
Image credit hudiemm/E +/Getty Images.

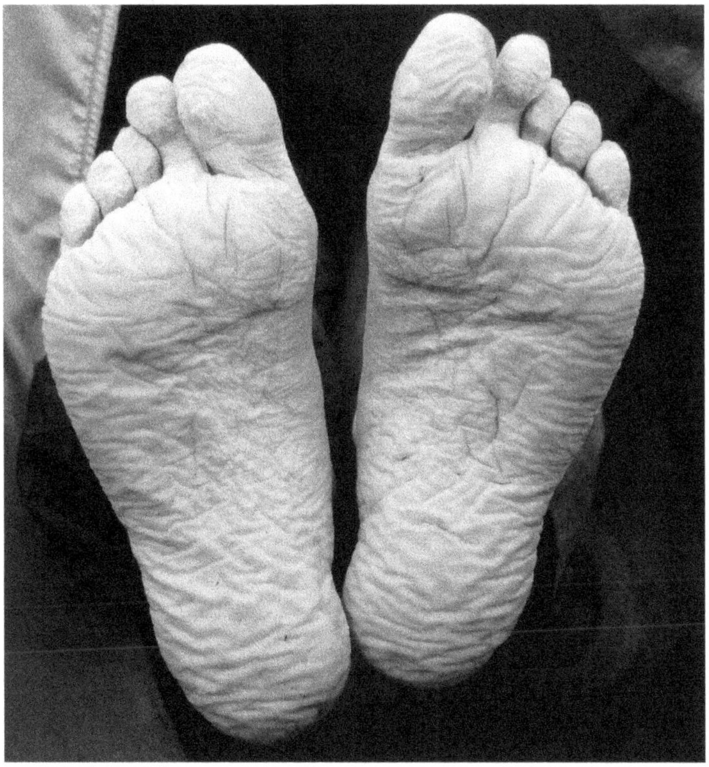

**Figure 19.2** Trench foot.
Image credit Mehmet Karatay, CC BY-SA 3.0 https://creativecommons.org/licenses/by-sa/3.0, via Wikimedia Commons.

## 6. ACTORS (CONFEDERATES) AND THEIR ROLES

- Patient or mannequin: sleepy, slow to respond, appears confused, shivering, describes burning pain in feet
- EMS: will stay for primary survey to answer questions and then will leave
- Nurse: assists team with administration and execution or orders
- Podiatry: may answer basic questions, but reports they are not an in-house consulting or admitting service and patient should be managed as per primary team recommendations

## 7. CRITICAL ACTIONS

- Evaluate for signs of cardiac or pulmonary compromise in a possible near-drowning patient scenario.
- Identify moderate hypothermia and initiate slow active rewarming, while being careful not to overly stimulate patient.
- Assess for secondary findings in hypothermia including evaluation of bloodwork, ECG, and maintaining on cardiac monitor.
- Give adequate pain control during rewarming process.
- Identify NFCI (trench foot), dry and slowly rewarm the extremities.
- Assess wounds for infection, recognize midfoot abscess, attempt I&D, and perform local wound care management.
- Initiate antibiotics for freshwater, nonsoil, or sewage contaminated skin infection, covering for staphylococci, streptococci, and *Pseudomonas* species.
- Admit the patient for monitoring and social services/safe disposition planning.

## 8. TIMELINE WITH TRANSITION POINTS

Initial stimulus: You are working at a small community hospital near a lower socioeconomic area in Miami, Florida. It is early winter, and due to heavy amounts of rainfall this season, there have been reports of flooding in several neighborhoods in the area. You receive initial notification that EMS has been called out to a patient trapped in a flooded one-story house with concern for possible near drowning.

### EMS Prehospital Report upon Arrival

A 70-year-old male with history peripheral vascular disease, DM, and bipolar disorder presenting found trapped inside his bedroom by an overturned dresser, wading through 3 feet of freshwater. Patient reports he had been trapped for over 24 hours, without access to food, water, warmth, or dry clothes. While initial report was for near drowning, EMS did not see any signs of drowning or note any immediate airway issues. They did, however, find the patient shivering in the cold, shoeless, with complaints of burning pain to both feet. No treatment was initiated.

### Time: Zero

VS: BP 100/70, HR 42, RR 12, O2 sat 97% on RA, temp 31°C (rectal)

**General Appearance**

Patient is awake, but somnolent, slow to respond to questioning, appears mildly confused. Complains of burning pain to both legs but difficult to get to answer other questions. He is shoeless and both his feet are white and swollen. His clothes are soaking wet.

### Primary Survey

- Airway: intact, phonating well, tolerating secretions
- Breathing: breathing comfortably, good air movement, and equal breath sounds bilaterally
- Circulation: normal cardiac sounds, bradycardic, pulses 4+ in all four extremities
- Disability: Glasgow Coma Scale (E4, V4, M5), answers questions but appears confused, pupils 3 mm bilaterally, patient moving all extremities
- Exposure: wet clothing removed. Patient fully exposed. Only abnormalities noted are feet.

### Initial Interventions

- IVs placed, preferably two large bores.
- Bloodwork sent, including chemistry, complete blood count, lactate, and CPK.
- Patient should be placed on cardiac monitor and have continual core temperature monitoring (such as a rectal probe).
- ECG may be performed due to bradycardia (see Figure 19.1).
- EMS will stick around and answer questions at this point. If they are not engaged by now, they will move on to another call.
  - If asked they will mention he lives alone. No family around. No obvious signs of trauma. No medications or advance directives (e.g., DNR/MOLST) were found. The room was filled with 3 feet of freshwater (uncontaminated by soil or sewage), in which his feet had been submerged for a prolonged period while he was lying in bed. He apparently couldn't find socks or his shoes. No signs of electrical or thermal burns.
- Patient should be actively rewarmed after exposed. Examples include warm blankets, forced air warming device, and heat packs in the groin and axilla.
- Providers should ask for IV fluids and to have them warmed/delivered through a fluid warmer (to 40–42°C).
  - Nurse will not hear the warmed fluids and will say aloud, "You want me to just hang a liter bolus?"
  - If provider specifies warmed fluids using closed-loop communication then it will be done.
  - If provider just says "yes" or doesn't close the loop then room-temperature fluids will be given (a point that could be brought up for discussion during the debrief).

## Time: Five Minutes – Transition Point 1

VS: BP 110/70, HR 50, RR 12, O2 sat 98% on RA, temp 33°C (rectal)

### Secondary Survey

- HEENT: PERRL, dry mucus membrane, normal pharynx
- Neck: supple, no midline cervical tenderness
- CV/chest: no signs of trauma, no tenderness, bradycardia, normal s1/s2, no MRG
- Pulmonary: clear and equal bilaterally
- Abdomen/pelvis: soft, nontender, nondistended. Pelvis stable.
- MSK: no signs of trauma. Both feet are white, swollen and macerated (see Figure 19.2). There are many small linear superficial lacerations on the bottom and dorsum of both feet. Some of the lacerations have surrounding erythema and some warmth. The right foot has a small area of fluctuance about the size of a nickel on the dorsum indicating an abscess, with surrounding cellulitis. Patient has decreased sensation to both feet, but good pulses.

### Further Actions

- At this point continued warming is indicated. Provider may escalate warming or continue.
  - If room-temperature saline given, providers may use this time to change it to warmed fluids.

- Providers should identify concern for NFCI (trench foot) to both feet.
  - Feet should be cleaned and dried. Providers may indicate slow rewarming either passively or actively.
- X-rays may be ordered (chest, pelvis, feet . . . etc.) and can either be normal or unavailable.
- Providers should identify overlying skin and soft tissue infection and abscess.
  - Providers may consider preparing for wound management and debridement of any dead or necrotic tissue or performance of bedside I&D.
- Providers should ask for IV antibiotics to cover for staphylococci, streptococci, and *Pseudomonas* species.

### Time: 15 Minutes – Transition Point 2

VS: BP 120/70, HR 55, RR 14, O2 sat 99% on RA, temp 35°C (rectal)

General appearance: Patient slowly becoming more alert. As feet become warmer the patient begins to ask for more and more pain medicine for burning numb pain.

Exam: unchanged except feet slowly becoming more hyperemic (red) during warming

**Further Actions**

- Providers should consider giving pain medicine during the course of rewarming. NSAIDs, opioids, and possibly amitriptyline are good options.
- Tetanus should also be updated.
- Labs, if ordered, are revealed (See 5. Images and Labs).
- Podiatry may be consulted. If so, they call back and give very basic instructions for trench foot (local wound care, drying and slow rewarming, managing infections) and indicate that they are not an in-house consulting or admitting service and that patient should be managed as per primary team recommendations.
- Social work may be involved (or can be deferred to admitting team).
- Patient will need to be admitted for continued rewarming, pain control, and wound care management.

## 9. STIMULI

See 5. Images and Labs.

## BIBLIOGRAPHY

Brown DJ, Brugger H, Boyd J, Paal P. Accidental hypothermia. *N Engl J Med.* 2012 Nov 15;367(20):1930–1938. doi:10.1056/NEJMra1114208. Erratum in: *N Engl J Med.* 2013 Jan 24;368(4):394. PMID: 23150960.

Diaz JH, Lopez FA. Skin, soft tissue and systemic bacterial infections following aquatic injuries and exposures. *Am J Med Sci.* 2015 Mar;349(3):269–275. doi:10.1097/MAJ.0000000000000366. PMID: 25374398.

Giesbrecht GG. Cold stress, near drowning and accidental hypothermia: a review. *Aviat Space Environ Med.* 2000 Jul;71(7):733–752. PMID: 10902937.

Thomas JR, Oakley HN. Nonfreezing cold injury. In: Pandolf KB, Burr RE, eds. *Medical Aspects of Harsh Environments.* Washington, DC: Office of the Surgeon General, United States Army; 2001: 467–490.

Ungley CC, Channell GD, Richards RL. The immersion foot syndrome. *Br J Surg.* 1946;33:17.

Vanden Hoek TL, Morrison LJ, Shuster M, et al. Part 12: cardiac arrest in special situations: 2010 American Heart Association Guidelines for Cardiopulmonary Resuscitation and Emergency Cardiovascular Care. *Circulation.* 2010 Nov 2;122(18 Suppl 3):S829–S861. doi:10.1161/CIRCULATIONAHA.110.971069. Erratum in: *Circulation.* 2011 Feb 15;123(6):e239. Erratum in: *Circulation.* 2011 Oct 11;124(15):e405. PMID: 20956228.

Wrenn K. Immersion foot: a problem of the homeless in the 1990s. *Arch Intern Med.* 1991 Apr;151(4):785–788. doi:10.1001/archinte.151.4.785. PMID: 2012466.

CASE 20

# Disaster Strikes Twice

## Managing a Dog Bite Injury in a Posthurricane Rescue

Colleen M. Donovan and Jennifer E. Geller

DISASTER PRINCIPLES

- Field stabilization, treatment, and transport
- EMS disaster operations
- Flooding
- Scene safety and security in the field
- Clinical diagnosis and treatment
- National disaster response
- Disaster Medical Assistance Teams (DMAT)
- National disaster management system
- Climate change and disaster medicine
- Information management/communications
- Field operations and logistics
- Disaster operations
- Vulnerable populations
- Search and rescue
- Hurricanes/cyclones/typhoons
- Care of animals

## 1. SCENARIO OVERVIEW

*This is a standardized patient (SP) scenario, with options for wound care/hemorrhage task trainer or mannequin, based on desired complexity. It takes place at the scene. The geographic location for this scenario is in a hurricane/flood prone coastal region.*

Lowell Rafferty is a 58-year-old male with a history of hypertension and type 2 diabetes, who was bitten by a large dog on the right arm at least 2 hours and 30 minutes prior to presentation. It is three days after a Category 5 hurricane made landfall, and there has been extensive flooding. Mr. Rafferty was acting as a civilian rescuer in his boat when he came across the wounded, stranded dog on the roof of a carport. The water level reaches the carport roof (~7–8 feet). He thinks he was bitten two or three times with significant force/head shaking; he had to kick the dog several times to get it to release his arm. In an attempt to free himself, he fell into the brackish flood water but was able to pull himself out. He is right-hand dominant and was unable to navigate his boat back to his home. He is now having significant pain/swelling of the right hand, wrist, and forearm, and can barely range any joints below the right elbow without intense pain. Using the radio in his boat, he was able to call for help. No details are known about the dog, and the dog escaped after biting him.

Learner(s) is/are physician member(s) of a standard six-person Federal Emergency Management Agency Type 3 Stillwater/Flood Search and Rescue (SAR) Team.[1] They are deployed to rescue Mr. Rafferty and arrive on scene to find him seated on the carport roof (e.g. the floor of any given simulation space). They are partnered with an emergency medical technician-basic (EMT-B). Learners should focus only on medical care for this scenario. After demonstrating situational awareness (SA)/inquiring about scene safety, they may assume that the carport has structural stability, that rest of the SAR team is standing by in the rescue boat, and that the team will ensure appropriate safe transport of the patient.

## 2. TEACHING OBJECTIVES AND DISCUSSION POINTS

### Clinical and Medical Management

a. SA, PPE, and scene safety
b. Evaluation of the bite wound patient for blunt trauma and penetrating injury to deeper anatomy including neuro/vascular structures.
c. Management of bite wound including irrigation, decontamination, dressing, and splinting.

### Communication and Teamwork

a. Discussion of plan with patient
b. Interprofessional communication with on-scene team member(s)
c. Communication with Incident Command or animal control regarding injured, potentially aggressive dog
d. Communication with receiving facility (casualty collection point [CCP], Disaster Medical Assistance Team [DMAT] field hospital, ED)

## 3. SUPPLIES

a. SP clothing: dirty, including long-sleeved shirt with shredded, blood-stained right sleeve
b. Personal equipment (e.g. stethoscope, PPE, wristwatch)
   i. Optional
      1. At the scene: life vests, helmets for added fidelity
      2. Two-way radios for communications with team/radio etiquette
c. Blood pressure cuff
d. Pulse oximeter
e. Glucometer
f. Wound care/hemorrhage task trainer: if planning to have learners demonstrate local anesthesia, wound exploration, or tourniquet placement
g. Wound care kit
   i. Example: *Auerbach's Wilderness Medicine*, Table 21-8, Wound Care First Aid Kit
      1. PPE, gloves, facemask with shield, etc.
      2. Tourniquet
      3. Wound irrigation: 60 cc syringe, various needles/blunt cannulas, saline or distilled water, povidone-iodine (e.g. Betadine), splash shield
      4. Suture material and instruments (not supposed to be used in this scenario but would be available in a field wound care kit. May help prompt discussion of contraindications to closure).
      5. Dressings: gauze, tape, gauze roll, flexible splint (e.g. SAM splint), elastic roll (e.g. ACE wrap), cravats, safety pins

6. Medications: lidocaine vials, 10 cc syringes, antibacterial ointment (e.g. Bacitracin), cephalexin 500 mg tabs in labeled pill bottle (green oval candy, such as Mike & Ikes), ciprofloxacin 500 mg tabs in labeled pill bottle (white oval candy, such as TicTacs)

## 4. MOULAGE

a. Multiple deep lacerations and puncture wounds to right forearm, oozing blood. The following article has a good photo for reference: https://jetem.org/k9-police-dog-bite/[3]

## 5. IMAGES AND LABS

None

## 6. ACTORS (CONFEDERATES) AND THEIR ROLES

a. Patient: SP, may be supplemented by wound care/hemorrhage control task trainer
b. EMT-B partner: assist with wound care props and prompt for appropriate care
c. Animal control officer/command staff (radio): discuss dog attack
d. Receiving physician at CCP/ED (radio): receives report, prompts for any missed critical actions

## 7. CRITICAL ACTIONS

a. Demonstrate SA, inquire about scene safety
b. Make contact and introduce self/team to SP
c. Obtain history
d. Perform focused physical exam of right upper extremity, including neurovascular evaluation
e. Consider and perform field management options (transport to CCP/field hospital/ED will take ~one hour)
   i. Irrigation
   ii. Dressing
   iii. Splint and sling
   iv. Optional: tourniquet placement (if including hemorrhage control task trainer)
f. Verbalize the need for advanced management
   i. Imaging for foreign bodies, fractures
   ii. More thorough irrigation
   iii. Need for antibiotics/postexposure prophylaxis
      1. May consider giving oral cephalexin and ciprofloxacin from kit if concern for delayed/long transport time is verbalized
      2. Review typical pathogens
      3. Consider brackish water pathogens (*Vibrio*)
      4. Tetanus and rabies prophylaxis
   iv. Consider additional evaluation for crush injury/compartment syndrome
   v. Consider surgical debridement/management
   vi. Discuss indications/contraindications for wound closure
g. Communications
   i. Discuss need for higher level of care with SP
   ii. Discuss transport with team

iii. Radio discussion with animal control about dog
iv. Radio discussion with receiving facility

## 8. TIMELINE WITH TRANSITION POINTS

### Time: Two Minutes – Prebrief

You are physician member(s) of a SAR team. It is three days after a Category 5 hurricane made landfall, and there has been extensive flooding. You are dispatched to rescue a 58-year-old male with a history hypertension and type 2 diabetes, who was bitten by a large dog on the right arm ~2.5 hours prior to patient contact. He is trapped on the roof of a carport; the water level reaches the carport roof (~7–8 feet). The patient was able to use his shirt as a makeshift bandage. You are partnered with an EMT-B SAR team member who is on their first ever deployment; the rest of the team is standing by in the boat. *Only if asked*: The dog's location is unknown at this time.

### Time: Zero – Arrival on Scene

a. Summary of initial presentation: Middle-aged man seated on the floor in his undershirt, right forearm wrapped in a blood-stained, partially shredded, long-sleeved shirt, shouting and waving to team on entry, "Over here!" He should attempt to move toward team very slowly, without success.
b. Initial interventions
   i. Advise patient to stay seated where he is
   ii. SA: inquire about roof structural integrity and location of dog
   iii. Ensure proper PPE is applied prior to approaching the patient
c. EMT partner: may prompt for SA
   i. "Ha ... this is probably the most dangerous thing I've ever done!" or "You know, I remember doing scenarios like this in sims ... what's the thing we're supposed to do before approaching the scene or the patient?," a prompt for "body substance isolation (BSI), scene safety."
      1. If learner states "BSI, scene safety," prompt for specific concerns, "like what?"
      2. EMT-B or facilitator may play audio files of structural creaking and dog barking
         a. Easily found via internet search for "creaking building sound effect," or "dog barking sound effect"
         b. May be played via EMT-B's phone or facilitator computer
      3. Facilitator: confirms (either overhead or via radio) that SAR teammates have ensured structural stability, the dog does not seem to be in the immediate area, and they will continue to monitor for changes

**Critical Actions**
- Demonstrate SA, inquire about scene safety
- Recognize need for PPE

### Time: Two Minutes – Transition Point 1 – Patient Contact and History

VS: BP 114/82, HR 99, RR 18, sat 94% RA, temp not available (no thermometer), but not hot to touch, fingerstick glucose 222 mg/dL (must ask)

a. Make contact and introduce self/team to SP
b. SP: "I'm so glad you are here. I'm Lowell Rafferty. I called hours ago – I thought you'd never come."
c. Obtain history
   i. SP: refuse exam until history complete
      1. S: multiple painful deep lacerations and puncture wounds to right forearm, oozing blood, makeshift bandage with shirt.
      2. A: NKDA
      3. M: metformin, amlodipine, aspirin
      4. P: type 2 diabetes, hypertension
      5. L: breakfast this morning: bagel and black coffee
      6. E: "I was out in my boat, just trying to check on neighbors and see if anyone needed help. I saw this big dog – not sure what kind, maybe part rottweiler? – on top of the roof here . . . he looked hurt – had a big wound on his back leg. He had a bright pink collar on, so I figured he was someone's stranded pet. He seemed friendly at first, but when I tried to get him into the boat, he started acting crazy! He did this to my arm.. . . I wrestled him but couldn't get him off me until we fell into the water. He let me go and swam away. I tried to fix it myself, but it hurts really bad. I can't make a fist to grip, can't steer the boat. My phone fell into the water and cell service is bad right now. I tried radioing my buddies, but none of them responded. That's when I really started to worry and called for you guys. My elderly dad is back at my home by himself, and I'm worried about him. I know he'll be wondering what happened to me.
   ii. EMT-B: pantomime obtaining VS
      1. Learner should direct EMT-B to use left arm
      2. EMT-B only report VS when asked

**Critical Actions**

- Make patient contact, introduce self/team
- Obtain history

### Time: Two to Four Minutes – Transition Point 2 – Physical Exam

a. Physical exam
   i. Learner should perform head-to-toe trauma exam; only pertinent positive finding is the RUE
   ii. General: initial relief, but still anxious, in severe pain. Patient alert and orientated ×4
   iii. Heart: regular rate and rhythm, unremarkable
   iv. Lungs: clear to auscultation bilaterally
   v. RUE: multiple deep lacerations and puncture wounds to right forearm, oozing blood, contaminated with debris/soil, exposed muscle, but no obvious exposure of tendon or bone
      1. Pulse: 2+ right radial pulse
      2. Motor: unable to move fingers, hand, wrist due to intense pain. Pain with both active and passive motion.
      3. Sensory: sensation to fingertips grossly intact
      4. The following article has a good photo for reference: https://jetem.org/k9-police-dog-bite[3]
   vi. Skin: scattered abrasions and contusions, but no other trauma

**Critical Actions**

- Perform physical exam, focusing on RUE neurovascular exam

### Time: 4–10 Minutes – Transition Point 3 – Field Management[2,4,5]

a. Consider and perform field management options – learners must demonstrate:
    i. Irrigation
        1. If using task trainer: must demonstrate local anesthesia administration
        2. If not using task trainer, must describe local anesthesia administration
    ii. Dressing
    iii. Splint and sling

**Critical Actions**

- Demonstrate field local anesthesia administration, irrigation, wound assessment and dressing, splint, and sling

### Time: 10+ Minutes – Transition Point 4 – Transport and Final Considerations

a. Transport: Local hospitals have been damaged and are on full facility divert.
    i. Transport to CCP/field hospital will take one to two hours
        1. DMAT Type 1 base load
            a. With some IV antibiotics, rabies immunoglobulin and vaccine, Tdap
            b. Currently without X-ray or surgical capability
    ii. Transport to the nearest hospital with surgical capability is in a neighboring state, minimum ~three to four hours by ground.
    iii. Air transport is not available due to windspeed and poor visibility.
b. Verbalize the need for advanced management
    i. Imaging for foreign bodies, fractures
    ii. More thorough irrigation
    iii. Need for antibiotics/postexposure prophylaxis
        1. Review typical pathogens
            a. Learners have access to oral cephalexin and ciprofloxacin in the would care kit – should consider giving oral doses due to prolonged transport times.
        2. Consider brackish water pathogens (*Vibrio*)
        3. Tetanus and rabies prophylaxis
    iv. Consider additional evaluation for crush injury/compartment syndrome
    v. Consider surgical debridement/management
        1. Discuss indications/contraindications for wound closure
c. SP: may help prompt verbalization of more detailed plan of care.
    i. "Thanks Doc – can you drop me at home? It's only 20 minutes from here. I need to get back to my dad. He's elderly and don't think he can take good care of himself without me . . ."
    ii. "You really think I need to go to the hospital? Aren't they in bad shape too, overwhelmed with people? I heard that the university hospital is partly underwater and running on backup generators."
    iii. "At the hospital/field hospital, they'll just stitch me up and send me on my way, right?"

iv. When plan adequately explained to SP, "Ok Doc, I understand. But please, can someone help get a message to my dad and my neighbor? They're both safe for now . . . our homes are on high ground, and we didn't get any damage to the houses, but someone needs to look in on him."

c. EMT-B: may help prompt for advanced management considerations
   i. "Doc – do you think it's broken?"
   ii. After discussion of complications from bite wound, time delay and antibiotics, "If only we had something to give him now . . . maybe there's something in the kit?"
   iii. "Why do you think the dog attacked like that?" (prompt discussion of rabies postexposure prophylaxis and tetanus)

**Critical Actions**

- Given long transport time, consider oral antibiotics from kit
- Verbalize the need for advanced management including imaging, lab work, IV antibiotics, source control/surgical management
- Communications
  i. Discuss need for higher level of care with SP
  ii. Discuss transport with team
  iii. Radio discussion with animal control about dog
  iv. Radio discussion with receiving facility

#### Curveball Inserts for Added Complexity

a. Twilight or night rescue (lights off in the sim space), requiring flashlights or headlamps
b. Active/arterial bleeding (if using a hemorrhage task trainer)
c. SP refuses transport to get back to his elderly dad

## REFERENCES

1. Federal Emergency Management Agency. *Resource Typing Definition for Response Mass Search and Rescue Operations*. Resource Typing and Library Tool. Washington, DC: Federal Emergency Management Agency; 2020:1–6. https://rtlt.preptoolkit.fema.gov/Public/Resource/ViewFile/8-508-1264?type = Pdf&q = still. Accessed July 3, 2022.
2. Jamshidi R. Wound management. In: Auerbach PS, Cushing TA, Harris NS, eds. *Auerbach's Wilderness Medicine*. 7th ed. Philadelphia: Saunders; 2017:440–450.
3. Han V, Marshall J. K-9 police dog bite. *J Educ Teach Emerg Med*. 2017;2(1). https://jetem.org/k9-police-dog-bite/. doi:10.21980/J8B88G.
4. Kassel MR, O'Connor T, Gianotti A. Splints and slings. In: Auerbach PS, Cushing TA, Harris NS, eds. *Auerbach's Wilderness Medicine*. 7th ed. Philadelphia: Saunders; 2017:492–517.
5. Phillips LL, Semple J. Bites and injuries inflicted by wild and domestic animals. In: Auerbach PS, Cushing TA, Harris NS, eds. *Auerbach's Wilderness Medicine*. 7th ed. Philadelphia: Saunders; 2017:617–645.

CASE 21

# When Rescuers Become Patients

## A Cold Immersion Injury Scenario from the DMAT Field Hospital

Colleen M. Donovan and Lekha Reddy

DISASTER PRINCIPLES

- Field stabilization, treatment, and transport
- EMS disaster operations
- Personal preparedness
- Flooding
- Scene safety and security in the field
- Clinical diagnosis and treatment
- National disaster response
- Disaster Medical Assistance Teams (DMAT)
- National disaster management system
- Displaced populations
- Climate change and disaster medicine
- Information management/communications
- Field operations and logistics
- Disaster operations
- Vulnerable populations
- Search and rescue

### 1. SCENARIO OVERVIEW

*This scenario can be done with a standardized patient (SP) or mannequin. It takes place at a field hospital. The geographic location for this scenario is in a cold weather, flood prone coastal region.*

Oedipus "Ed" Rafferty is a 38-year-old male without medical history who presents to the Disaster Medical Assistance Team (DMAT) field hospital with intense pain and swelling in both lower legs. It is eight days after a severe spring storm, and there has been extensive flooding.

Ed is a firefighter/emergency medical technician-basic (FF/EMT-B) and has been working long shifts (12 hours on, 12 hours off) as part of rescue and recovery efforts. Two days ago, 10 hours into their shift, Ed and his partner were dispatched to an elderly patient with a head injury – she had been clearing debris and sustained a superficial scalp laceration from a falling tree branch. She was on anticoagulation, and her scalp was initially bleeding "a lot." While evaluating the patient on scene, a local dam collapsed, causing a flash flood. Ed, his partner, and the patient were able to take shelter in her one-story home, but the flood water disabled their ambulance and trapped them with ~2 feet of flood water in the house and deeper water surrounding the property. The elderly patient's injury turned out to be superficial and the bleeding stopped with direct pressure and a bandage. Ed radioed for help, but due to safety issues, the Search and Rescue (SAR) team could not reach them for approximately 30 hours. They did have access to canned food and potable water, but no electricity or heat, and ambient temperatures ranged from 40–60°F.

The SAR team brought them to the DMAT, where the elderly patient was treated, and Ed and his partner were taken to a nearby internally displaced persons (IDP) shelter to debrief, clean up, and rest while transport home was being arranged. While taking off his uniform (including socks and boots), Ed noticed that his calves and feet were sore and crampy. The skin was pale, mottled, "pruney," and felt "weird," when he walked barefoot into the tiled shower stall, as if he still had shoes on, like "walking on a thick blanket." While taking a hot shower, he felt intense throbbing, burning pain in both lower legs and feet with rapid redness and swelling, forcing him to sit on the floor of the shower. He was able to crawl out of the shower stall and call for help. Shelter staff helped him dress and brought him back to the DMAT for evaluation.

Learner(s) is/are a physician or team at the triage/emergency tent of a DMAT field hospital. Mr. Rafferty is brought to them by the ICP staff. Learner(s) may assume they have access to a typical Type 1 DMAT base load/medical cache.

## 2. TEACHING OBJECTIVES AND DISCUSSION POINTS

### Clinical and Medical Management

- Appropriate diagnosis and management of mild hypothermia
- Appropriate differential diagnosis of prolonged, cold and wet exposure
- Appropriate diagnosis and management of nonfreezing cold injuries (NFCI)

### Communication and Teamwork

- Work as a team to appropriately manage a patient with NFCI
- Appropriate and timely discussion with receiving hospital for transfer

## 3. SUPPLIES

- IV fluids
- Blankets
- SP or mannequin with moulage described next

## 4. MOULAGE

- Wet socks, boots, EMT uniform
- Both feet are wrinkled with large, mottled white and red areas up the calves (signifies extreme vasoconstriction), with erythematous skin of the feet, scattered petechiae around the toes and early blistering – meant to simulate the transition from the prehyperemic phase to the hyperemic phase.

## 5. IMAGES AND LABS

- Point-of-care (POC) labs using a commercial portable/handheld blood analysis system
  - Sodium, potassium, calcium, chloride, total $CO_2$ or bicarbonate, glucose, BUN, creatinine
  - Hemoglobin, hematocrit
- Tests: ECG
- No imaging necessary

## 6. ACTORS

- Patient: mannequin or SP
- Nurse: should be knowledgeable and helpful

## 7. CRITICAL ACTIONS

- Identify and treat mild hypothermia
- Develop a differential diagnosis for the patient's lower extremity symptoms
- Recognize and treat the symptoms of NFCI
- Recognize that the patient requires inpatient care and transfer after stabilization

## 8. TIMELINE

### Time: Two Minutes – Prebrief

You are physician member(s) of a Type 1 DMAT field hospital team. It is eight days after a severe spring storm, and there has been extensive flooding. You receive notification via radio that a 38-year-old male with unknown medical history is coming in with staff from the nearby IDP shelter. He was recently rescued from a flooded home and is now complaining of bilateral leg pain so intense that he cannot walk.

### Time: Zero to Four Minutes – Patient Arrives at Field Hospital Triage/Emergency Tent, Initial Evaluation

VS: BP 90/50, HR 110, RR 20, $O_2$ sat 97% RA, T 34°C (temporal scan), ECG sinus tachycardia

Summary of initial presentation: Patient brought to field hospital by IDP shelter staff, with the history of prolonged cold-water immersion, delayed rescue, and subsequent pain several hours later while taking a shower. On arrival he is alert but crying in significant pain. He redressed in his damp clothing and is now shivering. Wet socks and boots are in a bag – he was in too much pain to put them back on.

- Initial interventions: expose patient skin, head-to-toe physical exam, place on monitor, POC glucose, establish peripheral IV access
- Physical exam
  - General: shivering, A&O ×3 but pain makes it difficult to provide full history
  - HEENT: atraumatic, pupils 3 mm and reactive, dry mucous membranes
  - Neck: supple
  - Chest: lungs clear to auscultation bilaterally, no chest wall trauma or bruising
  - Heart: sinus tachycardia
  - Abdomen: normal
  - Extremities: Distal lower extremities are cool in some places but hot over the feet with erythema and swelling. The soles of both feet are wrinkled and mottled with large asymmetric patchy white areas, two fluid-filled bullae on left foot, peripheral pulses are bounding, but capillary refill 4+ seconds, very painful to touch.
  - Skin: as detailed in extremities, otherwise general pallor, cool, wet
  - Neuro: Bilateral lower extremities have diminished sensation and 3/5 motor strength

- Nurse
  - Obtains IV access, POC glucose (informs team that glucose is 60), warm blankets for hypothermia.
    - Verbal cues: "Wow team – look at his feet! His body feels cool but his legs are hot. Did he get burned somehow? Why is this happening?"

**Critical Actions**

- Obtain history and perform physical exam
- Establish IV access
- Obtain POC glucose
- Identify and treat mild hypothermia
- Order POC chemistry, hemoglobin and hematocrit panels as part of hypothermia and NFCI workup
- Identify and consider differential diagnosis for lower extremity symptoms

### Time: Four to Six Minutes – Transition Point 1 – Rewarming and Fluid Resuscitation

VS: BP 105/55, HR 97, RR 18, $O_2$ sat 97% RA, T not rechecked

- Warm IV fluids will simultaneously improve the hypotension, tachycardia and treat NFCI
  - Prompt to consider strategies for warming IV fluids in the field
- Elevating lower extremities and leaving feet exposed will treat NFCI
- Consider dextrose containing fluids for relative hypoglycemia
- Tachypnea resolves with fluid administration and warming
- Patient stops shivering and some color returns to skin after warm blankets and IV fluids
- Nurse verbal cues: "What kind of fluid, doc? You know, one time, I had terrible gastro and had to go to the ED to get IV fluids.... I remember my arm got so cold and I was shivering so bad my IV almost came out! What is the temperature difference between human and room temp fluids anyway?"

**Critical Actions**

- Administer isotonic warm IV fluids
- Recognize hypoglycemia and consider dextrose containing fluids
- Recognize and treat NFCI
- Begin considering disposition/transfer

### Time: 6–10 Minutes – Transition Point 2 – Continued Monitoring, Rewarming, and Considerations for Medical Management

VS: BP 110/65, HR 85, RR 18, $O_2$ sat 97% RA, T 36.0°C (rectal), 35.5°C (oral)

- Hypotension and tachycardia resolve
- Hypothermia resolves with treatment
- Continue to expose and elevate lower extremities
- Nurse verbal cues
  - If asked for repeat temp: "How did you want me to check that doc?"

- "He seems like he is in a lot of pain – is there anything we can give him?"
- "His legs really don't look good – should we warm him more? Or faster? We can get hot bath water – wouldn't that warm him? Should we unroof those blisters?"
- "And I think I see cracks in his skin ... do we need to give him any kind of prophylaxis to prevent badness?"

**Critical Actions**

- Consider methods to monitor hypothermia (rectal versus oral temp)
- Consider tetanus prophylaxis
- Consider pain control
  - Prompt discussion for neuropathic pain agents (such as tricyclic antidepressants [TCAs]). Some DMATs do carry TCAs in their cache, along with acetaminophen, NSAIDs and opiates.

### Time: 10+ Minutes – Transition Point 3 – Transfer and Final Considerations

VS: BP 110/65, HR 85, RR 18, $O_2$ sat 97% RA, T 36.0°C (rectal), 35.5°C (oral)

- Verbalize the need for advanced management
  - Concern for tissue necrosis, reperfusion injury, monitoring for compartment syndrome (rare but possible) and soft tissue infections.
- Transport: Local hospitals have been damaged and are on full facility divert.
  - Transport to the nearest hospital with surgical capability is in a neighboring state, minimum ~three to four hours by ground.
  - Air transport is available (~1.5 hours), but with rapidly changing windspeed and visibility conditions
- Given the long transport time, discuss how to prevent lower extremities from warming too quickly, how to keep core warm but lower extremities cool during transport.
  - Continue to expose and elevate lower extremities, consider transport positioning
  - Cooling fan; light, sterile leg bandages and cooling with ice packs (requires close monitoring)
- Nurse verbal cues
  - "Hey Doc – I'm not sure we can care for him here. I think he might need more resources than we have."
  - "What's the fastest way to get him where he needs to go? What is the safest way?"
  - "Can he be transported sitting up? Could we just put him in a car?"
    - Prompt for supine transport with legs elevated above the level of the heart, protective cushioning while keeping the legs cool
- Receiving hospital physician (facilitator via radio) verbal cues:
  - "Sounds like he is in a lot of pain – how are you managing his pain?"
    - Prompt to consider neuropathic pain control, if not already done
  - "Are you sure he needs to come to us? What does he need that you don't have there? We're already swamped with overcrowding due to the floods."
  - When rationale for transfer is appropriately addressed: "Ah – I see your point. He sounds pretty bad although stable for now. The transport time will be long. How are you going to package him for transport, and how are you instructing your transport team?"
    - BONUS consideration: Who are you sending with him?
      - EMT, paramedic, mobile intensive care nurse, physician?

**Critical Actions**

- Verbalize the need for advanced management
- Consider transfer and transport
- Discuss how to transport patient safely while maintaining warm core and cool extremities
- Radio discussion with receiving facility/surgical/admitting team

## 9. STIMULI

- Initial ECG: sinus tachycardia
- Labs (Table 21.1)

**Table 21.1** Labs

| Parameter | Value | Comment |
|---|---|---|
| Hemoglobin | 8.0 | |
| Hematocrit | 11.1/39 | |
| Chemistries | | |
| Sodium | 135 | |
| Potassium | 4.9 | |
| Bicarbonate | 20 | |
| Chloride | 96 | |
| BUN | 28 | BUN:Cr > 20 with normal Cr signifies dehydration |
| Creatinine | 1.2 | |
| Calcium | 9.3 | |
| Glucose | 60 | |

## BIBLIOGRAPHY


Health and Medical Response System. Equipment and inventory: patient treatment cache (163–172); Team pharmaceutical equipment (173–182). In: *Response Teams Description Manual: Disaster Medical Assistance Team*. Washington, DC: US Department of Health and Human Services; 1999. www.odmt.org/docs/DMAT_OPS_NDMS.pdf. Accessed July 5, 2022.

Imray CHE, Handford C, Thomas OD, Castellani JW. Nonfreezing cold-induced injuries. In: Auerbach P, Cushing T, Harris NS, eds. *Auerbach's Wilderness Medicine*. 7th ed. Philadelphia: Elsevier; 2017:222–234.e3.

Zafren K. Nonfreezing cold injury (trench foot). *Int J Environ Res Public Health*. 2021;18(19):10482. doi:10.3390/ijerph181910482.

Zafren K. Nonfreezing cold water (trench foot) and warm water immersion injuries. In: Danzyl D, Ganetsky M, Post TW, eds. *UpToDate*. Waltham, MA: UpToDate; updated 2024, September 19. www.uptodate.com/contents/nonfreezing-cold-water-trench-foot-and-warm-water-immersion-injuries. Accessed July 5, 2022.

SECTION 5

# CLIMATOLOGICAL NATURAL DISASTERS

CASE 22

# Wildfire Chaos

## A Case of Trauma and Smoke Inhalation from Late Evacuation

Jonathan Gammel

DISASTER PRINCIPLES

- Clinical diagnosis and treatment
- Conventional standards of care
- Timing of medical and surgical interventions
- Heat emergencies
- Role of public health agencies in disaster medicine
- Field stabilization, treatment, and transport
- Transportation disasters
- Vehicle extraction
- Wildfires

### 1. SCENARIO OVERVIEW

A 42-year-old male with no known medical history is brought in by EMS to the ED trauma bay after a rollover motor vehicle accident while fleeing from a wildfire near his home. Per EMS, the patient was a restrained driver going approximately 60 mph when he ran through a red light and was struck by another vehicle attempting to evacuate the town. He lives near a heavily wooded area and initially refused to leave his home despite warnings from town officials to evacuate. Strong winds propelled the fire dangerously close to his home, with heavy smoke and approaching flames prompting him to rapidly evacuate the area. The patient is agitated and in distress, borderline hypotensive, and shouting that his leg is in excruciating pain. There is an obvious open tib-fib fracture on the right leg. On physical exam, the learner should identify carbonaceous sputum, bilateral wheezing, progressive hoarseness in the patient's voice, and right upper quadrant abdominal tenderness. Blood pressure continues to fall until blood products are given. Extended Focused Assessment with Sonography for Trauma (EFAST) exam reveals free fluid in Morrison's pouch. The patient is suffering from smoke inhalation injury and a liver laceration in addition to the open fracture. He will require airway management for anticipated progression of airway edema, orthopedic and trauma surgeon consultation, and open fracture management. Appropriate disposition is to the OR for positive EFAST with unstable vital signs. The scenario is complicated by patient agitation and acute stress reaction.

### 2. TEACHING OBJECTIVES AND DISCUSSION POINTS

1. The number of fatalities from wildfires has been increasing, driven by climate change as well as increasing development and populations in high fire prone environments.

2. The majority of wildfire fatalities in the past century occur during late evacuation. Early evacuation is key.
3. Motor vehicle accidents during evacuation are a significant cause of morbidity/mortality in wildfire disasters.
4. Late evacuation from wildfires is often complicated by difficult driving conditions, with poor visibility and traffic from other late evacuees.
5. Smoke-related disorders and bronchospasm are a significant cause of ED visits during wildfire disasters.
6. Patients showing signs of airway edema after smoke inhalation injury or burns should be intubated early.
7. Tetanus, antibiotics, and orthopedic consultation should be obtained for patients with open fractures.
8. Do not be distracted by dramatic but not acutely life-threatening injuries. The clinician must still perform a thorough trauma assessment looking for immediate life threats.
9. Understand when patients should be sent to CT versus directly to OR.

## 3. SUPPLIES

- Cervical collar
- Splinting material and wound dressings
- Ultrasound
- IV fluids
- PRBCs
- IV bags with medications (antibiotics)
- Syringes with medications (paralytics, sedatives, Tdap, push dose pressors)
- Noninvasive airway supplies (nasal cannula, NRB)
- Intubation supplies (BVM, suction, ETT, stylet, laryngoscope, bougie, backup airway device)
- Intubation capable mannequin, placed out of view or covered with sheet (or the patient can be a high-fidelity intubatable mannequin from the start)

## 4. MOULAGE

- Open tib-fib fracture to right leg
- Soot on face
- Minor abrasions scattered across body as desired

## 5. IMAGES AND LABS

- Portable CXR: unremarkable
- Portable pelvic XR: unremarkable
- ECG: sinus tachycardia
- Point-of-care ultrasound (POCUS): EFAST exam positive for free fluid in Morrison's pouch
- Labs: CBC, CMP, troponin, coags, type and screen, lactate, carboxyhemoglobin, cyanide level

## 6. ACTORS AND ROLES

- Patient: standardized patient or sim man, frightened and agitated although not confused, coughing from smoke inhalation injury, in pain and yelling about his leg, his concerns about his home and belongings etc.

- EMS: provide trauma report on arrival, unable to secure an IV, they have placed the patient in C-spine precautions
- Nurse: assists team by executing orders. Can prompt if team is not recognizing the smoke inhalation injury by saying "Why does his voice sound like that?"
- Trauma surgeon: will agree to bring patient to the OR once team discovers the positive EFAST with unstable vital signs. If desired, can have the trauma surgeon press team to send patient to CT despite positive FAST and hypotension.
- Orthopedics consultant: recommends administration of IV antibiotics and Tdap, requests placement of dressing over open wound and temporary splint for stabilization. Will join trauma team in the OR.

## 7. CRITICAL ACTIONS

- Demonstrates appropriate advanced trauma life support care
- Places patient on cardiac monitor and obtains IV access
- Maintains C-spine stabilization
- Recognizes signs and symptoms of impending airway compromise
- Recognizes positive EFAST
- Secures an advanced airway
- Administers antibiotics and Tdap for open fracture
- Administers blood products
- Consults orthopedics and trauma surgery
- Avoids sending patient to CT scanner

## 8. TIMELINE WITH TRANSITION POINTS

### Time: Zero

- Initial ED VS: BP 90/46 HR 112 RR 24 oral temp 98.6°F $SpO_2$ 96% on RA
- Summary of initial presentation: A 42-year-old male with no known medical history brought in by EMS to the trauma bay after a rollover motor vehicle accident while fleeing from a wildfire near his home. EMS reports that the patient was a restrained driver going approximately 50 mph when he ran through a red light and was struck by another vehicle attempting to evacuate the town. He lives near a heavily wooded area and initially refused to leave his home despite warnings from town officials to evacuate. Strong winds propelled the fire dangerously close to his home, with heavy smoke and approaching flames prompting him to rapidly evacuate the area. The patient is agitated and anxious, shouting that his leg is in excruciating pain.
- Physical exam
  - General: agitated, anxious, frightened. Voice is slightly hoarse, patient is coughing.
  - HEENT: pupils 3 mm bilaterally, PERRL. Soot and ash around mouth/nose. Carbonaceous sputum. No facial tenderness or crepitus. No hemotympanum. No scalp laceration or hematoma.
  - Neck: C-collar in place
  - Cardiovascular: tachycardic rate, regular rhythm, no MRG, no peripheral edema, intact pulses ×4
  - Pulmonary: mildly tachypneic, bilateral breath sounds with scattered wheezes, no accessory muscle use. Dry cough.
  - Chest wall: no tenderness, no crepitus
  - Abdomen: tenderness on palpation with guarding in the RUQ.

  - Extremities: obvious right lower extremity open tib/fib fracture with minor bloody oozing, no pulsatile bleeding, distal pulses intact
  - Skin: minor abrasions, otherwise unremarkable
  - Neuro: A&O ×4, anxious, agitated, no focal neuro deficits
- Initial intervention
  - Place on cardiac monitor and obtain initial set of vital signs
  - Perform primary trauma exam
  - Obtain IV access and begin fluid resuscitation
  - Provide appropriate pain control
  - Recognize potential for impending airway compromise

**Critical Actions**
- Place patient on monitor
- Obtain IV access and send labs
- Obtain history
- Perform primary trauma exam and appreciate signs of potential airway compromise

### Time: Three Minutes – Transition Point 1

- VS: BP 86/42 HR 116 RR 24 oral temp 98.6°F $SpO_2$ 96% on RA
- Physical exam: Patient is calmer after pain medication but hoarse voice is more pronounced. Continues to have guarding in right upper quadrant.
- Patient is now able to indicate that this is not the normal sound of his voice and it seems to be worsening
- If team does not recognize airway concern, RN can ask why his voice sounds strange
- Blood pressure does not respond to fluids until blood is given
- Team may choose to use push dose epi or start vasopressors as well to optimize for intubation

**Critical Actions**
- Begin PRBC transfusion
- Optimize patient and secure advanced airway
- Obtain CXR and pelvic X-ray
- Perform EFAST exam

### Time: Six Minutes – Transition Point 2

- VS: BP 98/56 HR 106 RR 16 $SpO_2$ 97% on ventilator
- Physical exam: intubated, sedated, vital signs improving with PRBC infusion
- Labs return and are relatively unremarkable
- Portable chest X-ray reveals ETT in good position, otherwise unremarkable
- EFAST reveals free fluid in Morrison's pouch

**Critical Actions**
- Consult trauma surgeon and orthopedic surgeon

### Time: Eight Minutes – Transition Point 3

- VS: BP 98/56 HR 106 RR 16 $SpO_2$ 97% on ventilator
- Physical exam: unchanged
- Orthopedic surgeon recommends placing sterile dressing over open wound and temporary splint, IV antibiotics, and tetanus if not already done. Will join trauma team in the OR.
- Trauma surgeon will agree to bring patient to the OR. If desired, trauma surgeon can be argumentative and demand sending patient to CT scanner first

## 9. STIMULI

ECG: sinus tachycardia
Portable CXR: unremarkable
Portable pelvic XR: unremarkable
POCUS: EFAST reveals free fluid in Morrison's pouch
Labs

- CBC: WBC 13, Hgb 12, hematocrit 36, platelets 210
- BMP: sodium: 141, potassium 4.0, chloride 102, bicarbonate 24, BUN 18, creatinine 0.9, glucose 126 calcium 9.5
- LFTs: ALT 32, AST 28, alkaline phosphatase 84, Tbili 0.9
- Troponin: <0.01 ng/mL
- INR: 0.9
- PTT: 28
- Type and screen: A+
- Lactate: 2.6
- UA: color yellow, specific gravity 1.010, glucose 0, protein 0, ketones 0, nitrite neg, leukocyte esterase neg, urine WBC 0–3, urine RBC 0–2, bacteria none

## BIBLIOGRAPHY

Balmes JR. Where there's wildfire, there's smoke. *N Engl J Med.* 2018 Mar 8;378(10):881–883. doi: 10.1056/NEJMp1716846. Epub 2018 Jan 31. PMID: 29384719.

Haynes K, Short K, Xanthopoulos G, et al. Wildfires and WUI fire fatalities. In: Manzello SL, ed. *Encyclopedia of Wildfires and Wildland-Urban Interface (WUI) Fires.* Cham: Springer; 2020:1073–1088.

Shusterman D, Kaplan JZ, Canabarro C. Immediate health effects of an urban wildfire. *West J Med.* 1993;158(2):133–138.

SECTION 6

# BIOLOGICAL NATURAL DISASTERS

CASE 23

# Critical Management of Ebola Virus Disease in the Emergency Department

Matthew Carlisle

DISASTER PRINCIPLES

- Clinical diagnosis and treatment
- Timing of medical and surgical interventions
- Recognition and clinical treatment
- National disaster management system
- Role of public health agencies in disaster medicine
- Public health surveillance
- Biological disasters
- Category A bioterrorism agents
- MCI triage and considerations for biological agents
- Biological safety
- Epidemiologic and medical countermeasures
- Personal protective equipment (PPE)
- Quarantine/isolation
- Information management/communications
- Viral hemorrhagic fevers

## 1. SCENARIO OVERVIEW

Patient is a 55-year-old male brought in by EMS for weakness, fever, vomiting, and diarrhea. Patient returned from West Africa after completing a medical mission trip. Upon his return, he discovered the Centers for Disease Control and Prevention (CDC) is evaluating the hospital for an outbreak of fever and diarrheal illness. He reports symptoms started as fevers, chills, and myalgias 5 days ago and progressed to nausea, vomiting, and diarrhea. He had one episode of bloody stools this morning. He has been quarantining at home but reports he was so weak this morning that he could not get out of bed and called EMS. Per EMS, patient appeared lethargic, but arousable, with tachycardia, tachypnea, and decreased blood pressure. On arrival to the emergency department, patient is in overt shock requiring IV fluids and ultimately vasopressor support. As patient is resuscitated, he develops pulmonary edema along with worsening respiratory muscle fatigue leading to respiratory failure requiring intubation. If patient is not resuscitated in an appropriate timeframe, he may decompensate with worsening hypotension, PEA/Vfib/V-tach arrest. Complete physical exam will reveal a petechiae and conjunctivitis. Laboratory studies show leukopenia, thrombocytopenia, transaminitis, prolonged PT, PTT, elevated BUN, elevated creatinine, hypokalemia, hyponatremia, and metabolic acidosis. Patient should be placed in isolation and dispositioned to the ICU.

## 2. TEACHING OBJECTIVES AND DISCUSSION POINTS

a. Complete assessment with ABCs
b. Provide appropriate resuscitation and treatment in the setting of hypovolemic/ septic shock (IVF, pressors, antibiotics)
c. Discuss appropriate PPE in a patient with suspected Ebola
d. Evaluate and reassess airway status of dynamic, critically ill patients
e. Discuss appropriate labs in setting of Ebola including coagulation studies
f. Discuss risk factors for Ebola infection
g. Discuss disposition, notification of state and local health departments in setting of a patient under investigation for Ebola

## 3. SUPPLIES

a. PPE for droplet/ bodily fluid protection
b. Cardiac monitor, $SpO_2$
c. Noninvasive airway supplies such as NC, NRB, HFNC, BiPAP
d. Intubation supplies: BVM, ETT, stylet, blade, suction

## 4. MOULAGE

a. Petechial rash (may also have maculopapular rash)

## 5. IMAGES AND LABS

a. CXR showing pulmonary edema
b. Labs: CMP, CBC, PT/INR, PTT, lactic acid
c. ABG
d. ECG
e. May consider head CT, troponin

## 6. ACTORS (CONFEDERATES) AND THEIR ROLES

a. Nurse: place on monitors, draw labs, give IVF, medications
b. Respiratory therapist: set up noninvasive oxygenation, assist with intubation

## 7. CRITICAL ACTIONS

a. Complete initial survey and recognize shock state
b. Fluid resuscitate patient with goal mean arterial blood pressureof 65
c. Obtain appropriate history to determine underlying diagnosis
d. Don appropriate PPE for droplet/bodily fluid protection and isolate the patient
e. Recognize respiratory failure and appropriately intubate
f. Obtain appropriate laboratory studies including coagulation studies
g. Disposition to ICU

## 8. TIMELINE WITH TRANSITION POINTS

### Time: Zero

a. Patient in shock, hypotensive, tachycardic, febrile, altered tachypneic with shallow respirations due to muscle weakness
   i. Vital signs: BP 85/60, HR 120, RR 30, temp 39.5°C oral, sat 96% RA, point of care glucose 100 (if requested)
   ii. Summary of initial presentation: A 55-year-old male with past medical history of hypertension brought in by EMS for weakness, fever, vomiting, and diarrhea. Patient returned from West Africa after completing a medical mission trip. Upon his return, he discovered the CDC is evaluating the village for an outbreak of fever and diarrheal illness. He reports symptoms started as fevers, chills, and myalgias five days ago and progressed to nausea, vomiting, and diarrhea. He had one episode of bloody stools this morning. He has been quarantining at home, but reports he was so weak this morning that he could not get out of bed and called EMS.
   iii. Initial physical exam
      1. General: ill appearing, lethargic, arouses to verbal stimuli
      2. HEENT: atraumatic, normocephalic, conjunctival injection, mucous membranes dry, no tonsillar exudates/erythema
      3. Neck: supple, trachea midline, no midline spinal tenderness
      4. Chest: tachypneic, mild crackles at bases, no tenderness of ribs or chest wall
      5. Cardiac: tachycardia, regular rhythm
      6. Abdomen: soft, mild diffuse tenderness to palpation, no rebound or guarding, bowel sounds hyperactive
      7. Genitourinary: gross blood on rectal, circumcised penis, no testicular abnormalities
      8. Musculoskeletal, back: no midline spinal tenderness, no costovertebral angle tenderness, full range of motion all extremities, no obvious deformities, edema
      9. Skin: petechial rash noted to arms, face, chest, abdomen; pale, diaphoretic, cap refill delayed.
      10. Neuro: Glasgow Coma Scale (GCS) 14–15, oriented ×3, global weakness, no focal deficits
   iv. Initial intervention
      1. IV placement, large bore (18 G or larger), bilateral upon request
      2. Labs drawn including coagulation studies, type and screen, blood cultures
      3. Placed on cardiac monitor and $SpO_2$
      4. IV fluids: 30 cc/kg bolus

**Critical Actions**

- Complete primary survey with ABCs
- Obtain initial vital signs
- Begin resuscitation with IVF
- Start oxygen therapy
- Obtain exposure history
- Don appropriate PPE

### Time: 5–10 Minutes – Transition Point 1

a. Blood pressure improves with IVF, but respiratory status worsens secondary to pulmonary edema
b. VS: BP 95/70, HR 120, RR 30, sat 85% RA → 92% on NRB
c. CXR shows pulmonary edema
d. Interventions
   i. Give increased oxygen (noninvasive positive pressure ventilation will temporarily stabilize the patient)
   ii. Give additional fluids or start vasopressors
e. Nurse sends labs

**Critical Actions**

- Reevaluation of vital signs
- Recognition of respiratory distress and need to increase oxygenation, provide noninvasive positive pressure ventilation (NIPPV)
- Give additional hemodynamic support (additional IV fluids, vasopressors)

### Time: Two Minutes – Transition Point 2

a. Patient becomes increasingly altered, worsening respiratory function, GCS decreased to 8
b. VS: BP 105/72, HR 109, RR 20, sat 90% NIPPV, NRB
c. Interventions
   1. Intubation
d. Critical actions
   1. Reevaluation of clinical status, vital signs
   2. Intubation for respiratory failure, expected clinical course
e. Alternative transition: may consider dropping blood pressure if pressors are not started prior to intubation

### Transition Point 3: Final Disposition

a. VS: BP 110/75, HR 101, RR 16, sat 96% 100% $FiO_2$
b. Labs with normal Hgb, WBC count of 3.1, platelets 65K. Chemistry with creatinine of 4.5 and K+ of 6.8.
c. Consult medical ICU for admission
d. May consider advanced imaging (CT head, CT abdomen/pelvis)
e. Contact state and local health departments

**Critical Actions**

- Reevaluation of vital signs after intubation
- Consult medical ICU
- Contact state and local health departments

## 9. STIMULI

a. ECG with sinus tachycardia
b. CXR with pulmonary edema

c. CBC with WBC of 2 000, Hgb 10, platelets 75 000
d. CMP with Na 129, K 2.5, Cl 95, $CO_2$ 15, Cr 3.0, BUN 65, AST 400, ALT 300
e. PTT 60, INR 3
f. Lactate 5.0
g. ABG with pH 7.2

**Discussion Points**

1. Management of critically ill patient with hemorrhagic fever
   a. Fluid resuscitation
   b. Monitoring or electrolytes (often have derangements of potassium in particular with both hyper- and hypokalemia observed)
   c. Airway management
2. Exposure risk for staff. What should be done for clinical staff, registration, and anyone else who came in contact with the patient (at minimum, logging who was present, whether they had unprotected exposure, quarantine, follow-up).

## BIBLIOGRAPHY

Centers for Disease Control and Prevention. *Clinical Guidance for Ebola Disease.* Atlanta: Centers for Disease Control and Prevention; 2025, January 30. www.cdc.gov/ebola/hcp/clinical-guidance/. Accessed April 8, 2025.

Chertow D, Bray M, Palmore T. Clinical manifestations and diagnosis of Ebola virus disease. In: Hirsch M, ed. *UpToDate.* Waltham, MA: UpToDate; 2022. www.uptodate.com/contents/clinical-manifestations-and-diagnosis-of-ebola-disease. Accessed March 24, 2025.

Gesch J. New and emerging infections. In: Swadron S, Nordt SP, Mattu A, Johnson W, eds. *CorePendium.* Burbank, CA: EM:RAP; updated January 10, 2025. www.emrap.org/corependium/chapter/reczdVssp61r9033j/New-and-Emerging-Infections. Accessed April 7, 2025.

CASE 24

# From Cabin Cleanup to Critical Care

## Managing Hantavirus Infection

Matthew Carlisle

DISASTER PRINCIPLES

- Clinical diagnosis and treatment
- Timing of medical and surgical interventions
- Recognition and clinical treatment
- Biological disasters
- MCI triage and considerations for biological agents
- Biological safety
- Epidemiologic and medical countermeasures
- Personal protective equipment (PPE)
- Quarantine/isolation
- Information management/communications

### 1. SCENARIO OVERVIEW

Patient is a 45-year-old male presented to the ED with chief complaint of shortness of breath. He has been in his usual state of health until five days ago when he developed myalgias, fever, chills, and two episodes of nonbloody, nonbilious emesis. This morning he woke up with a dry cough and severe shortness of breath. Patient was recently hiking two weeks ago in Yellowstone National Park where he was staying in cabins. The patient and his friends were the first people to use the cabin since the winter, so they had to clean it up including sweeping, removing debris, and disposing of rodent nests and feces. He reports several other friends who went with him on the trip are having similar symptoms. On arrival to the emergency department, patient is hypoxic requiring supplemental oxygen and/or positive pressure ventilation. Patient quickly declines requiring intubation and vasopressor support. If patient is not resuscitated in an appropriate time frame, he may decompensate with worsening hypotension, PEA/Vfib/V-tach arrest. Laboratory studies show diagnostic triad of marked leukocytosis, immunoblasts, and thrombocytopenia. Patient should be dispositioned to the ICU.

### 2. TEACHING OBJECTIVES AND DISCUSSION POINTS

a. Complete assessment with ABCs
b. Provide appropriate resuscitation and treatment in the setting of hypoxia and cardiovascular collapse
c. Discuss route of transmission for hantavirus cardiopulmonary syndrome (HCPS) (murine, not person to person)

d. Evaluate and reassess airway status of dynamic critically ill patients
e. Discuss diagnostic triad of leukocytosis, immunoblasts, and thrombocytopenia in HCPS
f. Discuss disposition, notification of state and local health departments

## 3. SUPPLIES

a. Cardiac monitor, $SpO_2$
b. Noninvasive airway supplies such as NC, NRB, HFNC, BiPAP
c. Intubation supplies: BVM, ETT, stylet, blade, suction

## 4. MOULAGE

a. None

## 5. IMAGES AND LABS

a. CXR showing bilateral infiltrates
b. Labs: CMP, CBC, PT/INR, PTT, lactic acid
c. ABG
d. ECG
e. May consider troponin, BNP

## 6. ACTORS (CONFEDERATES) AND THEIR ROLES

a. Nurse: place patient on monitors, draw labs, give IVF, medications
b. Respiratory therapist: set up noninvasive oxygenation, assist with intubation

## 7. CRITICAL ACTIONS

a. Complete initial survey and recognize respiratory distress
b. Obtain appropriate history to determine underlying diagnosis
c. Recognize respiratory failure and appropriately intubate
d. Recognize hypotension and resuscitate with IVF, pressors
e. Obtain appropriate laboratory studies
f. Disposition to ICU

## 8. TIMELINE WITH TRANSITION POINTS

### Time: Zero – Patient in Moderate Respiratory Distress, Hypoxic, Alert, and Oriented

a. Vital signs: BP 130/80, HR 120, RR 30, temp 39.5°C oral, sat 89% RA, point of care glucose 100 (if requested)
b. Summary of initial presentation: A 45-year-old male with no past medical history who presented for shortness of breath that started this morning. Patient reports five-day history of fevers, chills, myalgias that progress to nonproductive cough and shortness of breath this morning. He reports returning from a hiking trip two weeks ago in Yellowstone National Park. Several friends who went with him on the trip have similar symptoms. No history of tick bites. Patient denies ever having these symptoms before and was in good health prior to his trip.

c. Initial physical exam
   i. General: actively coughing, in moderate respiratory distress
   ii. HEENT: atraumatic, normocephalic, PERRL, oropharynx unremarkable
   iii. Neck: supple, trachea midline, no midline spinal tenderness
   iv. Chest: tachypneic, diffuse rales throughout, no tenderness of ribs or chest wall
   v. Cardiac: tachycardia, regular rhythm, no murmurs, rubs,
   vi. Abdomen: soft, nontender, nondistended, no rebound or guarding, bowel sounds normal
   vii. Genitourinary: normal
   viii. Musculoskeletal, back: no midline spinal tenderness, no costovertebral angle tenderness, full range of motion all extremities, no obvious deformities, edema
   ix. Skin: no rashes, wounds, lesions. Capillary refill <3 seconds
   x. Neuro: Glasgow Coma Scale (GCS) 15, oriented $\times$3, global weakness, no focal deficits
d. Initial intervention
   i. IV placement, large bore (18 G or larger), bilateral upon request
   ii. Labs drawn
   iii. Placed on cardiac monitor and $SpO_2$
   iv. Give supplemental oxygen

**Critical Actions**
- Complete primary survey with ABCs
- Obtain initial vital signs
- Provide supplemental oxygen (NC, NRB, BiPAP, high-flow $O_2$)
- Obtain exposure history

### Time: 5–10 Minutes – Transition Point 1

a. Oxygenation improves slightly, but patient develops hypotension
b. VS: BP 85/60, HR 120, RR 30, sat 85% RA→92% on NRB, 98% on BiPAP
c. CXR shows pulmonary edema
d. Interventions
   i. Give fluids, consider vasopressors
e. Nurse sends labs

**Critical Actions**
- Reevaluation of vital signs
- Recognition of hemodynamic instability
- Give additional hemodynamic support (IV fluids, vasopressors)

### Time: Two Minutes – Transition Point 2

a. Patient becomes increasingly altered, worsening respiratory function, GCS decreased to 8
b. VS: BP 95/65, HR 109, RR 24, sat 90% noninvasive positive pressure ventilation, NRB
c. Interventions
   i. Intubation

d. Critical actions
    i. Reevaluation of clinical status, vital signs
    ii. Intubation for respiratory failure, expected clinical course
e. Alternative transition: may consider dropping blood pressure if pressors are not started prior to intubation
g. CXR difficult to distinguish from acute respiratory distress syndrome, team should consider management with lung-protecctive ventilation protocol (low volume, high pressure) and patient should be difficult to oxygenate unless positive end-expiratory pressure (PEEP) is increased
g. Team may consider potential need for extracorporeal membrane oxygenationif appropriate ventilation not achieved despite increasing PEEP, consideration of proning, etc.

### Transition Point 3: Final Disposition

a. VS: BP 110/75, HR 101, RR 16, sat 96% 100% $FiO_2$
b. Consult medical ICU for admission
c. May consider advanced imaging (CT chest)
d. Contact state and local health departments

**Critical Actions**
- Reevaluation of vital signs after intubation
- Consult medical ICU
- Contact state and local health departments

## 9. STIMULI

a. ECG with sinus tachycardia
b. CXR with bilateral infiltrates
c. CBC with WBC of 32 000, band, neutrophil predominance, 15% immunoblasts, platelets 75 000
d. CMP with Na 135, K 2.5, Cl 100, $CO_2$ 15, Cr 1.8
f. Lactate 4.0

## BIBLIOGRAPHY

Centers for Disease Control and Prevention. *Clinician Brief: Hantavirus Pulmonary Syndrome (HPS).* Centers for Disease Control and Prevention; 2024, May 23. www.cdc.gov/hantavirus/hcp/clinical-overview/hps.html. Accessed April 7, 2025.

Hjelle B. Hantavirus cardiopulmonary syndrome. In: Hirsch M, ed. *UpToDate.* Waltham, MA: UpToDate; 2024. www.uptodate.com/contents/hantavirus-cardiopulmonary-syndrome. Accessed March 24, 2025.

CASE 25

# Medical Response in Crisis

## Pediatric Diarrhea and Shock in Refugee Camps

Matthew A. Tovar LT, MC, USN and James P. Phillips

DISASTER PRINCIPLES

- Clinical diagnosis and treatment
- Timing of medical and surgical interventions
- Crisis standards of care
- Scarce resource allocation protocols
- International systems
- Nongovernmental organizations (NGO)
- Displaced populations
- Field operations and logistics
- Disaster operations
- Medical care for refugee populations
- UN cluster system
- Emergency medical teams and World Health Organization
- Role of public health agencies in disaster medicine
- Public health surveillance
- Needs assessments
- Sphere standards; water, sanitation, and hygiene (WASH)
- Complex public health emergencies
- Epidemiology



### 1. SCENARIO OVERVIEW

A male child appearing to be 3–4 years old presents to the refugee clinic with his father in northern Kenya after passing out while playing outside. He and his father speak only Swahili and the camp interpreter is not immediately available. He appears stuporous and pale on initial physical exam. Physical exam is significant for a 100.4°F oral temp, tachycardia, and hypotension. Following the arrival of the interpreter, his father reveals that the patient has had near-constant nonbloody diarrhea for the past four or five days. The patient will require volume resuscitation and initiation of antibiotic therapy for undifferentiated infectious diarrhea. The ultimate disposition will be a MEDEVAC to the nearest hospital for continued management and IV fluid support.[1,2]

## 2. TEACHING OBJECTIVES AND DISCUSSION POINTS

### Clinical and Medical Management

- Identification of pediatric shock in a resource-limited environment
- Initiation of appropriate volume resuscitation in a pediatric patient with hypovolemic shock
- Administration of appropriate antibiotics for presumed infectious diarrhea
- Administration of zinc as an adjunctive therapy

### Communication and Teamwork

- Early identification of the need for an interpreter
- Communication with concerned father to address his concerns
- Reassessment of a critically ill patient
- Delivery of a MEDEVAC patient transfer report

## 3. SUPPLIES

- Broslow tape
- Ultrasound
- IV fluid: 1 000 mL, 500 mL, 250 mL
- IV start supplies: tourniquet, chlorhexidine swab, Tegaderm, IV extension set, IV tubing, tape
- Antibiotics
- Zinc tablets
- Table with sterile blue towel (makeshift exam table)
- Mosquito netting (prop)
- Telephone/satellite phone for interpreter

## 4. MOULAGE

- Makeup to simulate ashen grey appearance

## 5. IMAGES AND LABS

- Focused Assessment with Sonography for Trauma/Rapid Ultrasound in Shock and Hypotension (FAST/RUSH) ultrasonography: no evidence of intraperitoneal bleeding on FAST views. No evidence of pneumothorax on thoracic views. Cardiac view shows a hyperdynamic left ventricle. The IVC diameter is small and compresses with inhalation.
- 12-lead ECG: unavailable
- Labs: Basic iSTAT labs are available but in low supply. iSTAT BMP will show hyperkalemic metabolic alkalosis.

## 6. ACTORS

- Patient: actor or SimJunior simulator, not able to communicate due to clinical status and language barrier.

- Father: actor, not able to communicate due to language barrier.
- Interpreter (voice): helpful demeanor but not available for the first portion of the case. Translates from Swahili to English.
- Nurse: assists team with administration and execution of orders. Provides guidance when physician is confused. Questions physician orders when they seem inappropriate.

## 7. CRITICAL ACTIONS

- Identify hypovolemic shock within 60 seconds of patient presentation.
- Recognize need to obtain IV access and begin fluid resuscitation at a dose of 20 cc/kg (estimated 18–20 kg/40–44 lb given age)
- Initiate appropriate antibiotics for infectious diarrhea: doxycycline 4.4 mg/kg (estimated 18 kg/40 lb given age)
- Initiate treatment with zinc

## 8. TIMELINE

### Time: Zero – Initial Presentation to Initiation of IV Fluid Resuscitation

Background: You are working in a refugee clinic in the northern territory of Kenya. You are part of a team of 10 physicians who serve a population of approximately 200 000 refugees, many of whom have fled civil war and conflict in Somalia. You are the only physician in the eastern sector of the camp and have basic supplies including IV fluid, ultrasound, antibiotics, analgesics, and basic procedural supplies. You do not have access to subspecialist support and the closest hospital is two hours away by helicopter.

Summary of initial presentation: A Swahili-speaking father carries his child into the clinic. He appears frantic and the child is unresponsive, somnolent, and pale. The child appears to be 3–4 years old but his exact age is unclear. No further information is available given the language barrier. Case branch points are discussed in Table 25.1.

VS: BP 75/60, HR 162, RR: 28, sat 100% on room air, temp: 38.2°C (100.8°F)

- Physical exam
  - General: somnolent, pale appearing child. He does not respond to verbal stimuli. Moans and pushes away painful stimuli.
  - HEENT: dry mucous membranes. Pupils equal, round, and reactive to light. Posterior oropharynx without erythema or exudate.
  - Neck: supple and without lymphadenopathy
  - Chest: lung fields clear to auscultation bilaterally
  - Heart: tachycardic rate, regular rhythm, ejection murmur appreciated at the left lower sternal border
  - Abdomen: soft and nontender, no organomegaly
  - Skin: cool and clammy
  - Neuro: pediatric Glasgow Coma Scale (pGCS 9) E2 V2 M5
- Initial interventions
  - Gain appropriate exposure and initiate physical examination
  - Use of ultrasound to appreciate signs of hypovolemic shock, including collapsible IVC and hyperdynamic left ventricle.
  - Large-bore IV placement

**Table 25.1** Changes and case branch points 1

| Action/time point | Change in case | Additional information |
|---|---|---|
| Provider attempts to speak to father. | Father motions that he cannot understand provider. | |
| Provider calls for interpreter. | Provider is notified that in-person interpreter was airlifted from the refugee camp two days ago due to exposure to bad water. | Provider is notified that tele-interpreter will be available as soon as possible. Interpreter will be available approximately five minutes after the initial request. |
| Provider attempts to start IV before an interpreter is reached.<br>OR<br>Provider attempts to start IV without informing father. | Parent rushes to resuscitation table yelling in Swahili, blocking the learner's attempts to initiate IVF resuscitation. | Parent continues to yell and physically interfere until the learner requests an interpreter, explains the reasoning for the procedure, and asks the parent to not interfere with medical care. |
| Provider asks for ECG. | Nurse informs provider that ECG is not available | |
| Provider asks for iSTAT BMP. | Nurse questions provider's choice, saying "Doc, we have only two more iSTAT cartridges until our resupply in five days, are you sure you want to use one? | The provider should still elect to use an iSTAT cartridge for this patient due to their high acuity.<br>If the provider chooses to continue with the iSTAT BMP, the nurse will indicate that the results will be ready in about 10 minutes (in stage 1 of the simulation). |
| Provider attempts to intubate child. | Nurse informs provider that the patient is maintaining their own airway and that airway team is on the other side of the refugee camp | |
| Provider fails to initiate IVF resuscitation within five minutes of presentation. | After five minutes the vital signs will continue to worsen:<br>5:30: BP 70/58, HR 135, RR: 24<br>6:00: BP 66/57, HR 96, RR: 15<br>6:15: bradycardia to PEA arrest | The provider should initiate CPR according to PALS protocol at this point. They should be notified that they have limited cardiopulmonary resuscitation supplies.<br>Should the simulation come to this point, the provider should be coached to think through their H/T algorithm, stopping at hypovolemia as a causative etiology of cardiac arrest. |

**Table 25.1** (*cont.*)

| Action/time point | Change in case | Additional information |
|---|---|---|
| | | The provider should be coached to initiate volume resuscitation. After initiation of volume resuscitation, the patient achieves return of spontaneous circulationand the simulation ends. |
| Provider successfully recognizes hypovolemic shock, achieves IV access, and initiates appropriate fluid resuscitation within five minutes of presentation. | Blood pressure improves to 85/64 and heart rate decreases to 144 after first 360–400 cc fluid bolus. Provider proceeds to stage 2. | |

- Use of Broselow tape to approximate appropriate fluid dosing: approximate weight 18–20 kg
- Initiation of fluid resuscitation at 20 cc/kg (360–400 cc)
- Optional: Administration of Tylenol for mild fever: 10–15 mg/kg PR (200–300 mg)

### Transition Point 1: Initial Fluid Resuscitation through Delivery of MEDEVAC Report

VS: BP 85/64, HR 144, RR: 20, sat 100% on room air, temp: 38.2°C (100.8°F)

An interpreter is now available by voice. The provider is instructed to communicate to the patient's father via the interpreter:

Name of child: "Raj"
Chief complaint: "My son passed out while playing outside."
When did this happen?: "About 10 minutes ago."
Events leading up to incident: "I don't know, I was watching him play through the window, turned around, and then everybody started yelling for me to come."
Prior incidents?: "No, this has never happened before."
Any seizure-like activity? "No, I don't think so."
How does he look to you since the incident?: "He looks really pale."

Have you noticed anything else with him recently?: "Well, he has been pooping a lot in the last few days." There have been 10–12 nonbloody stools per day for the last four or five days. The patient has had abdominal pain immediately prior to the stool. The father has tried at-home remedies without relief. No vomiting. No other known sick contacts in the household. The patient likes to play around a pond. It is unknown if he drinks the pond water.

Past medical history: "I don't think he has any problems. He's usually healthy but we can't go to a doctor because we are refugees."
Allergies: "I don't think he's allergic to anything."
Surgeries: "He hasn't had any surgery."

Social history: Patient lives in a cloth tent with his father and older two sisters. His mother died from postpartum hemorrhage after delivering patient. Water and food access is limited. Father feels somewhat safe in his current living situation, but is hopeful that things might improve in the next few weeks.

### Nurse Interrupts Interview Conversation, Stating that the Patient Is Starting to Deteriorate

Subsequent branch points are addressed in Table 25.2.

VS: BP 80/62, HR 154, RR: 22, sat 100% on room air, temp: 38.2°C (101.5°F)

- Physical exam
  - General: somnolent, pale appearing child. Somewhat responsive to verbal stimuli, improved from prior examination.
  - HEENT: dry mucous membranes. Unchanged from previous examination.
  - Neck: supple and without lymphadenopathy. Unchanged from previous examination.
  - Chest: lung fields clear to auscultation bilaterally. Unchanged from previous examination.
  - Heart: tachycardic rate, regular rhythm, with resolved ejection murmur
  - Abdomen: soft and nontender, no organomegaly. Unchanged from previous examination.
  - Skin: cool and clammy
  - Neuro: pGCS 11 (E3 V3 M5), improved from prior examination
- Interventions
  - Administer another 20 cc/kg bolus (360–400cc bolus)
  - Administer Tylenol for fever
  - Begin antibiotics: Doxycycline is the preferred regimen of choice for suspected *Vibrio cholerae* at a dose of 4.4 mg/kg (80–100 mg).
  - Optional: begin zinc supplementation

After antibiotics are hung, the iSTAT BMP results are:

Na: 134 K: 6.0 HCO3: 16 Cl: 100 BUN: 28 Cr: 1.2 Glu: 85

Interpretation: hyperkalemic metabolic acidosis with prerenal azotemia

Nurse: "Doc, what are we going to do with this kid?"

Disposition: MEDEVAC to the nearest hospital for hypovolemic shock with metabolic derangement and evidence of end-organ damage.

Nurse: "Alright, let me radio the authorities to see what I can do"

[. . .]

"Alright patch them through"

Humanitarian evacuation coordinator: Ground site Beniuji how do you copy?

[. . .]

Ground site Beniuji this is Big Bertha – Charlie-One-Niner. We are 1-2-0 minutes away from your location, spinning up our bird from Nairobi to your location at ______ latitude-tac-_____longitude. What is the patient's status?

Prompt the provider to deliver a MIST report, or equivalent

Ideal report:

Big Bertha – Charlie-One-Niner this is Ground Site Beniuji. At our facility we have a critically ill refugee child, approximately 4–5 years in age, presenting after a syncopal episode and subsequently found to be in hypovolemic shock likely secondary to profuse diarrhea in the preceding four or five days. He has received two fluid boluses for a total of 800 mL IVF. We also have antibiotics and analgesics running. iSTAT BMP with evidence of a hyperkalemic metabolic

**Table 25.2** Changes and case branch points 2

| Action/time point | Change in case | Additional information |
|---|---|---|
| Provider does not continue fluid resuscitation. | After five minutes the vital signs will continue to worsen:<br>5:30: BP 70/58, HR 135, RR: 24<br>6:00: BP 66/57, HR 96, RR: 15<br>6:15: bradycardia to PEA arrest | The provider should initiate CPR according to PALS protocol at this point. They should be notified that they have limited cardiopulmonary resuscitation supplies.<br>Should the simulation come to this point, the provider should be coached to think through their H/T algorithm, stopping at hypovolemia as a causative etiology of cardiac arrest.<br>The provider should be coached to initiate volume resuscitation.<br>After initiation of volume resuscitation, the patient achieves return of spontaneous circulation and the simulation ends. |
| Provider attempts to initiate vasopressor support. | Nurse remarks that they don't have pressors or IV titration equipment at their site. | |
| Antibiotics other than doxycycline are initiated. | Nurse questions provider's choice, saying that she's seen cases of infectious diarrhea be treated with a different regimen, she thinks the drug might have started with a "D." | |
| Antibiotics are NOT started. | Nurse remarks that something should probably be done for the fever. If the provider orders just antipyretics the nurse should remark that she thinks this is a GI bug. | |
| Provider suggests disposition to remain at the refugee clinic. | Nurse remarks that they don't have the supplies to continue to care for the patient. They suggest that the nearest hospital is two hours by helicopter but she remembers the flight paramedics picked up someone with similar symptoms about a week ago. | |

acidosis and prerenal azotemia. Working diagnosis is hypovolemic shock secondary to infectious diarrhea. He likely needs continued IV fluid support and antibiotics at your facility. Over.

Coordinator: Copy. Any other civilian transports? Over.

"He will be accompanied by his father."

Coordinator: Copy. Expect a crew to your location in 1-2-0 minutes. Bertha-Charlie-One-Niner clear radio traffic.

## 9. STIMULI

Ultrasound: hyperdynamic left ventricle, collapsible IVC
Labs: BMP: Na: 134, K: 6.0, HCO3: 16, Cl: 100, BUN: 28, Cr: 1.2, Glu: 85

## BIBLIOGRAPHY

Farmer P, Ivers L. Cholera in Haiti: please do not forget zinc – authors' reply. *The Lancet.* 2011;377(9779):1746–1747. doi:10.1016/S0140-6736(11)60731-9.

Nelson EJ, Nelson DS, Salam MA, Sack DA. Antibiotics for both moderate and severe cholera. *N Engl J Med.* 2011;364(1):5–7. doi:10.1056/NEJMp1013771.

World Health Organization. Cholera. Updated December 5, 2024. www.who.int/news-room/fact-sheets/detail/cholera. Accessed March 24, 2025.

CASE 26

# Resource Management during a Pandemic Surge in a Small Hospital

Christopher Hayden

DISASTER PRINCIPLES

- Clinical diagnosis and treatment
- Information management/communications
- Timing of medical and surgical interventions
- Recognition and clinical treatment
- Role of public health agencies in disaster medicine
- Quarantine/isolation
- Emergency operations plans for the healthcare environment
- Medical surge capacity
- Mass-casualty incidents
- Pandemics/emerging infectious diseases
- Epidemiology
- Mass care during pandemics
- Pandemic triage
- Personal protective equipment

## 1. SCENARIO OVERVIEW

Evaluation of multiple patients who present with worsening respiratory distress syndromes can be difficult for the practitioner. Difficulty arises not only from narrowing down the cause but also in determining which patients will benefit most from advanced therapy. This scenario will challenge the participants to manage numerous ED presentations of patients with illnesses having common signs and symptoms with progressive worsening respiratory distress that overwhelms conventional operations.

### Background

A small cruise ship is pulling into port. Onboard are around 100 people from the United States who are stopping to see the sights. The news has been briefly discussing a new respiratory virus that is affecting multiple people, but this location has had no cases and is not under lockdown. The community hospital near the port is a 30-bed hospital with a 10-bed ED that has limited critical capabilities. Patients are often transferred to a hospital about 3 hours flight by fixed wing. The ED is double coverage with a physician and an advanced practice provider (APP) with two additional physicians (one surgeon and one family medicine physician) and one APP who live in the surrounding community. There is a general internist who manages the floor patients and there is a two-bed ICU with one patient who is an 86-year-old male on the ventilator. There are three additional ventilators in the hospital that can also be used for BiPAP or CPAP.

## 2. TEACHING OBJECTIVES AND DISCUSSION POINTS

### Teaching Objectives

1. Recognized the initial assessment and stabilization of patients presenting in respiratory distress
2. Recognized the need to and employ emergency management resources as the ED transitions its operations from conventional, though contingency operations, to crisis management.
3. Demonstrate ability to mass triage and treat patients based on likelihood of survival
4. Recognize the need to limit the spread of the virus and limit exposure by utilizing personal protective equipment (PPE)
5. Recognize the need for more resources while following the organization's established program to call in additional providers

### Discussion Points

1. This scenario is intended to reinforce the recognition of a potential acute viral respiratory disease. The participant will demonstrate awareness to anticipate the need for advanced airway support in a setting of limited resources. Some patients will need intubation, some may be fine on nonrebreather or BiPAP.
2. Upon recognition that all are struggling from the same respiratory disorder, it will be important to investigate resources that may be required.
3. As more patients present the participant must recognize the transition of conventional ED operation to contingency and beyond by calling the house supervisor for extra resources, to initiate transfer processes, and evaluate hospital's ICU capabilities become overwhelmed.

## 3. SUPPLIES

- Oxygen delivery masks
- Pulse oximeter equipment
- Intubation equipment: endotracheal tubes, laryngoscopes, bougies, laryngeal mask airways, bag-valve masks
- Suction
- $ETCO_2$
- IV equipment
- Thermometers
- ECG
- Cardiac monitor
- Customary emergent airway management drugs
- Standard provider PPE to include N95 masks

## 4. IMAGES AND LABS

- Full lab capacity
- Venous blood gas/ABG
- Chest X-ray
- CT machine
- Bedside ultrasound

## 5. ACTORS

Six patients (Nnmber adjusted according to desired scope of disaster and length of scenario) aged 15–92 with varying levels of respiratory distress and neurological responses who are all family and friends on the same cruise to celebrate the birthday of their elderly grandmother. The patients share a similar story in that they have been on the cruise for about a week. Two days prior to evaluation the patients all relate they have been developing a cough, subjective fevers, and respiratory distress, which has been worsening over the last two days. Currently, there are three patients in the ED. Patient 1 is undergoing workup following an MVC, Patient 2 is being evaluated for abdominal pain, and Patient 3 is being evaluated for chest pain and is on oxygen.

## 6. MOULAGE

Patients should appear diaphoretic and pale or have cyanosis.

## 7. TIMELINE

### Time: Zero – Patient 1

EMS called about a 45-year-old male patient with history of hypertension and diabetes complaining shortness of breath, cough, and worsening exertional dyspnea. EMS states the patient is found to have a pulse ox of 80% on RA, pulse 120, BP 150/76 RR 24 and appears to be breathing shallowly and in distress. He is alert and oriented, anxious, and obeys all commands. Pulse ox improves to 88% when you place him on an NRB at 10 LPM. EMS relates they are five minutes away from your facility.

### Time: One Minute – Patient 2

EMS called about a 47-year-old female with history of asthma and HTN complaining of shortness of breath, cough, and wheezing. States she has been taking her rescue inhaler without changes in her condition. Pulse ox 84% on RA with pulse 110, BP 100/76, RR 30 and appears with some distress. She is alert and orientated, anxious, and obeys all commands. Pulse ox increases to 91% on 10 LPM NRB. EMS states they are six or seven minutes away from your facility.

### Time: Two Minutes – Patient 3

A patient presents to triage. He is a 22-year-old male with no medical history who states he has exertional shortness of breath with a cough.

- Vital signs: BP 120/76 HR 72, RR 16 pulse ox 94% on RA, with temperature of 99.8°F
- General: states he feels well, states his parents are coming by ambulance and he wanted to be seen as well, he has an occasional cough, answer questions appropriately without distress and is mildly febrile.
- HEENT: no signs of infection
- Neck: supple, nontender, no JVD, no stridor
- Chest: clear bilateral breath sounds
- Heart: regular rate no murmurs
- Abdomen: soft nontender
- Extremity: all pulses present with good strength in all extremities
- Neuro: alert and orientated with no signs of weakness
- Skin: warm to the touch with no rash and nondiaphoretic

**Desired Interventions**

If obtained ABG there it is normal.

- CXR with bilateral pulmonary infiltrates noted to lower lobes
- Labs unremarkable
- This is the third patient from a cruise ship with similar symptoms. There should be some discussion about whether this is a viral/bacterial/biochemical concern and what type of equipment should be utilized to keep the providers and other patients safe.

## Time: Five Minutes – Patient 1 Arrives

On initial presentation the appears to be stated as previously. He is speaking in two- to three-word sentences, he is tired.

- Vitals: BP 136/96, HR 120, RR 28, pulse ox 95% at 10 LPM temp 103.5°F
- General: Patient is in severe distress but is responding to command speaking in two- to three-word sentences.
- HEENT: no signs of infection
- Neck: supple, nontender, no JVD, no stridor
- Chest: crackles noted lower lobes with signs of increased respiratory effort
- Heart: regular rate no murmurs
- Abdomen: soft nontender
- Extremity: all pulses present with good strength in all extremities
- Neuro: alert and orientated with no signs of weakness
- Skin: warm to the touch with no rash and nondiaphoretic

**Desired Interventions**

An alert patient with respiratory distress with increased work of breathing would benefit from BiPAP starting at 10/5 (or basic starting levels) and adjusting to decrease work of breathing and to ensure adequate tidal volumes.

- ABG (if ordered): pH 7.30, $PaO_2$ 55 $PaCO_2$ 48 $HCO_2$ 23
- IV fluids +/–
- Monitor: sinus tachycardia
- CXR: bilateral pulmonary infiltrates noted to lower lobes
- Bedside echo (if available): negative for signs of heart failure, pulmonary embolism, pleural effusion, and pericardial effusion.
- Labs: unremarkable with blood sugar 103

## Time: Eight Minutes

Patient 2 arrives and is speaking in one- to two-word sentences, is sitting tripod and is pulling off her NRB mask.

- Vitals: BP 160/90, HR 130, RR 32, $SPO_2$ 78% on NRM, temp 102.5°F
- General: Patient is in obvious distress, is diaphoretic, and pulling at her oxygen mask
- HEENT: no obvious signs of infection
- Neck: supple nontender, no JVD, no stridor
- Chest: crackles and wheezing noted throughout with signs of impending respiratory failure
- Heart: regular rate no murmurs

- Abdomen: soft nontender
- Extremity: all pulses present with pulses noted to all extremities
- Neuro: Patient is agitated and confused and not responding to questions with no meningeal signs
- Skin: warm to the touch with diaphoresis and no rashes present

**Desired Interventions**

This patient with altered mentation, pulling of her oxygen mask, and in severe respiratory distress should be intubated.

- Patient placed on ventilator with settings conducive to lung protective strategy
- ABG (if ordered): pH 7.19, $PaO_2$ 41 $PaCO_2$ 68 $HCO_2$ 24
- IV fluids +/–
- Monitor: sinus tachycardia
- CXR: bilateral pulmonary infiltrates with ETT 2 cm above the carina
- Bedside echo (if available): negative for signs of HF, pericardial effusion, pulmonary embolism, pneumothorax, pleural effusion abdominal aortic aneurysm, and FAST negative
- Labs: unremarkable with blood sugar 110

### Time: 10 Minutes – Patient 4

EMS calls and states they are en route with a patient in cardiac arrest. States the patient is a 78-year-old female with multiple medical comorbidities who was reported to be from a cruise ship. They state the patient was found in severe respiratory distress and shortly after their arrival suffered cardiac arrest. EMS states she has a supraglottic airway, she has been given three rounds of epi via IV, and remains in PEA, they are five minutes out.

### Time: 11 Minutes

At this time in the scenario, the participant should recognize the need to bring in additional resources to help. This should include the family medicine physician from upstairs and contacting the charge nurse to call for assistance from the community.

### Time: 12 Minutes – Patient 5 Arrives

Patient from the community is presenting to the ED to be evaluated for left arm pain that started earlier this am. Patient is an 86-year-old male with history of HTN, DM, HLD, previous MI, smokes two packs a day, states he has been experiencing pain to the left arm for the last 4 hours. States the pain is dull in nature, radiating to his neck, 7/10, nothing makes the pain worse, and nothing makes the pain better. States he has never had the pain in the past. States he has noted similar pain over the last couple of weeks while walking up the stairs.

- Vitals: BP 190/100, HR 66, RR 16 pulse ox 99% on RA, temp 98.7°F
- General: Patient is in no acute distress but while speaking keeps moving his shoulder around
- HEENT: no signs of infection
- Neck: supple, nontender, no JVD, no stridor
- Chest: clear bilateral breath sounds
- Heart: regular rate with holosystolic murmur noted at the mitral position
- Abdomen: soft nontender
- Extremity: all pulses present with good strength in all extremities

- Neuro: alert and orientated with normal strength without numbness or tingling
- Skin: warm to the touch with no rash and nondiaphoretic

**Desired Interventions**

- IV, $O_2$ not necessary at this time, and patient placed on the monitor
- ABG (if ordered): pH 7.4, $PaO_2$ 41 $PaCO_2$ 40 $HCO_2$ 24
- IV fluids +/–
- Monitor: sinus with elevations on the ECG
- 12-lead ECGif ordered: anterior wall MI noted on the 12 lead
- CXR: no abnormal pathology noted
- Bedside echo (if available): mitral valve regurgitation with decreased movement noted on the anterior septal walls of the heart, and moderately deceased contractility
- Labs: Troponin elevated patients should be given nitro, aspirin, ticagrelor (or other P2Y12 antagonists), and thrombolytics could be initiated. If thrombolytics are not available, a heparin drip should be initiated and discussion should be made with receiving hospital to establish transfer.

## Time: 15 Minutes – Patient 4 Arrives

On arrival EMS states the patient obtained her pulse shortly after they finished the report. Patient overall received 4 mg of epi with a liter of fluid and 25 g of D50 because her initial blood sugar was 52.

- Airway: being maintained by supraglottic airway
- Breathing: being controlled via BVM at a rate of 18
- Circulation: Patient has weak thready pulses to the extremities, she is cool to the touch, with strong carotid
- Deformity: Patient's pupils are 8 mm and nonresponsive to light with no response to painful stimulation
- Vitals: BP 70/40, HR 130 RR 18 pulse ox 95% on 100% oxygen via supraglottic airway with temp 97.0°F
- General: Patient is nonresponsive with no signs of trauma
- HEENT: no signs of infection
- Neck: supple, nontender, no JVD, no stridor
- Chest: bruising and redness noted to the sternum with decreased lung sounds bilaterally
- Heart: tachycardic with no murmurs noted
- Abdomen: soft with no signs or bruising or rashes
- Extremity: IO noted to the left upper shoulder, no bruising with thready weak pulses to all extremities
- Neuro: patient not responsive to painful stimuli, no blink reflexes, no stratal reflexes, and unable to assess gag due to supraglottic airway placement.
- Skin: cool to the touch with no rashes present

**Desired Interventions**

- Exchange the supraglottic airway for an endotracheal tube
- Patient should be placed on the ventilator with lung protective strategy
- IV, $O_2$ and monitor
- ABG (if ordered): pH 7.02, $PaO_2$ 30 $PaCO_2$ 86 $HCO_2$ 10
- IV fluids +/–
- Monitor: sinus tachycardia
- 12-lead ECG if ordered: sinus tach with no ST elevation

- CXR: following intubation shows bilateral interstitial edema, multiple rib fractures, an endotracheal tube 4 cm from the carina and an IO in the right humerus.
- Bedside ultrasound (if available): shows normal cardiac activity without signs of pericardial effusion or tamponade, pulmonary embolism, or pneumothorax.
- Labs: troponin: 4.1, lactate: 13, anion gap metabolic acidosis

## Time: 20 Minutes – Abdominal Pain Patient

The patient being evaluated for abdominal pain labs and imaging returned, and she is suffering from appendicitis. There is a local surgeon on another island, and he cannot come to the hospital. Would discuss transfer to that hospital while placing the patient on antibiotics and admitting until the plan can be arranged.

## Time: 21 Minutes

If the participant asked for assistance before now, the local family medicine physician who also works in the ED has also arrived to provide support. This physician can be used in any way to assist the participant.

## Time: 22 Minutes – Patient 1

You are alerted by the nurse to come and evaluate Patient 1. The nurse states the patient is no longer responding like he was earlier.

When you evaluate Patient 1 you notice that he is lethargic, minimally responsive to questions, has "gasping" respirations and his oxygen saturation is now 82% on BiPAP. His BP is 116/98, HR 120, RR 26 and shallow; he is cool to the touch with thready pulses bilaterally, with minimal air movement bilaterally when assessing lung sounds.

### Desired Interventions

Based on the patient's sudden decline in mental status and increased oxygen requirements, he will need to be intubated.

Postintubation chest X-ray will show endotracheal tube 2 cm above the carina with OG tube in the stomach (if this was placed).

ABG: pH 7.10 $PaO_2$ 46 $PCO_2$ 46 $HCO_3$ 14

Bedside echo without signs or pneumothorax, normal cardiac function, no concern for PE, no pericardial or pleural effusion appreciated.

## Time: 25 Minutes – Patient 6

A car pulls up with someone banging on the door of the ED. Staff run outside to see a patient barely breathing slumped over in the front passenger seat of a cab.

It is reported the patient was on their way back to the cruise ship from an island excursion when they "just stopped speaking." The patient's family states the patient has been having trouble breathing for the last two days and since they finished their snorkeling about an hour ago the respiratory distress has become much worse. The patient's family states that the patient stopped speaking to them about two minutes ago, which is when the driver of the cab came to the hospital. The patient is reported to have a history of HTN, DM, CKD 4, HLD, depression, and systolic heart failure with the most recent echocardiogram six months ago showing EF 50%.

- Airway: Patient's airway is opened by head tilt chin lift with no vomitus or blood noted.
- Breathing: being ventilated by BVM, lung sounds
- Circulation: pulses are present in all extremities
- Deformity: Patient's pupils are 3 and equal bilaterally and she groans in pain while withdrawing her upper extremities.
- Patient is rolled and quickly evaluated with no obvious signs of injury or trauma.
- Patient placed on the monitor, pulse ox and IV started
- Vital signs: BP 102/50 HR 100 RR 8, pulse ox 74% on room air (if being ventilated then 87% with BVM), skin is warm to the touch, with temperature 98.6°F

### Desired Intervention

Patient with decreased responsiveness and hypoxia will need to be intubated.

The question for the provider will be how the patient will be ventilated given that all ventilators are currently in use.

This is a difficult scenario in which we must try to make the best decision based on resources and current care being required by other patients in the hospital.

Questions that could be asked are:

- Should we discontinue care for the postcardiac arrest patient who has no meaningful responses?
- Is there a way to double ventilate from one machine?
- Is there a transport service in the area that will provide a ventilator for use?
- Do we have the staff to provide ventilation via BMV using $ETCO_2$ to monitor rate and tidal volume?
- Can we ventilate for a little bit until the patient can be transported to another facility?
- There are numerous ways for this to be handled and I believe it best to be discussed as a team to obtain different opinions and consider how in their treatment environment they would address this situation.
- At this time, the case can be continued by either adding additional patients with conditions determined by the agency reviewing the scenario of the scenario can be discontinued.

## BIBLIOGRAPHY


ARDSNet. Ventilation with lower tidal volumes as compared with traditional tidal volumes for acute lung injury and the acute respiratory distress syndrome. The Acute Respiratory Distress Syndrome Network. *N Engl J Med.* 2000 May 4;342(18):1301–1308.

Brown CA 3rd, Walls RM. The decision to intubate. In: *The Walls Manual of Emergency Airway Management.* 5th ed. Philadelphia: Lippincott Williams & Wilkins; 2018:3–8.

Hathaway WR, Peterson ED, Wagner GS, et al. Prognostic significance of the initial electrocardiogram in patients with acute myocardial infarction. GUSTO-I Investigators. Global Utilization of Streptokinase and t-PA for Occluded Coronary Arteries. *JAMA.* 1998; 279:387–391.

Kirk MA, Deaton ML. Bringing order out of chaos: effective strategies for medical response to mass chemical exposure. *Emerg Med Clin North Am.* 2007 May;25(2):527–548; abstract xi. doi: 10.1016/j.emc.2007.02.005. PMID: 17482031.

Lee CL. Disaster and mass casualty triage. *Virtual Mentor.* 2010;12(6):466–470. doi:10.1001/virtualmentor.2010.12.6.cprl1-1006.

Luce JM, Alpers A. Legal aspects of withholding and withdrawing life support from critically ill patients in the United States and providing palliative care to them. *Am J Respir Crit Care Med.* 2000 Dec;162(6):2029–2032. doi: 10.1164/ajrccm.162.6.1-00. PMID: 11112108.

Navalesi P, Fanfulla F, Frigerio P, Gregoretti C, Nava S. Physiologic evaluation of noninvasive mechanical ventilation delivered with three types of masks in patients with chronic hypercapnic respiratory failure. *Crit Care Med.* 2000 Jun;28(6):1785–1790. doi: 10.1097/00003246-200006000-00015. PMID: 10890620.

Parshall MB, Schwartzstein RM, Adams L, et al. An official American Thoracic Society statement: update on the mechanisms, assessment, and management of dyspnea. *Am J Respir Crit Care Med.* 2012;185:435.

Pavli A, Maltezou HC, Papadakis A, et al. Respiratory infections and gastrointestinal illness on a cruise ship: a three-year prospective study. *Travel Med Infect Dis.* 2016 Jul-Aug;14(4):389–397. doi: 10.1016/j.tmaid.2016.05.019. Epub 2016 Jun 15. PMID: 27320130.

Tonetti T, Zanella A, Pizzilli G, et al. One ventilator for two patients: feasibility and considerations of a last resort solution in case of equipment shortage. *Thorax.* 2020;75:517–519.

Ward KA, Armstrong P, McAnulty JM, Iwasenko JM, Dwyer DE. Outbreaks of pandemic (H1N1) 2009 and seasonal influenza A (H3N2) on cruise ship. *Emerg Infect Dis.* 2010;16:1731–1737.

SECTION 7

# TECHNOLOGICAL DISASTERS

CASE 27

# Medical Management of Chlorine Gas Exposure Following a Freight Train Derailment

Colleen M. Donovan, Mary G. McGoldrick, and Denise Fernandez

DISASTER PRINCIPLES

- Scene safety and security in the field
- Conventional standards of care
- Clinical diagnosis and treatment
- Information management/communications
- Personal protective equipment (PPE)
- Fireground safety
- Timing of medical and surgical interventions
- Field operations and logistics
- Organizational preparedness and resiliency
- Business continuity
- Community preparedness and resiliency
- Transportation disasters
- Choking agents
- Chlorine
- Chemical agents
- Recognition and clinical treatment
- MCI triage and considerations for chemical agents
- Chemical safety
- Decontamination

## 1. SCENARIO OVERVIEW

This is a hybrid scenario, beginning with a standardized patient (SP), and transitioning to a mannequin as the case progresses. It takes place in a community hospital in the United States, as the scenario is built with US Department of Transportation (DOT) references and Codes of Federal Regulations.

Samir Green is a 47-year-old male with a past medical history of hypertension and hyperlipidemia who was acting as a freight engineer for a train transporting 17 rail tankers of industrial chemicals. Due to a track defect, the train derailed in a rural but populated area at approximately 0300. At least one tank was punctured, and its contents spilled. The weather is rainy and warm, and the derailment site is uphill and upwind from a moderately sized mill town. Mr. Green was one of many people in the immediate area of exposure in the derailment. He was able to self-extricate from the engine and contacted emergency services, along with several town residents who drove out to investigate the loud crash.

A HAZMAT team was dispatched and is currently securing the scene and initiating evacuation within a one-mile radius of the crash. Paramedics on scene evaluated Mr. Green, who sustained multiple abrasions/lacerations and reports a burning sensation in his eyes and throat. He was triaged with a green tag using START criteria and was transported to a community hospital for further evaluation.

The setting is a community hospital. The ED is experiencing a surge of patients, including injured first responders and residents from within the exposure radius. Other patients include worried well residents and residents from other nearby communities with potential exposure and vague symptoms. At ED triage, Mr. Green is initially anxious and, in addition to eye and throat burning, now complains of mild nausea and cough. There is a strong bleach-like odor. He is assigned to a hallway bed. Learners can assume the other patients are being cared for and that Mr. Green is their primary patient. They are evaluating him one hour after exposure.

The learners will obtain a history and physical exam and send Mr. Green to be decontaminated. Shortly after decon, Mr. Green will decompensate. His intubation and resuscitation will be complicated by laryngeal edema, pulmonary edema, and acute respiratory distress syndrome (ARDS). The team will have to manage his airway, stabilize him, and admit him to the ICU, thus ending the scenario.

## 2. TEACHING OBJECTIVES AND DISCUSSION POINTS

### Clinical and Medical Management

- Identify hazardous materials from US DOT mandatory labeling requirements, such as placards
- Diagnose, decontaminate, and manage a chlorine exposure patient
- Discuss the mechanism of injury for chlorine and appropriate level of suspicion for inhalation injury
- Manage the difficulty airway in a patient with presumed laryngeal edema, noncardiogenic pulmonary edema, and ARDS

### Communication and Teamwork

- Work as a team to appropriately manage a decompensating patient with chlorine exposure
- Call on resources: toxicologist/poison control and ICU

## 3. SUPPLIES

- Personal equipment (e.g. stethoscope, PPE)
- Standard patient clothing: undershirt and work pants/boots, triage tag with green designation
- Small volume of diluted bleach and a cloth towel
- Mannequin clothing: hospital gown
- Mannequin equipment (bedside monitor, etc.)
- 18 G IVs
- Oxygen delivery equipment: NRB mask, nasal cannula
- Medications: albuterol-ipratropium (nebulized), sodium bicarb (nebulized), dexamethasone (IV)
- Intubation equipment: suction, BVM, laryngoscope handles/blades, video laryngoscope with stylet, bougie, ETT size 6.5–8.0, 10 cc syringe, $ETCO_2$ monitor
- Edematous airway model: inflammation of the arytenoids, epiglottis, trachea

## 4. MOULAGE

- Abrasion to right shoulder
- Bleach odor: pour a small amount of bleach onto a cloth towel and set aside

## 5. IMAGES AND LABS

- ECG: sinus tachycardia, but otherwise unremarkable
- CXR: diffuse pulmonary edema, ETT positioned correctly above the carina
- Labs: within normal limits if requested, except for ABGs (see Transition Points 1 and 3)

## 6. ACTORS

- SP: patient Samir Green, supplemented with mannequin or airway model
- Nurse: at bedside, prompts for appropriate care
- Toxicologist/poison control/critical care physician: available via telephone, receives report, prompts for any missed critical actions

## 7. CRITICAL ACTIONS

- Obtain history and physical exam, identify chlorine as the likely industrial toxin
- Order decontamination
- Recognize decompensation after decon and resuscitate appropriately
- Administer appropriate medications (humidified oxygen, inhaled bronchodilators) and adjunct therapies (high-dose corticosteroids, nebulized sodium bicarbonate)
- Anticipate difficult airway with primary and backup plans, perform intubation. As first pass attempt is likely to be unsuccessful, second attempt must demonstrate modification and rationale
- Confirm intubation, ensure postintubation sedation, reassess patient
- Verbalize appropriate ventilator management, including ARDS-like lung protective settings
- Clearly communicate with all confederates and admit patient to the ICU

## 8. TIMELINE

### Time: Two Minutes – Prebrief

You are the physician team at a community hospital that is the closest facility to a nearby train derailment. The ED is currently experiencing a surge of patients as the train was transporting tanks of industrial chemicals. It is unclear which chemicals were being transported at this time. HAZMAT is on scene. Patients are occupying all rooms and hallway beds are being utilized for patient care. Your patient is Samir Green, a 47-year-old male with a past medical history of hypertension and hyperlipidemia who was operating the train during the derailment. He was exposed to the chemicals prior to arrival of emergency services. He presents via EMS approximately one hour after exposure with complaints of eye and throat burning. He has developed mild nausea en route to the ED. You are evaluating him in an open hallway with his assigned nurse. Mr. Green has not yet been decontaminated.

### Time: Zero to Four Minutes – Arrive at Bedside

VS: HR 101, BP 161/84, RR 20, $SPO_2$ 98% on room air, temp 98.4°F

- Summary of initial presentation: Middle-aged man on a stretcher in his undershirt/work clothes with green triage tag around his neck. There is a strong odor of bleach. *This may be simulated by pouring a small amount of bleach onto a cloth towel. The towel may be placed nearby, or the SP may hold the towel in his hands.*

- Initial interventions: introduce self/team to SP, obtain history and physical exam
- History
  - SP: "I was operating the train when we went off the tracks. The engine I was in stayed upright; I just got tossed around a little trying to keep it under control. Some of the cars overturned. I was able to get out and called 911."
  - Pain: "After I got out my eyes and throat started to feel a little scratchy and I've been coughing. Right now, my eyes feel a little bit better but my throat's a still sore. Can't seem to clear my throat."
  - Time: "About an hour ago, maybe two."
  - Pertinent positives: "I can see ok; it just feels like there's something in my eyes, and my nose is running. I can swallow but it's a little scratchy. I do have a little pain in my chest when I take a deep breath, but I think it's just because I got jostled around – my right shoulder hurts a bit too. I've just started with this nagging, cough – it feels like I can't clear my throat. I do feel nauseated, and I threw up once in the ambulance. I'm still queasy but it's a bit better now. And my clothes STINK – I think that's making everything worse."
    - *If the learners do not ask about the odor, the SP may prompt them by having them smell the bleached cloth.*
  - This should prompt the learners to ask what chemicals were in the tanker cars. SP: "I'm not 100% sure because I don't know which tankers were leaking, but I took this photo of the crash. This placard was on several of the rear cars." (Figures 27.1 and 27.2 may be uploaded to the SP's phone. For added complexity, show only the crash photo, do not show the placard.)
- Pertinent negatives: "I don't think I hit my head – it doesn't really hurt, although I do feel a little dizzy. I didn't pass out or anything." No fever or neck pain, no trouble breathing.
- PMH: HTN, HLD
- Medications: losartan, rosuvastatin
- Allergies: none
- Social: 1 pack per week smoking history, social EtOH, no drug use
- Physical exam: primary survey followed by more detailed relevant exam
- Primary survey
  - Airway: phonating, mildly hoarse
  - Breathing: symmetric breath sounds bilaterally
  - Circulation: intact pulses, appropriate HR and BP
  - Disability: Glasgow Coma Scale 15
  - Exposure: limited due to hallway bed location
- Detailed relevant exam
  - HEENT: normocephalic, atraumatic, + conjunctival injection, vision is 20/30 in both eyes, nares with erythema and some rhinorrhea, mucous membranes moist, no malocclusion or intraoral injury, + pharyngeal erythema, no pooling of secretions, trachea midline
  - Cardiac: borderline tachycardic, regular, no MGR
  - Respiratory: symmetric chest expansion, faint coarse breath sounds at lung bases, intermittent dry cough that temporarily clears coarse sounds
  - Abdomen: soft, nondistended, nontender
  - Extremities: mild tenderness to palpation of the acromioclavicular joint of the right shoulder, with moulaged abrasion, otherwise full ROM and normal extremities
  - Neuro: A&O ×3, strength and sensation intact and symmetric

- Nurse: verbal cues
  - "Geez. That crash photo looks awful. What are those diamond shaped things on the tanker cars?"
  - "Aren't there supposed to be some sort of safety sheets or something that list what to do in case of exposure?"
    - Prompts to look up Material Safety Data Sheets (MSDS or SDS) for chlorine
  - "I'll have the tech take Mr. Green to be decontaminated. Maybe we can look up those MSDSs while he's getting cleaned up.... What do they say we should do? Anything we need to be on the lookout for? Is there anyone we should call?"
    - Prompt to call toxicologist/poison control (800-222-1222) and/or National Response Center (800-424-8802)
- "When he gets back from decon, what are your orders?"
  - Management decisions
    - Labs and imaging
      - ECG, CXR (CBC, CMP if desired at this point)
        - ECG sinus tachycardia, otherwise within normal limits
        - CXR currently normal
        - Labs pending, if requested
      - Medications (optional at this point)
        - Supplemental $O_2$ for comfort
        - Albuterol-ipratropium nebulizer

**Critical Actions**
- Obtain history, including clues to chemical exposure
- Identify chlorine as the likely industrial toxin
- Perform physical exam including detailed eye, pharynx, and lung exams
- Order decontamination
- Evaluate for trauma, given crash history

## Time: Four to Six Minutes – Transition Point 1 – Return from Decon and Symptoms Worsen

*Time-in-scenario has advanced 30 minutes. Mr. Green has been decontaminated, but during the process, his respiratory symptoms have worsened. At this time, we transition from the SP to the mannequin.*

- Reevaluation initiated by nurse: "Doc, can you come take another look at Mr. Green? He doesn't look so good."
  - Repeat primary survey
    - A: stridulous, tripoding
    - B: diffuse wheezes and crackles, tachypneic, increased work of breathing
    - C: tachycardic, intact pulses
- Repeat vitals
  - HR 110, BP 171/82, RR 28, $O_2$ 80% on room air, 89% on NRB mask
- Immediate interventions
  - Move patient to a resuscitation area
  - Supplemental humidified oxygen with NRB mask
  - Establish IV access if not already in place (bilateral, large bore)

  - First-line medication
    - Albuterol-ipratropium ($O_2$ improves to 92%)
  - Consider adjunct therapies
    - High-dose corticosteroids
    - Nebulized sodium bicarbonate
  - Call for respiratory therapy for a trial of noninvasive ventilation (optional)
  - Plan for intubation
    - RN can prompt interventions while awaiting additional support or moving the patient
    - Team should recognize need for likely intubation given airway compromise
    - If requested: ABG on NRB: pH: 7.22, $PaO_2$ 40 mmHg, $PaCO_2$ 50 mmHg, lactate 6.5

**Critical Actions**

- Recognize need for emergency reevaluation
- Repeat primary survey and identify airway and breathing compromise
- Ensure IV access, oxygen supplementation, cardiac monitoring/pulse oximetry
- Administer appropriate medications, including humidified oxygen and inhaled bronchodilators
- Consider adjunct therapies including high-dose corticosteroids and inhaled sodium bicarbonate
- Note: Empiric antibiotics are not recommended

### Time: 6–10 Minutes – Transition Point 2 – Failure to Improve, Laryngeal Edema, Pulmonary Edema and ARDS Suspected

*Despite initial therapies, Mr. Green does not improve and requires intubation due to pulmonary edema/acute lung injury and ARDS. Mannequin or task trainer should be set for laryngeal edema, with pulmonary edema if possible (e.g. https://jetem.org/pulm_edema_sim/)*

VS: HR 110, BP 96/56, RR 33, 82% on NRB mask

#### Emergent Airway Management

- Intubation
  - Preparation with supplemental oxygen, suction, BVM, end-tidal $CO_2$ monitor, respiratory therapist contacted, vent available
  - Verbalize airway plan
    - Inform patient of the need to intubate
    - Equipment selection – learners should opt for video to increase first pass success, state backup plans (direct, bougie, surgical airway)
    - Learners should not need to progress to surgical airway if initial intubation fails
- Sedation and paralytics
  - Ketamine and rocuronium at appropriate weight-based dosing
- Performing the intubation
  - If utilizing video laryngoscope will note edematous airway, tracheal narrowing
  - ETT size 7.5 and greater should not pass, and $O_2$ sat should drop

- Learner should recognize failed first attempt, remove laryngoscope and bag and reoptimize patient
- Verbalization of backup plan
- Can ask surrounding team members for advice, who may recommend using a bougie or smaller ETT
- Successful intubation on second attempt using verbalized backup
- Confirmation of intubation on $ETCO_2$ and with breath sounds

**Critical Actions**

- Anticipate difficult airway with primary and backup plans
- Clearly communicate with team and patient
- Reassess patient after unsuccessful first pass attempt
- Perform intubation. As first pass attempt is likely to be unsuccessful, second attempt must demonstrate modification (use of bougie, change of technique (e.g. direct to video laryngoscopy), smaller ETT, change intubators, etc.)
- Confirm intubation and ensure postintubation sedation

### Time: 10+ Minutes – Transition Point 3 – Stabilization and Final Considerations

- Reevaluation
- Repeat vital signs (BP 136/74, $O_2$ 100%, bag ventilations at rate of 20, HR 90)
- Repeat CXR
  - Confirms tube placement appropriately above the carina
  - Demonstrates diffuse pulmonary edema not present on previous CXR
  - Ventilator settings: lung protective strategy, low tidal volume (6 mL/kg ideal body weight), positive end-expiratory pressure 5 or greater
- Obtain additional labs and imaging
  - ABG after intubation ($FiO_2$ 100%): pH: 7.35, $PaO_2$ 215 mmHg, $pCO_2$ 55 mmHg
  - Lactate: 4.4
  - CT chest (optional), also consistent with pulmonary edema and ARDS
- Disposition
- Contact medical ICU and provide warm handoff

**Critical Actions**

- Repeat vital signs, reassess
- Verbalize appropriate ventilator management, including ARDS-like lung protective settings
- Recognition of the need for critical care and disposition to the ICU

## 9. STIMULI

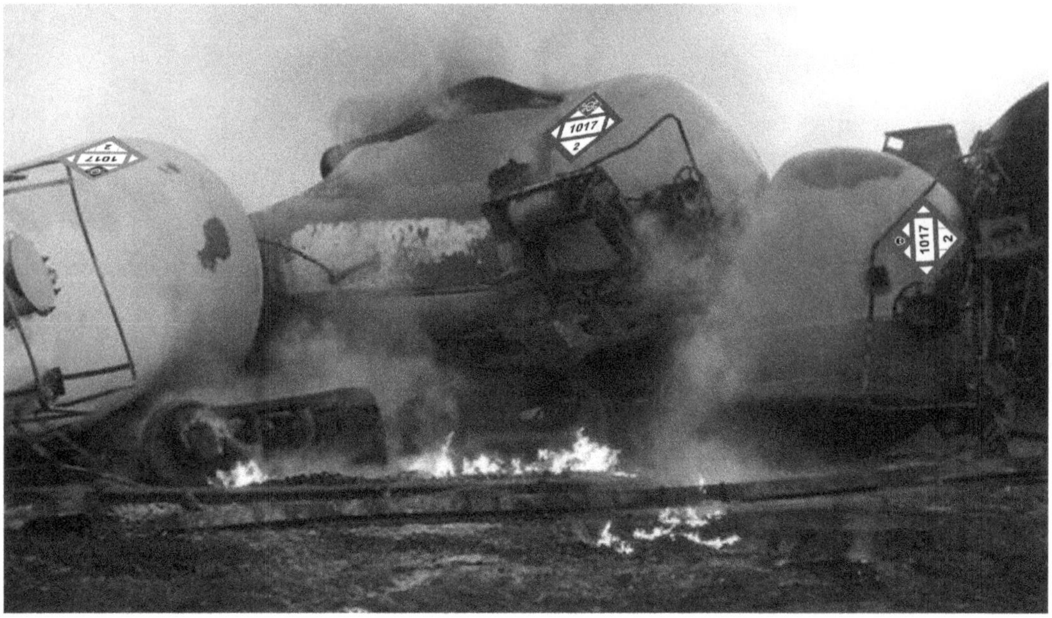


**Figure 27.1** Rail tanker crash with placards.
Adapted from "Part of the tank car pileup and residual fire resulting from the train collision near Casselton, North Dakota" by NTSBgov. https://commons.wikimedia.org/wiki/File:2013_NTSB_Casselton,_ND_train_crash.jpg. Public Domain Mark 1.0. To view the terms, visit https://creativecommons.org/publicdomain/mark/1.0/?ref=openverse.

**Figure 27.2** Chlorine placard.
Drawn by author Colleen M. Donovan in Microsoft PowerPoint, January 28, 2023.

## BIBLIOGRAPHY

Achanta S, Jordt S. Toxic effects of chlorine gas and potential treatments: a literature review. *Toxicol Mech Methods.* 2021;31(4):244–256. doi:10.1080/15376516.2019.1669244.

Centers for Disease Control and Prevention. Public health consequences from hazardous substances acutely released during rail transit: South Carolina, 2005; selected states, 1999–2004. *MMWR Morb Mortal Wkly Rep.* 2005;54(03):64–67. www.cdc.gov/mmwr/preview/mmwrhtml/mm5403a2.htm. Accessed March 24, 2005.

Dunning AE, Oswalt JL. Train wreck and chlorine spill in Graniteville, South Carolina. *Transportation Research Record.* 2007;2009(1):130–135. doi:10.3141/2009-17.

Gresham C, LoVecchio F. Chapter 204: industrial toxins. In: Tintinalli JE, Ma OJ, Yealy DM, et al., eds. *Tintinalli's Emergency Medicine: A Comprehensive Study Guide.* 9th ed. New York: McGraw-Hill Education; 2020:1318–1322.

Harvey RR, Boylstein R, McCullough J, et al. Fatal chlorine gas exposure at a metal recycling facility: case report. *Am J Ind Med.* 2018;61(6):538–542. doi:10.1002/ajim.22847.

Heather Starmer Research Lab. Head & neck surgery: Lymphedema. 2022. https://med.stanford.edu/starmer-lab/research/lymphedema.html. Accessed March 24, 2025.

Huynh Tuong A, Despréaux T, Loeb T, et al. Emergency management of chlorine gas exposure: a systematic review. *Clin Toxicol (Phila).* 2019;57(2):77–98. doi:10.1080/15563650.2018.1519193.

Mastenbrook J, Hughes N, Fales W, Overton D. An innovative inexpensive portable pulmonary edema intubation simulator. *J Educ Teach Emerg Med.* 2020;5(2):I9–I20. doi:10.21980/J8MM1R.

Nelson LS, Odujebe OA. Simple asphyxiants and pulmonary irritants. In: Nelson LS, Howland MA, Lewin NA, et al., eds. *Goldfrank's Toxicologic Emergencies* 11th ed. New York: McGraw-Hill Education; 2019:1651–1662.

New Jersey Department of Health. *Right to Know: Hazardous Substance Fact Sheet. Chlorine.* Trenton: New Jersey Department of Health; 2015. https://nj.gov/health/eoh/rtkweb/documents/fs/0367.pdf. Accessed April 4, 2025.

Pipeline and Hazardous Materials Safety Administration. *DOT chart 17: Markings, labeling, and placarding guide.* Washington, DC: US Department of Transportation; 2022. www.phmsa.dot.gov/training/hazmat/dot-chart-17-markings-labeling-and-placarding-guide. Accessed April 4, 2025.

Wang L, Wu D, Wang J. Chlorine gas inhalation manifesting with severe acute respiratory distress syndrome successfully treated by high-volume hemofiltration. *Medicine (Baltimore).* 2018;97(30): e11708. doi:10.1097%2FMD.0000000000011708.

CASE 28

# Treating Life-Threatening Injuries with Limited Resources while at Sea

Cody Johnson

DISASTER PRINCIPLES

- Scarce resource allocation protocols
- Clinical diagnosis and treatment
- Information management/communications
- Timing of medical and surgical interventions
- Organizational preparedness and resiliency
- Business continuity
- Transportation disasters
- Recognition and clinical treatment
- Field stabilization, treatment, and transport

## 1. SCENARIO OVERVIEW

You are the medical officer contracted by a large commercial fishing vessel that is returning to port after collecting a large haul of Dungeness crabs. About an hour prior to reaching port, a large metal crate filled with crabs is swung on its crane striking a crew member on deck on his left side and subsequently throwing him to the ground. You are called to the scene from your position in the infirmary and arrive in less than five minutes after the incident.

On arrival you find a 25-year-old man who gasps out that he has no medical history or allergies and takes no medications. He last ate at breakfast that morning more than eight hours prior. He complains of severe left-sided chest and side pain, worse with inspiration and associated with mild shortness of breath.

The ship carries few medical supplies, mostly what is necessary for life-saving treatments: a basic first aid kit, a chest tube kit, a cricothyrotomy tray, intubation equipment, IV supplies, cervical collars, a small volume of crystalloid, and two units of uncrossmatched blood. Proctor decides if portable ultrasound is available.

The patient is traumatized as described and develops a left-sided hemopneumothorax and spleen laceration. He is hemodynamically unstable and will require a chest tube (not a needle decompression) and emergent blood transfusion, all without labs or advanced imaging.

## 2. TEACHING OBJECTIVES AND DISCUSSION POINTS

- Reevaluation of patients and identification of occult trauma
- Management of trauma in an austere environment

  - Pneumothorax and rib fractures
  - Spleen laceration
- Rapid activation of prehospital resources

## 3. SUPPLIES

- Portable ultrasound
- Chest tube tray
- IV supplies
- Uncrossmatched O-negative blood
- Intubation supplies

## 4. MOULAGE

- Abrasions to the left arm and side
- Bruising over the left chest (approximately intercostal spaces 5–8)
- Later bruising on the left flank

## 5. IMAGES AND LABS

- If the proctor decides to include portable ultrasound, ultrasound will show an absence of lung sliding on the left with a left pleural effusion (hemothorax) and a positive Focused Assessment with Sonography for Trauma (FAST) exam in the LUQ.

## 6. ACTORS (CONFEDERATES) AND THEIR ROLES

- The patient who is in acute pain
- Bystanders who are panicked (optional)

## 7. CRITICAL ACTIONS

- Identification of obvious and occult trauma
- Management of immediately life-threatening pathology in the austere setting
- Alert the shore to have EMS ready on arrival

## 8. TIMELINE AND TRANSITION POINTS

### Time: Zero

1. 25-year-old patient
   VS: BP 80/palp, HR 120, RR 33, O2 sat 90%, temperature 38°C
   The patient is evaluated immediately on the deck of the ship.

**Physical Exam**
General: appears ill. Participatory with exam but opens eyes only when asked
HEENT: no apparent trauma, no septal hematoma noted, no midline C-spine tenderness to palpation
Heart: regular tachycardia, no murmurs/rubs/gallops
Lungs: no breath sounds noted on the left, normal breath sounds on the right.

Chest: severe tenderness along the left chest at the mid-axillary line between intercostal spaces 5–8. Slight bruising over intercostal space 5-8 at the MAL. Normal chest wall excursion. No open wounds.

Abdomen: soft, nondistended, severe tenderness to palpation in the LUQ with rebound, bruising to flank as described later

Extremities: no gross deformities, cool to the touch ×4

Skin: ecchymosis to left chest and flank

Neuro: Glasgow Coma Scale 14 (E3 V5 M6), A&O ×4, follows commands with all extremities (LUE limited by pain), no focal deficits

**Actions**

- The learner will perform their evaluation as if they are on deck and their supplies are in the infirmary. They have only brought equipment to check vital signs.
- If the learner attempts to perform a resuscitation procedure without calling for supplies from the infirmary, they will be made to wait a short period while supplies are obtained.
- If the learner attempts needle decompression, there will be no improvement in vital signs or exam. A chest tube will result in a hiss of air when the pleura is entered and approximately 100 cc of blood once the tube is placed.
- If the learner does not attempt some form of chest decompression the patient will lose consciousness.
- If the learner intubates the patient without some form of chest decompression, the patient will arrest until decompressed and then regain pulses.
- After chest decompression, the patient's blood pressure will remain low and unstable until he is transfused at least one unit of uncrossmatched blood.

**Critical Actions**

- Rapidly call for supplies from the infirmary
- Identify obvious trauma multiple rib fractures without flail chest and treat pneumothorax
- Suspect occult trauma (spleen laceration)
  - Empirically transfuse with an emphasis on blood over crystalloid
- Have someone call to shore to arrange transfer to an EMS crew for immediate transportation to a hospital

## 9. STIMULI

M-Mode image of absent lung sliding and positive LUQ FAST if instructor decides to allow ultrasound, otherwise none

## BIBLIOGRAPHY

Littlejohn LF. Treatment of thoracic trauma: lessons from the battlefield adapted to all austere environments. *Wilderness Environ Med.* 2017;28:S69–S73.

Stancil SA. Development of a new infusion protocol for austere trauma resuscitations. *Air Med J.* 2017;36:239–243.

CASE 29

# Outbreak at Sea

## Managing Acute Gastroenteritis on a Cruise Ship

Cody Johnson

DISASTER PRINCIPLES

- Scarce resource allocation protocols
- Clinical diagnosis and treatment
- Information management/communications
- Timing of medical and surgical interventions
- Organizational preparedness and resiliency
- Business continuity
- Recognition and clinical treatment
- Contingency standards of care
- Public health surveillance
- Complex public health emergencies
- Quarantine/isolation
- Medical surge capacity
- Mass-casualty care in the field
- Operational continuity
- MCI triage and considerations for biological agents
- Biological safety

### 1. SCENARIO OVERVIEW

You are the senior medical officer on a large commercial cruise ship. The passenger log consists of approximately 3000 people with an age distribution of approximately 20% children, 50% adults ages 18–65 years old, and 30% geriatric passengers older than 65 years. There are approximately 750 crew members on board. The ship has robust medical capabilities including 10 sick bays for patient observation with suction setups, five telemetry packs, and one isolated negative pressure room with built-in ICU level bed. Equipment includes most over-the-counter medications, common prescription medications including ample crystalloids, narcotic analgesia, a 12-lead ECG machine, an X-ray machine, and two ventilators.

On the third day of what is intended to be a nine-day journey you are seeing a six-year-old, otherwise healthy male patient with more than five episodes each of vomiting and diarrhea in the last three or four hours. There has been no blood in any of his emissions, but he has been unable to keep down any of the electrolyte solution his parents had brought with them. While you're evaluating this patient, your junior medical officer tells you there are two additional patients coming in with nausea, vomiting, and diarrhea, one 21-year-old who is celebrating a recent marathon win and one 70-year-old who has been shouting that it's not related to his gallbladder, which he recently had removed.

The captain calls to ask if you've been made aware of multiple sick passengers complaining of nausea and vomiting; she's being told by managers that multiple crew members are sick and housekeeping reports nearly 100 passengers have developed severe nausea and vomiting since departure. She wants to know what to do about this. Multiple patients are sick with a viral gastroenteritis. No one is significantly dehydrated or has electrolyte derangements. The physician must recognize the outbreak and potential to be overwhelmed at sea and take action in conjunction with the captain to minimize the spread of the illness. The captain will not turn around, as no one is likely to die, and it is days to the next port.

## 2. TEACHING OBJECTIVES AND DISCUSSION POINTS

- Management of acute viral GI illness (this should be a minor point)
- Differential diagnosis of severe nausea, vomiting, and diarrhea in each presenting age group
- An "outbreak" is defined as >3% of passengers developing acute gastroenteritis[1]
- Basic infection control measures

## 3. SUPPLIES

- IV fluids
- Medications (blister packs or vials)
- POC chemistry analyzer and cartridges

## 4. MOULAGE

- Artificial emesis (optional)

## 5. IMAGES AND LABS

All may be obtained or omitted; history and exam should be sufficient

- POC chemistry
- Abdominal X-ray
- ECGs

## 6. ACTORS (CONFEDERATES) AND THEIR ROLES

- Pediatric mannequin
  - actor or proctor to act as parent and provide history
  - Parents are very worried
- Junior medical officer as voice over the phone or in person
- Two additional actors as patients all with acute viral gastroenteritis who are very vocal about their symptoms and how it is ruining their cruise
  - The elderly patient may or may not have a spouse with them; if no spouse, then patient will demand cruise be turned around.
- Captain: over the phone from the bridge

**Critical Actions**
- Treatment of acute GI illness
- Consideration of more emergent pathologies (e.g. volvulus, SBO)
- Identification of potential endemic
- Initiation of basic public health actions

## 7. TIMELINE AND TRANSITION POINTS

### Time: Zero

- An 8-year-old patient
  VS: BP 95/60, HR 115, RR 30, O2 sat 99%, temperature 38°C
  Brought in by parents for ongoing nausea and vomiting in their cabin as described previously.

**Physical Exam**
- General: appears irritable. Appropriate with exam and minimally participatory with conversation
- HEENT: dry oral mucosa, otherwise unremarkable
- Heart: regular tachycardia, no murmurs/rubs/gallops
- Lungs: clear to auscultation bilaterally, no increased work of breathing
- Abdomen: soft, nondistended, mild diffuse tenderness with deep palpation without rebound or guarding, bowel sounds are present
- Extremities: unremarkable
- Skin: no rashes
- Neuro: A&O ×4, follows commands, no focal deficits

Patient will respond to either PO or IV medication and fluids.

**Critical Actions**
- Obtain focused H&P including severity of dehydration, if present
- Accurately diagnose gastroenteritis
- Trial ODT antiemetic and oral rehydration therapy or place IV and give IV antiemetic and crystalloid bolus

### Time: Five Minutes

- A 21-year-old patient
  VS: BP120/80, HR 55, RR 18, O2 sat 99%, temperature 37.2°C
  Presenting after small blood streaking in his vomitus after many episodes of emesis in his cabin.
  Patient will deny blood thinner use, chest pain, shortness of breath

**Physical Exam**
- General: well-appearing
- HEENT: dry oral mucosa, normal conjunctiva without pallor, no sublingual pallor, otherwise unremarkable
- Heart: regular rate and rhythm, no murmurs/rubs/gallops, no Hamman sign
- Lungs: clear to auscultation bilaterally, no increased work of breathing, no crepitus on palpation of chest wall

- Abdomen: soft, nondistended, mild diffuse tenderness with deep palpation without rebound or guarding, bowel sounds are present
- Extremities: unremarkable
- Skin: no rashes, petechiae, or purpura
- Neuro: A&O ×4, follows commands, no focal deficits

Patient will respond to either PO or IV medication and fluids.

- A 70-year-old patient
  VS: BP 100/70, HR 90, RR 30, O2 sat 99%, temperature 38°C
  Brought in by husband after developing mild diffuse abdominal pain in the setting of multiple episodes of vomiting and diarrhea

**Physical Exam**

- General: appears irritable. Appropriate with exam and minimally participatory with conversation.
- HEENT: dry oral mucosa, otherwise unremarkable
- Heart: irregularly irregular, no murmurs/rubs/gallops
- Lungs: clear to auscultation bilaterally, no increased work of breathing
- Abdomen: soft, nondistended, no apparent tenderness to palpation. Bowel sounds are present.
- Extremities: unremarkable
- Skin: no rashes
- Neuro: A&O ×4, follows commands, no focal deficits

Patient will respond to either PO or IV medication and fluids. The husband will demand that the boat be turned around. If asked, the patient or spouse will confirm A-Fib is chronic and well managed by their home cardiologist.

**Critical Actions**

- Obtain focused H&P of each patient
- Accurately diagnose gastroenteritis with consideration of more emergent pathology
- Trial ODT antiemetic and oral rehydration therapy or place IV and give IV antiemetic and crystalloid bolus

## Time: 15 Minutes

The captain calls to the medical bay and updates the doctor about the status of the ship with many symptomatic passengers and some crew as detailed. They are requesting recommendations on what to do about this.

Captain will appreciate and implement any (reasonable) recommendations; she will not divert the ship or return to port.

**Critical Actions**

- Consider as many modes of transmission as possible including foodborne, environmental persistence, and person-to-person spread
- Make appropriate recommendations, for example, isolation of ill persons, paid sick leave for crew, reeducation of staff regarding food handling, informing passengers and promotion of hand washing

## 8. STIMULI

- X-ray with nonobstructive bowel gas pattern for any of the patients and no acute findings
- POC chemistry strips with normal (or abnormal) electrolytes and kidney function at the discretion of the proctor for any of the patients
- An ECG will show:
  - Sinus tachycardia on the pediatric patient
  - Normal sinus rhythm on the young adult
  - Atrial fibrillation without rapid ventricular response on the older patient

## REFERENCES

1. Isakbaeva ET, Widdowson MA, Beard RS, et al. Norovirus transmission on cruise ship. *Emerg Infect Dis.* 2005;11:154–158.
2. Minooee A, Rickman LS. Infectious diseases on cruise ships. *Clin Infect Dis.* 1999;29:737–743; quiz 744.
3. Dahl E. Dealing with gastrointestinal illness on a cruise ship. Part 1: description of sanitation measures. Part 2: an isolation study. *Int Marit Health.* 2004;55:19–29.
4. Jenkins KA, Vaughan GH, Jr, Rodriguez LO, Freeland A. Acute gastroenteritis on cruise ships: Maritime Illness Database and Reporting System, United States, 2006–2019. *MMWR Surveill Summ.* 2021;70:1–19.

CASE 30

# Illness on the High Seas

## Navigating a Gastrointestinal Outbreak 50 Miles from Shore

Rashed Al Remeithi and Natalie Sullivan

DISASTER PRINCIPLES

- Scarce resource allocation protocols
- Clinical diagnosis and treatment
- Information management/communications
- Timing of medical and surgical interventions
- Organizational preparedness and resiliency
- Business continuity
- Recognition and clinical treatment
- Public health surveillance
- Complex public health emergencies
- Quarantine/isolation
- Medical surge capacity
- Mass-casualty care in the field
- Operational continuity
- MCI triage and considerations for biological agents
- Biological safety

### 1. SCENARIO OVERVIEW

Over the past two days, several passengers aboard a cruise ship 50 miles from Key West, Florida, share a common complaint of frequent diarrhea and abdominal pain. The cases vary in severity. Most patients report relatively mild symptoms and appear stable; however, several patients are reporting high fevers, severe diarrhea, and lethargy. There are three beds in the cruise ship medical facility. Available staff include one physician, two nurses and two technicians, and some nonmedical support staff.

### 2. TEACHING OBJECTIVES

- Develop familiarity with cruise ship chain of command and the declaration of an outbreak at sea
- Recognize early signs of possible foodborne illness and establish incident report team to investigate the index case
- Discuss when to enact quarantine rules and isolate confirmed and suspected cases
- Implement hygiene rules and contact precautions in the cruise ship environment
- Initiate environmental cleaning and disinfection protocols

- Manage available medical supplies and stockpile
- Ensure early detection of the outbreak and any decompensated patients
- Plan for transportation of patients in need of emergent hospitalization

## 3. SUPPLIES

- Three hospital beds and one examination room
- IV fluids (limited supply)
- Contact precautions supplies: gloves, and gowns (limited)
- Antibiotics (limited supply)

## 4. MOULAGE

- No significant moulage needs.

## 5. IMAGES AND LABS

- Vital signs: temperature, BP, HR, RR, $O_2$
- Labs: CBC, basic metabolic panel and stool immunoassay kits (for *Clostridium diff* antigen and toxin)
- Signage

## 6. ACTORS

- Passengers: cruise passengers coming to the onboard medical facility complaining of symptoms
- Crew members: establish hygiene rules and begin disinfection process, can assist with nonmedical tasks
- Captain: calls in and requests updates on the patient status and if there is a need for patient transportation
- Nurses/technicians: assist with surge of cases and medical management
- Harbormaster: in contact with the captain, to receive any plans for transportation

## 7. CRITICAL ACTIONS

- Declare status of outbreak of gastroenteritis at sea and inform the captain of the incident
- Convene with onboard medical team and crew member for incident report and investigation of source
- Triage and allocate beds appropriately for sick patients
- Identify *C. diff* infection upon taking detailed history and ordering confirmatory immunoassay testing kits
- Allocate resources (IV fluids) to patients in need of volume resuscitation
- Identify patient in need of transport and facilitate urgent hospitalization urgent hospitalization

## 8. TIMELINE AND TRANSITION POINTS

### Time: Zero

A crew member informs the medical team that several people have begun reporting frequent diarrhea on board the ship. The exact number of affected individuals is unclear. No patients have yet arrived at the medical area but they expect that some patients may arrive soon. There is a crew member present to answer any initial questions the provider may have.

### Time: Two Minutes – Provider Actions

- Identifies the need for key information regarding a potential outbreak including any suspected location or causation and whether an index case is known
  - *Index case:* One of the kitchen personnel had suffered from runny diarrhea and abdominal cramps in the last two days. Upon further history, he reports a recent course of Clindamycin as a treatment for a skin abscess. He was involved in food handling and preparation in the kitchen.
- Requests information regarding the line of communication between the medical unit, the captain, and the cabin crew
- Establishes a team to investigate the outbreak, look for any similar signs and symptoms. Start contact tracing and record cases.
- Enacts and defines quarantine rules for suspected and confirmed cases.
  - *Quarantine* should consist of confinement to room isolation with dedicated toilet, strict contact precaution (no direct skin-skin contact or exposure to bodily fluid)
- Considers the future need to announce outbreak to passengers and offer advice on hygiene rules
- Initiates full cleaning and disinfection of the kitchen surfaces
- Ensures all providers are familiar with appropriate PPE

### Time: 10 Minutes – Transition Point 1

Seven patients arrive at the medical unit in rapid succession.

- Patient 1, vital signs: 80/55 BP, 121 HR, 20 RR, sat 97%, T 102°F
  - A 67-year-old female, with a history of hypertension and coronary artery disease who reports diarrhea that is loose and has occurred more than five times in the past 24 hours. Stool is nonbloody and associated with diffuse abdominal pain, fever, and chills.
  - Physical exam: Patient appears in moderate distress with signs of dehydration: > 2-second capillary refill, dry axilla, and mucous membranes. Mild diffuse abdominal tenderness, no distention, no guarding, no rebound tenderness, and no organomegaly. Normal heart sounds, regular pulse, and no peripheral swelling. Lung sounds are clear bilaterally.
- Patient 2, vital signs: 110/65 BP, 95 HR, 18 RR, sat 100%, T 99°F
  - A 58-year-old male with a history of type 2 diabetes presents with mild nonbloody diarrhea that has occurred three times in the past 24 hours associated with fatigue but no fever or chills.
  - Physical exam: Patient is in no distress. He has no signs of dehydration: <2-second capillary refill, normal skin turgor. Abdominal soft, nontender, and no organomegaly. Normal heart sounds, regular pulse, and no peripheral swelling. Lung sounds are clear bilaterally.
- Patient 3, vital signs: 115/78 BP, 90 HR, 18 RR, sat 100%, T 97.5°F
  - A 49-year-old male with no significant past medical history, complains of mild diarrhea (runny, three times in the last 24 hours) with no blood
  - Physical exam: Patient is in no distress. No signs of dehydration: <2-second capillary refill, normal skin turgor. Abdominal soft, nontender and no organomegaly. Normal heart sounds, regular pulse, and no peripheral swelling. Bilateral air entry, no lung sounds.
- Patient 4, vital signs: 90/60 BP, 125 HR, 22 RR, sat 98%, T 102.5°F
  - A 52-year-old male with a history of GERD who reports four episodes of nonbloody watery and mild abdominal pain.

  - Physical exam: Patient appears in mild distress, signs of dehydration: <2-second capillary refill, dry mucous membrane. Abdomen is soft, nondistended with epigastric tenderness, no rebound or rigidity. Normal heart sounds, regular pulse, and no peripheral swelling. Lung sounds are clear bilaterally.
- Patient 5, vital signs: 105/75 BP, 89 HR, 15 RR, sat 99%, T 97.7°F
  - A 39-year-old, with a history of hypertension who presents with four or five episodes of nonbloody diarrhea and no abdominal pain.
  - Physical exam: Patient appears in no distress and has no signs of dehydration. Abdomen is soft, nondistended, no organomegaly. Normal heart sounds, regular pulse, and no peripheral swelling. Lung sounds are clear bilaterally.
- Patient 6, vital signs: 82/58 BP, 109 HR, 19 RR, sat 98%, T 101.5°F
  - A 44-year-old male complains of more than seven episodes of nonbloody diarrhea.
  - Physical exam: Patient appears in mild distress with signs of dehydration: >2-second capillary refill, dry mucous membranes. Mild diffuse abdominal tenderness, no distention, no guarding, no rebound tenderness, and no organomegaly. Normal heart sounds, regular pulse, and no peripheral swelling. Lung sounds are clear bilaterally.
- Patient 7, vital signs: 110/80 BP, 92 HR, 18 RR, sat 99%, T 101.7°F
  - A 60-year-old female with a history of osteoarthritis, macular degeneration and lupus who complains of four episodes of nonbloody diarrhea without blood. No PMHx.
  - Physical exam: Patient appears in mild distress. No signs of dehydration: < 2-second capillary refill, normal skin turgor. Abdomen soft, nontender, and no organomegaly. Normal heart sounds, regular pulse, and no peripheral swelling. Lung sounds are clear bilaterally.

### Time: 11 Minutes – Provider Actions

- Conducts a brief HPI and physical examination for each of the patients focusing on the ABCs
- Triages the patients and allocates the available beds to the sickest patients (1, 4, and 6)
- Identifies that the other patients are stable enough for room quarantine. Discusses management and contact precautions. Identifies need for a patient monitoring system and plan for transport between rooms and the medical unit.
- Initiates fluid resuscitation only on those who are unstable or cannot tolerate oral hydration
- Orders appropriate diagnostic testing for the remaining patients

### Time: 20 Minutes – Transition Point 2

The captain calls for an update and repeat vital signs and updates are available to the provider (if requested) on the patients still in the unit. Lab results become available.

- Patient 1, vital signs: 85/58 BP, 117 HR, 20 RR, sat 99%, T 101.2°F
  - If the provider gave the order, the patient received intravenous fluid resuscitation, blood was drawn for lab testing and a stool sample taken for toxin assay.
  - Patient is still hypovolemic but some vitals are improving with mild clinical improvement.
- Patient 2, vital signs: 103/70 BP, 96 HR, 18 RR, sat 100%, T 101.5°F
  - If the provider gave the order, the patient received intravenous fluid resuscitation, blood was drawn for lab testing, and a stool sample taken for toxin assay.
  - Patient vitals normalize with significant clinical improvement.

- Patient 3, vital signs: 108/74 BP, 92 HR, 16 RR, sat 98%, T 101°F
  - If the provider gave the order, patient received intravenous fluid resuscitation, blood drawn for lab testing, and stool sample taken for toxin assay.
  - Patient vitals normalize with mild clinical improvement.

### Time: 25 Minutes – Provider Actions

- Summarizes and provides status update
  - *Report status:* Three beds are occupied. There is clinical improvement of two of the three sick patients, and one is still in need of close monitoring. Management and lab investigation is ongoing.
- Analyzes laboratory results
  Expresses concern for *C. diff* and starts antibiotics

### Time: 27 Minutes – Transition Point 3

Staff report that the IV fluid supply is decreasing. Only 3 L of fluid remain on board. Another patient update is available (if the provider requests).

- Patient 1, vital signs: 89/63 BP, 109 HR, 19 RR, sat 99%, T 101°F
  - Patient has received ongoing volume resuscitation with IV fluids, and oral vancomycin.
  - Patient is not responding to fluid treatment and continues to be hypotensive.
- Patient 2, vital signs: 110/77 BP, 87 HR, 16 RR, sat 100%, T 100.2°F
  - Patient has had significant clinical improvement and is tolerating water.
- Patient 3, vital signs: BP, 115/75 HR, 81 RR, sat 100%, T 99.5°F
  - Patient has had significant clinical improvement and feels much improved.

### Time: 35 Minutes – Provider Actions

- Considers transfer of Patient 1 to a higher level of care
- Transitions Patient 2 to oral hydration and transfer to room for quarantine
- Transitions Patient 3 to oral hydration and transfer to room for quarantine
- Updates the captain on the current status and the need for onshore medical facility for Patient 1

### Time: 40 Minutes – Transition Point 4 and Conclusion – Transportation Planning Takes Place

- The provider initiates a call between the medical unit, the captain, and the harbormaster to report status of sick patient and arrange transportation via helicopter or rescue boat to an onshore medical facility to receive appropriate care.

## 9. STIMULI

- Labs
  - Patient 1 Na: 134, K: 3.5, Cl: 94, $CO_2$: 19, BUN: 40, Cr: 1.8. Stool immunoassay kit positive for *C. diff* toxin.

- Patient 2 Na: 140, K: 4, Cl: 99, $CO_2$: 21, BUN: 30, Cr: 1.2. Stool immunoassay kit positive for *C. diff* toxin.
- Patient 3 Na: 139, K: 3.9, Cl: 101, $CO_2$: 21, BUN: 28, Cr: 1.1. Stool immunoassay kit positive for *C. diff* toxin.

## BIBLIOGRAPHY

Cramer EH, Blanton CJ, Blanton LH, et al.; Vessel Sanitation Program Environmental Health Inspection Team. Epidemiology of gastroenteritis on cruise ships, 2001–2004. *Am J Prev Med.* 2006; 30(3):252–257.

Jenkins KA, Vaughan GH Jr., Rodriguez LO, Freeland A. Acute gastroenteritis on cruise ships: Maritime Illness Database and Reporting System, United States, 2006–2019. *MMWR Surveill Summ.* 2021; 70(No. SS-6):1–19. doi:10.15585/mmwr.ss7006a1.

Kelly CR, Fischer M, Allegretti JR, et al. ACG clinical guidelines: prevention, diagnosis, and treatment of *Clostridioides difficile* infections. *Am J Gastroenterol.* 2021;116(6):1124–1147.

Kelly CR, Pothoulakis C, LaMont JT. *Clostridium difficile* colitis. *New Engl J Med.* 1994;330(4):257–262.

McDonald LC, Gerding DN, Johnson S, et al. Clinical practice guidelines for *Clostridium difficile* infection in adults and children: 2017 update by the Infectious Diseases Society of America (IDSA) and Society for Healthcare Epidemiology of America (SHEA). *Clin Infect Dis.* 2018;66(7):e1–e48.

Norovirus Working Group, Health Protection Agency, & Maritime and Coastguard Agency. *Guidance for the Management of Norovirus Infection in Cruise Ships.* London: Health Protection Agency; 2007. https://assets.publishing.service.gov.uk/government/uploads/system/uploads/attachment_data/file/362998/2007_guideline_norovirus_cruiseships.pdf. Accessed April 4, 2025.

Widdowson M-A, Cramer EH, Hadley L, et al. Outbreaks of acute gastroenteritis on cruise ships and on land: identification of a predominant circulating strain of norovirus – United States, 2002. *J Infect Dis.* 2004;190(1):27–36.

CASE 31

# Riot Control Fallout

## Surge due to Chemical Irritant Exposures

Rashed Al Remeithi and Natalie Sullivan

DISASTER PRINCIPLES

- Clinical diagnosis and treatment
- Information management/communications
- Timing of medical and surgical interventions
- Recognition and clinical treatment
- Medical surge capacity
- Mass-casualty care in the field
- Emergency operations plans for the healthcare environment
- Command center operations
- Mass-casualty incidents
- Hospital preparedness
- Field operations and logistics
- Field disaster triage
- Field stabilization, treatment, and transport
- Chemical agents
- Chemical safety
- Decontamination

### 1. SCENARIO OVERVIEW

There is a large protest in progress in the city. Thousands of protestors and counterprotestors congregate in one area. During this period both law enforcement and civilians have reportedly deployed riot control agents (RCAs). Subsequently, the ED receives a surge of patients arriving both by EMS and by privately operated vehicle from the protest event. Chief complaints range from eye pain and skin irritation to cough, and shortness of breath. One patient en route to the hospital via EMS reports severe dyspnea and chest tightness.

### 2. TEACHING OBJECTIVES

- Demonstrate understanding of prehospital preparation and management in the setting of a potential mass casualty event
- Differentiate between pepper spray, tear gas, and their physiological effects
- Describe the initial setup and process for a decontamination station
- Summarize the proper environment, PPE, and technique for RCA decontamination

- Triage and identify patients with severe symptoms and potential critical illness.
- Recognize and resuscitate the critically ill patient affected by RCA and the need for a secure airway
- Execute appropriate treatment of both minor and major symptoms of RCA exposure
- Obtain dermatological/ophthalmological consultation for complicated cases
- Determine the appropriate disposition plan for each patient

## 3. SUPPLIES

- Whiteboard or paper to draw diagram of outdoor "decontamination stations"
- Sealable bag for clothing
- Intravenous crystalloid
- Morgan lens for eye irrigation
- Normal saline for eye irrigation
- Eye wash station
- Oxygen source, nasal cannula
- Supplies for noninvasive airway: nasal trumpet, NRB face mask
- Supplies for intubation: laryngoscope handle, Macintosh/Miller blade, ET tube, stylet, BVM, suction, and $CO_2$ detector
- Syringes with medication
- Eye drops (to simulate tetracaine)

## 4. MOULAGE

- Eye reddening drops if available
- Red face makeup

## 5. IMAGES AND LABS

- Vitals: temperature, BP, HR, RR, $O_2$
- Chest X-ray showing pulmonary edema
- Labs: VBG/ABG for the patient in respiratory distress

## 6. ACTORS

- Crowd: in the waiting room complaining of eye pain
- Patient A: medium-acuity pepper spray exposure
- Patient B: low-acuity tear gas exposure
- Patient C: high-acuity exposure in respiratory distress
- EMS: presenting a case of patient with severe respiratory decompensation
- ED tech/nurse: assistance with decontamination, and management
- Security: securing area, assisting with outdoor decontamination

## 7. CRITICAL ACTIONS

- Prehospital planning and role assignment
- Setting up
- Allocating beds for sick patients

- Manage patient with low oxygen saturation
- Obtaining VBG/ABG
- Securing airway in compromised patient
- Obtaining dermatological/ophthalmological consult for complicated cases

## 8. TIMELINE

### Time: Zero

EMS radio report describes multiple casualties at large protest following the use of unspecified riot control agents by both police and protesters. Report they are in the process of extricating a patient in respiratory distress and that there are multiple patients en route. EMS states they will call back with further details.

### Time: Five Minutes – Provider Actions

- Notifies the hospital emergency manager that they may expect a large influx of patients.
- Assigns roles to the staff who are available.
- Notifies security and request assistance with setting up and securing the outdoor decontamination area
- Outlines a plan for triage of EMS patients outside and plan for immediate decontamination
- Describes plan for decontamination and that all patients will need decontamination prior to entering the ED
- Instructs staff on appropriate PPE

### Time: Six Minutes – Transition Point 1

Patient A arrives as a walk-in and reports severe eye and skin pain. His behavior is hysterical and distracting.

- Vital signs: 130/84 BP, 95 HR, 14 RR, sat 100%, T 98.5°F
  - A 23-year-old male with no significant past medical history. He reports that he was a protester and that the police doused him with pepper spray approximately 20 minutes prior to his arrival. He states he was with friends who are also en route to the hospital in a private vehicle with the same exposure. He denies any shortness of breath, chest pain, coughing, or throat swelling.
  - Physical exam: Patient is behaviorally agitated but in no respiratory distress. He has obvious contamination on his face and his shirt. There is no active airway or breathing concern. Airway is patent. Breath sounds are clear to auscultation bilaterally. Circulation is intact. Conjunctiva are severely erythematous. He has a large amount of tearing. The skin on his face is also erythematous and irritated.

### Time: 10 Minutes – Provider Actions

- Conducts a brief HPI and physical examination covering the ABCs
- Sends patient outside for decontamination
- Updates staff to expect more patients
- Verbalizes that this is a possible mass casualty incident (MCI) but do not yet activate an MCI plan

### Time: 12 Minutes

The triage nurse reports that four more patients have checked in with similar though mild-appearing symptoms.

### Time: 13 Minutes – Transition Point 2

Patient B arrives via ambulance. She states that she was exposed to an unknown gas by a counter-protestor. The patient is not able to give further detail regarding the type of chemical. If asked, the paramedics report they believe she was exposed to tear gas. They also report that this patient came from a separate group of people many of whom were also exposed to the gas and may seek treatment. Her vital signs are stable.

- Vital signs: 112/74 BP, 78 HR, 14 RR, sat 99%, T 98.8°F
  - A 30-year-old female with a history of seasonal allergies. She states that she was exposed to an unknown gas by a counterprotestor. The patient is not able to give further detail regarding the type of chemical. If asked, the paramedics report they believe she was exposed to tear gas. They also report that this patient came from a separate group of people, many of whom were also exposed to the gas and may seek treatment.
  - Physical exam: Patient is crying quietly but in no respiratory distress. She also has evidence of contamination on her hair and clothing. There is no active airway or breathing concern. Airway is patent. Breath sounds are clear to auscultation bilaterally. Circulation is intact. Conjunctiva are severely erythematous. She has a large amount of tearing. The skin on her face is also erythematous and irritated.

### Time: 15 Minutes – Provider Actions

- Conducts a brief HPI and physical examination covering the ABCs
- Sends patient outside for decontamination
- Considers activation of the MCI procedure with emergency manager

### Time: 20 Minutes

Patient A returns from decontamination and is agitated and disruptive.

### Time: 21 Minutes – Provider Actions

- Reexamine the patient. Check ABCs. Confirm that decontamination is complete
- Recommend thorough eye irrigation – Morgan lens or eye station
- Consider tetracaine for pain relief
- Counsel the patient on the treatment plan
- Ask for visual acuity testing following eye irrigation

### Time: 26 Minutes – Transition Point 3

EMS calls back. They have an ETA of three minutes with a patient in acute respiratory distress following exposure to one of these agents. They report they believe the patient was exposed to an extensive amount of tear gas about 15 minutes ago.

### Time: 27 Minutes – Provider Actions

- Prepares for a critically ill patient by assigning roles
- Prepares materials for possible airway intervention and oxygen supplementation given report of respiratory distress
- Simultaneously addresses the needs of Patient A who remains agitated and disruptive

### Time: 29 Minutes – Transition Point 4 – Patient C Arrives

- Vital signs: 187/99 BP, 117 HR, 28 RR, sat 92% on NRB, T 97.9°F
    - A 42-year-old obese male with a history of asthma. He is acutely short of breath and is only able to speak one word at a time. EMS reports that he was cornered by counter protestors in a bus stop and was exposed to a large amount of tear gas. Upon EMS arrival the patient was hypoxic to 90%. They placed him on an NRB mask and his saturation is now 92%.
    - Physical exam: Patient is in respiratory distress. Airway appears to be patent as patient is able to say single words and his voice is unchanged. On auscultation he is wheezing and there are crackles in the bases of his lungs bilaterally. He is tachycardic and hypertensive. There is no evidence of trauma. Similar to the other patients, his conjunctiva are severely erythematous. He is tearing and the skin on his face, neck, and arms is erythematous and irritated.

### Time: 35 Minutes – Provider Actions

- Conducts a brief HPI and thorough physical examination focusing first on the ABCs
- Elects not to send patient outside for decontamination given breathing compromise and instructs a support staff person to expose the patient and attempt dry decontamination
- Orders albuterol nebulizer treatment and discusses possible need for airway intervention – can start with BiPAP
- Orders portable chest X-ray, blood gas (optional)

### Time: 40 Minutes – Transition Point 5 and Conclusion

CXR returns and shows pulmonary edema. Patient C exhibits signs of worsening respiratory distress. Meanwhile, Patient A has completed eye irrigation and has improved. Patient B has returned from decontamination and wants to see the doctor.

### Time: 41 Minutes – Provider Actions

- Conducts rapid sequence intubation on Patient C
- Admits Patient C to the ICU
- Recommends discharge for Patient A
- Reexamines Patient B. She has evidence of a corneal ulcer and will need close ophthalmology follow-up

## 9. STIMULI

- Chest X-ray with pulmonary edema
- Venous blood gas
- Consider photos of patient appearance if adequate moulage is unavailable

## BIBLIOGRAPHY


Agrawal Y, Thornton D, Phipps A. CS gas: completely safe? A burn case report and literature review. *Burns.* 2009;35(6):895–897.

Barry JD, Hennessy R, McManus JG. Jr. A randomized controlled trial comparing treatment regimens for acute pain for topical oleoresin capsaicin (pepper spray) exposure in adult volunteers. *Prehosp Emerg Care.* 2008;12(4):432–437.

Bessac BF, Sivula M, von Hehn CA, et al. Transient receptor potential ankyrin 1 antagonists block the noxious effects of toxic industrial isocyanates and tear gases. *FASEB J.* 2009;23(4):1102–1114.

Gerber S, Frueh BE, Tappeiner C. Conjunctival proliferation after a mild pepper spray injury in a young child. *Cornea.* 2011;30(9):1042–1044.

Haar RJ, Iacopino V, Ranadive N, Weiser SD, Dandu M. Health impacts of chemical irritants used for crowd control: a systematic review of the injuries and deaths caused by tear gas and pepper spray. *BMC Public Health.* 2017;17(1):831.

Horton DK, Burgess P, Rossiter S, Kaye WE. Secondary contamination of emergency department personnel from O-chlorobenzylidene malononitrile exposure, 2002. *Ann Emerg Med.* 2005;45(6):655–658.

Olajos EJ, Salem H. Riot control agents: pharmacology, toxicology, biochemistry and chemistry. *J Appl Toxicol.* 2001;21(5):355–391.

Rothenberg C, Achanta S, Svendsen ER, Jordt S-E. Tear gas: an epidemiological and mechanistic reassessment. *Ann N Y Acad Sci.* 2016;1378(1):96–107.

Toprak S, Ersoy G, Hart J, Clevestig P. The pathology of lethal exposure to the riot control agents: towards a forensics-based methodology for determining misuse. *J Forensic Leg Med.* 2015;29(January):36–42.

Vaca FE, Myers JH, Langdorf M. Delayed pulmonary edema and bronchospasm after accidental lacrimator exposure. *Am J Emerg Med.* 1996;14(4):402–405.

CASE 32

# Emergency Management of Blast Trauma from Refinery Explosion

Meghan Maslanka

DISASTER PRINCIPLES

- Clinical diagnosis and treatment
- Timing of medical and surgical interventions
- Recognition and clinical treatment
- Information management/communications
- Decontamination
- Conventional standards of care
- Scene safety and security in the field
- Fireground safety
- Blast injuries

## 1. SCENARIO OVERVIEW

A 42-year-old male with no significant PMHx presents to a large academic ED with hearing loss, shortness of breath, abdominal pain, and burns after an explosion at an oil refinery. He arrived by EMS who reports that no other victims were injured in the incident. The patient is alert but is unable to hear questions/instructions, which makes the history and physical difficult. The patient has multiple injuries from the blast including bilateral perforated tympanic membranes, basilar skull fracture, subdural hematoma, right-sided pneumothorax, bowel perforation, liver laceration, left wrist fracture, right ankle fracture with neurovascular compromise, and superficial flash burns. The patient is stable on arrival and requires decontamination. On initial exam, the patient's right ankle is pulseless due to a fracture and requires emergent reduction. Shortly after, the patient's respiratory status declines due to a developing tension pneumothorax and necessitates a chest tube placement. CT imaging obtained after stabilization reveals additional injuries that require consult to specialty services.

## 2. TEACHING OBJECTIVES AND DISCUSSION POINTS

### Clinical and Medical Management

- Perform patient decontamination
- Assess for primary, secondary, tertiary, and quaternary blast injuries
- Emergently reduce a fracture resulting in neurovascular compromise
- Perform chest tube insertion to manage a tension pneumothorax

### Communication and Teamwork

- Coordinate with EMS to identify HAZMAT concerns prior to patient arrival

## 3. SUPPLIES

- Radios
- Decontamination room/area and supplies
- Chest tube kit and chest tube
- Chest tube insertion trainer
- Syringes with medications
- SAM splint ×2
- Coban
- ACE bandage
- Silk tape

## 4. MOULAGE

- Superficial burns to exposed skin (face and arms)
- Occipital hematoma
- Left wrist deformity
- Right ankle deformity

## 5. IMAGES AND LABS

- X-ray chest (before chest tube): moderate right pneumothorax
- X-ray chest (after chest tube): successful chest tube placement with interval improvement in pneumothorax
- X-ray left wrist: distal radius fracture.
- X-ray right ankle: distal tib/fib fracture with significant displacement.

## 6. ACTORS (CONFEDERATES) AND THEIR ROLES

- Patient: actor or mannequin

## 7. CRITICAL ACTIONS

- Assess for HAZMAT risks
- Decontaminate patient
- Perform emergent ankle reduction
- Insert chest tube for tension pneumothorax
- Obtain appropriate imaging to assess for injuries from blast

## 8. TIMELINE WITH TRANSITION PPOINTS

### Time: Zero

- Report given via radio: EMS is en route with a 42-year-old male with no PMHx who presents with hearing loss, chest pain, forearm fracture, tib/fib fracture, head injury, and facial burns after an explosion at the oil refinery where he works. Vitals are BP 110/70, HR 85, RR 18, $O_2$ sat 98%, 98°F. ETA two minutes.

- Team should ask additional questions to gather additional information about the patient and scene.
  - Additional injured or ill patients (none)
  - Information about substance exposure (occurred at oil refinery)
  - Signs of illness concerning for chemical exposure (no obvious signs at this time)
  - Decontamination completed prior to transport (none)
- Team should plan to decontaminate the patient on arrival.

### Time: Two Minutes – Transition Point 1

VS: BP 110/70, HR 85, RR 18, $O_2$ sat 98%, 98°F

- Summary of initial presentation: A 42-year-old male with no significant PMHx arrives by EMS with multiple complaints after an explosion at work. He is unable to hear after the incident but is able to respond to written questions. He is shouting very loudly, "I can't hear you but everything hurts, especially my leg." The patient is wearing a work T-shirt and pants. He has areas of dark substance on his hands, arms, neck, back, and in his hair.
- Initial intervention
  - Remove the patient's clothing and perform decontamination. The students can verbalize that they would decontaminate the patient.
  - Consider other possible chemical/toxic exposures.

### Time: Seven Minutes – Transition Point 2

VS: BP 110/70, HR 95, RR 20, $O_2$ sat 97% (slightly less stable)

- Physical exam
  - General: shouting due to hearing loss
  - Skin: superficial burns to exposed skin (face and hands). No intraoral burns.
  - HEENT: occipital hematoma. Bilateral perforated tympanic membranes.
  - Neck: trachea midline. No JVD. No injuries. No tenderness.
  - Chest: decreased right lung sounds
  - Heart: sinus tachycardia
  - Abdomen: diffuse tenderness with guarding
  - FAST exam with trace free fluid in the RUQ and diminished lung sliding on the right. No other abnormalities.
  - Musculoskeletal
    - LUE: deformity of the wrist. Hand neurovascularly intact.
    - RLE: deformity of the ankle. No pulse. Unable to wiggle toes. No sensation.
  - Neuro: Glasgow Coma Scale 4E 4V 6M. Alert. Loss of motor and sensation in right foot. Moving all other extremities.
- Team should recognize the need to emergently reduce the right ankle due to neurovascular compromise.

### Time: 10 Minutes – Transition Point 2

VS: BP 90/55, HR 120, RR 32, $O_2$ sat 90%

- Physical exam: The patient becomes more tachypneic and says, "It's getting hard to breathe." Right-sided breath sounds are absent. JVD and mild tracheal deviation are present.

- Team should ensure no intraoral burns if this has not already been assessed.
- Team should assess for signs of chemical exposure (none present).
- Team should recognize tension pneumothorax and insert a chest tube.
- A chest X-ray should be obtained to confirm placement.

### Transition Point 3: Final Actions

VS: BP 110/75, HR 80, RR 16, $O_2$ sat 99%

- Physical exam: The patient's respiratory status improves after chest tube placement.
- Team should obtain advanced imaging upon stabilization to further evaluate injuries from the blast.
  - CT head: basilar skull fracture and small subdural hematoma without midline shift
  - CT max/face: no acute findings
  - CT cervical spine: no acute findings
  - CT chest: s/p right chest tube placement with interval improvement in pneumothorax. Small bilateral pulmonary contusions.
  - CT abdomen/pelvis: small amount of free air and colonic contusion. Grade 2 liver laceration.
  - CTA right lower extremity: distal tib/fib fracture without vascular disruption
  - X-ray left wrist: distal radius fracture
  - X-ray right ankle: distal tib/fib fracture with significant displacement
- Team should initiate treatment based on results.
  - Antibiotics for suspected tympanic perforation
  - Update tetanus vaccine
  - Bacitracin for burns
  - Consult trauma/general surgery
  - Consult neurosurgery
  - Consult orthopedic surgery

## 9. STIMULI

- Imaging optional to use as stimuli

## BIBLIOGRAPHY

American College of Emergency Physicians. Bombings: Injury patterns and care. 2022. www.acep.org/imports/clinical-and-practice-management/resources/ems-and-disaster-preparedness/disaster-preparedness-grant-projects/bombings-injury-patterns-and-care/. Accessed July 26, 2022.

Nawrocki P, Jasani G. Emergency preparedness and disaster response. In: Swadron S, Nordt SP, Mattu A, Johnson W, eds. *CorePendium*. Burbank, CA: CorePendium, LLC; updated August 26, 2024. https://www.emrap.org/corependium/chapter/recgpYnQ06urUjv7Q/Emergency-Preparedness-and-Disaster-Response#h.sz1l4cgbjvrj. Accessed March 31, 2025.

SECTION 8

# TERRORISM-RELATED DISASTERS

CASE 33

# Navigating Care after Detonation of a Radioactive Incendiary Device

Sukhshant Atti, Ritu Sarin, and Ziad Kazzi

DISASTER PRINCIPLES

- Local disaster response
- Clinical diagnosis and treatment
- Conventional standards of care
- Timing of medical and surgical interventions
- Scene safety and security in the field
- Hospital preparedness
- EMS disaster operations
- Decontamination
- Radiation/nuclear events
- Acute radiation syndrome
- Timing of medical and surgical interventions
- Contamination and irradiation
- Medical countermeasures for radiation contamination
- MCI triage and considerations for radioactive/nuclear events
- Blast injuries

## 1. SCENARIO OVERVIEW

A 23-year-old male with no significant past medical history arrives at the ED as a casualty after being in the vicinity of an explosion at a marathon. There is word from EMS that the explosion involved a radioactive detonation device, a device designed to spread radioactive material for the purpose of harming others. On arrival, the patient is vomiting and complaining of "ringing" in his ears and appears to be in respiratory distress. The patient has wounds on his legs that appear to be contaminated with shrapnel from the explosion.

## 2. TEACHING OBJECTIVES AND DISCUSSION POINTS

- Isolation and decontamination of a patient with external radiation contamination
- Recognition of blast injury and appropriate evaluation and management
- Recognition of a contaminated patient with radioactive material
- Recognition of need for appropriate PPE for health personnel
- Recognition of need for decontamination
- Recognition of need for an antidote for radiation exposure

## 3. SUPPLIES

- Level C PPE includes an air purifying respirator or a high-efficiency particulate air (HEPA) filter. An N95 mask or a surgical mask are acceptable if a respirator is not available.
- Geiger counter and personal dosimeter
- Needle decompression and tube thoracostomy kits
- Sealable bag for PPE after doffing
- Water for decontamination
- Forceps to remove radioactive shrapnel
- Sealed box to store radioactive shrapnel

## 4. MOULAGE

- Wounds to legs with embedded shrapnel, superficial abrasions on arms and legs

## 5. IMAGES AND LABS

- Images: CT images of head, cervical spine, chest, abdomen, and pelvis
- Labs: CBC, chemistry

## 6. ACTORS (CONFEDERATES) AND THEIR ROLES

- Resident physician (main physician)
- Nurse (help with obtaining IV lines, place on monitor, decontamination)
- Radiation officer (to provide Geiger counter)
- Medical toxicologist (actor to answer poison center phone call)

## 7. CRITICAL ACTIONS

- Emergency needle decompression and chest thoracostomy for right-sided pneumothorax from primary blast injury prior to decontamination of the patient
- Donning and doffing of personal protective equipment with proper technique. Donning of PPE is before evaluation of the patient, no matter how critically ill they appear.
- Contact radiation safety officer to obtain a radiation survey device such as a Geiger Muller counter for patient radiation contamination detection and for a personal dosimeter.
- Decontamination of the patient until radiation is less than or equal to two times background radiation.
- Discussion of patient with the poison center medical toxicologist for need for medical countermeasures/antidotes.
- Recognize need to complete blast evaluation of patient.
- Admit patient for further observation given blast injuries and radiation exposure.

## 8. TIMELINE

### Time: Zero

Summary of initial presentation: A 23-year-old male who is brought in by EMS from the scene of an explosion at a marathon. He was in the vicinity of an explosion that is believed to be a "dirty bomb," or a radiation dispersal device, causing an explosion that spread radioactive material. On exam, the patient appears to be in respiratory distress. He was within 15 feet of the explosion in an open space. He is now presenting with complaints of headache, tinnitus in both ears, loss of hearing, vomiting, shortness of breath and burns and wounds to his legs. He was brought to the ED by EMS personnel.

**Initial Evaluation and Interventions**

1. Isolate patient in decontamination room
2. Obtain Level C PPE for all healthcare personnel involved in patient's care. Level C PPE includes an air purifying respirator or a HEPA filter.
3. Emergency medicine resident dons Level C PPE. Donning procedure as follows:
   a. Perform hand hygiene.
   b. Put on shoe covers.
   c. Put on a gown.
   d. Put on respirator (either powered air-purifying respirator or N95).
   e. Put on eye protection.
   f. Put on gloves.
4. Treat life-threatening injuries prior to decontamination.
5. Contact radiation safety officer to obtain a radiation survey device such as a Geiger Muller counter for patient radiation contamination detection and for a personal dosimeter.
6. Disrobe the patient completely including undergarments (removes 90% of contamination) and put patient's garments into a double bag and seal.
7. Place patient into a gown and cover patient with a sheet
8. Obtain 18 G IV placement in bilateral arms
9. Administer ondansetron, 4 mg IV for vomiting and 100 mcg of fentanyl for pain.
10. Give patient a normal saline bolus

Vital signs: BP: 98/72 HR 130 bpm sinus tachycardia, RR is 16, O2 sat 80% on RA, temperature 98.4°F

1. Primary survey
   a. Airway: Patient is speaking in short sentences, breathing fast, and gasping for air.
   b. Breathing: Patient is in moderate respiratory distress and decreased breath sounds are heard on the right. Normal breath sounds on the left. Mild tracheal deviation to the left.
   c. Circulation: Patient has normal capillary refill in extremities, which are cool to touch. Distended neck veins.
2. Assess need for lifesaving interventions.
3. Perform lifesaving interventions (in the case of radiologic material contamination, lifesaving interventions should be performed prior to complete decontamination as the risk to healthcare personnel from exposure to radioactive contamination is much less likely to be life threatening than in other types of contamination events).
   a. Place patient on an NRB mask
   b. Perform needle decompression (audible air after insertion of the needle) followed by tube thoracostomy
   c. Two large-bore peripheral IV lines obtained
   d. Resident also prepares for emergent intubation (in case this is needed)

On reassessment after needle decompression and thoracostomy, the patient's vitals have improved: BP 122/83, HR 110 bpm, RR 14, temperature 37.9°C, sat 98%.

Physical exam

- General: agitated, anxious, and vomiting on exam. Holding his bilateral ears with his hands. Appears to be breathing fast.

- Skin: mild diaphoresis, no cyanosis, no pallor, small areas of superficial abrasions on bilateral arms and legs
- HEENT: Pupils 3 mm, equal and reactive briskly to light, bilateral tympanic membrane rupture, trachea midline, no stridor
- Neck: supple, C-collar in place (placed by EMS), no midline cervical spine tenderness
- Heart: regular rate and rhythm, normal heart sounds, no murmurs
- Lungs: clear lung sounds bilaterally, tube thoracostomy in right chest wall
- Abdomen: soft, nondistended, nontender
- Neuro: Repeated attempts are necessary to get patient to follow commands secondary to loss of hearing, but is A&O ×4 and has normal strength and sensation in all extremities
- MSK: bilateral lower legs with 2.25% BSA burns overlying each anterior aspect. Both lower extremities with one superficial open wound on each side, measuring 4 cm × 2 cm on the right leg and 3 cm × 2 cm on the left leg. There is embedded shrapnel in bilateral anterior lower extremities.
- Back: no midline thoracic or lumbar spine tenderness

## Time: Five Minutes – Transition Point 1

BP: 125/70 HR 105 bpm sinus tachycardia, RR 16, O2 sat 99% on RA, temperature 98.0°F

- Perform radiation survey from head to toe using an appropriate survey instrument with a probe for beta/gamma radiation such as a Geiger-Muller counter.
- The probe should be held ½ inch to 1 inch from the body and move at 1 inch/second.

**Priorities of Radiation Survey**

- First survey open wounds on the patient (bilateral lower extremities in this case)
- Then survey the head, face, nose, mouth, neck and intact skin
- Any areas that give readings of greater than two times the background radiation should be outlined with a permanent marker and covered with clean gauze pads (for later decontamination)

## Time: 10 Minutes – Transition Point 2

- Start dry decontamination; for simplicity, in this exercise only the wounds with embedded areas of shrapnel on the legs will require decontamination (i.e. no need for washing of hair, total body wet decontamination).
- Employ shielding of skin wounds with embedded radioactive shrapnel to create some shielding for healthcare workers.
- Start dry decontamination by removing visible pieces of radioactive contaminant materials by using masking tape. Can also use a brush to remove debris contamination to remove shrapnel materials.
- Reperform radiological survey after each dry decontamination to ensure radiation is falling below or equal to two times normal of background radiation levels.
- Areas that do not achieve the target of equal to or less than two times normal of background radiation levels upon initial dry decontamination efforts × 2 will require "survey-wash-rinse" cycles. This is further decontamination using focal spot decontamination by irrigating with copious saline or water, at low pressure, along with one of the following methods:
    - Clean with liquid soap and then use copious water or saline to rinse
    - Wipe down with a soapy wet cloth

  - Spray with soapy water and wipe thereafter
  - Use wet wipes
- After each wash and rinse cycle, survey with a radiation detector to ensure that the target of equal to or less than two times normal of background radiation levels is achieved. Swab applicators can also be applied to wounds after decontamination and then surveyed to detect for contamination.
- Ensure that the emergency medicine resident does not repeat this survey-wash-rinse cycle more than three times to prevent too vigorous attempts at decontamination that may push the contamination material further into tissue to create internal decontamination.

Once the survey-wash-rinse cycles have obtained a target of equal to or less than two times normal of background radiation levels using dry and spot decontamination, it's time to move on and manage blast injury aspects of the patient's presentation.

**Critical Actions**

- Timely and appropriate management of open wounds with radioactive material is critical to prevent significant absorption and systemic toxicity.

### Time: 20 Minutes – Transition Point 3

BP: 125/80 HR 100 bpm sinus tachycardia, RR 16, O2 sat 99% on RA, temperature 98.1°F

- The emergency medicine resident should recognize that the patient has signs of primary blast injury that need to be evaluated further.
- The patient needs to undergo trauma scans next to assess for other signs of barotrauma including intracranial, pulmonary, and hollow viscous injury with CT imaging.
- The patient's vomiting is a possible sign of acute radiation sickness and blood work, including CBC, CMP should be obtained.
- Now that the patient is decontaminated, the emergency medicine resident should remove their PPE
  - Doff PPE into a bag to be double sealed
    a. Remove shoe covers
    b. Remove gown and gloves together
    c. Perform hand hygiene
    d. Remove eye protection
    e. Remove respirator
    f. Perform hand hygiene
  - Order CT imaging of the head, cervical spine, chest, abdomen/pelvis, thoracic and lumbar spines
  - Obtain CBC and CMP lab tests
  - Patient is rolled away to CT imaging
  - Patient is brought back from CT imaging
  - Repeat physical examination; remains unchanged
  - Lab results are within normal limits
    a. CBC: WBC 6.6, Hb 14.0, hematocrit 42, platelets 270
    b. CMP: $Na^+$ 136, $K^+$ 4.0, $Cl^-$99, $HCO3^-$ 24, BUN 12, Cr 0.9
  - CT imaging results with no signs of intracranial, pulmonary injury or hollow viscous injury

### Time: 40 Minutes – Transition Point 4

BP: 120/80 HR 95 bpm sinus rhythm, RR 16, O2 sat 99% on RA, temperature 98.1°F

There is word now that the patient may have been contaminated by cesium from this radiation dispersal device based on police and radiation officer investigation on the ground. This information has been relayed to the emergency department.

The resident physician should recognize that the local poison center needs to be contacted to speak to a medical toxicologist to discuss further management of Cesium radiation exposure. Poison center is called using the number: 800-222-1222 and the case is discussed with an on-call toxicologist who recommends that in the case of cesium poisoning that an antidote be administered. Resident physician should clarify dose and total daily dose of 9 g divided into 3 g, three times per day. The resident physician will also be informed by the toxicologist that Prussian Blue is part of the US Strategic National Stockpile and is accessed by contacting the Centers for Disease Control and Prevention emergency response hotline: 770-488-7100.

Patient will need admission for observation for delayed presentations of blast injury (i.e. pulmonary contusions) and for ongoing repeat lab work for assessment of acute radiation sickness and for signs of internal radiation contamination. Patient will also need wound care.

- Reassess the patient and look for any signs of changes in his mental status or physical examination, including vitals. Patient will remain stable for the purpose of this exercise.
- Admit patient to a monitored floor for ongoing assessments to evaluate for delayed pulmonary effects of blast injury
- Patient will require 24-hour stool and 24-hour urine collection for assessment of internal contamination
- Patient will require serial blood work to look for signs of acute radiation sickness

### Time: 45 Minutes – Transition Point 5

The resident physician and healthcare workers who helped manage this patient should also undergo a radiation survey now with a Geiger counter to ensure there has not been any contamination with ionizing radiation.

### Case Ends

#### Notes

Blast injury considerations from detonation of a radiation dispersal device is of primary concern when managing a patient with such exposure. The explosion of a bomb or detonation device generates a blast wave that spreads out from a point source. The blast wave consists of two parts including a shock wave of high pressure, followed closely by a blast wind, or air in motion. Types of blast injury include primary, secondary, tertiary and quaternary blast injury. The patient in this case initially had many signs of primary blast injury: vomiting, bilateral hearing loss and tinnitus from bilateral tympanic membrane rupture, a tension pneumothorax. Time, distance and shielding are the best methods for reducing radiation exposure from a source external to the body to levels that are as low as reasonably achievable (ALARA). For example, radiation exposure rates decrease greatly (by the square of the distance) as you increase the distance from the source, in addition to shielding. Typically, the amount of radiation released from a radioactive detonation device is not significant enough to cause acute radiation syndrome, but patients should be monitored for effects of radiation.

Attention should be paid to life-threatening injury in patients needing resuscitation and lifesaving procedures should be performed in the "hot zone" prior to decontamination. Concomitant physical trauma such as thermal burns or wounds may produce a synergistic effect with harmful doses of radiation. These physical injuries can lead to prolonged recovery time and increased morbidity and mortality.

## BIBLIOGRAPHY


Ashkenazi I, Olsha O, Turegano-Fuentes F, Alfici R. Tympanic membrane perforation impact on severity of injury and resource use in victims of explosion. *Eur J Trauma Emerg Surg.* 2017;43(5):623–626.

Bushberg JT, Kroger LA, Hartman MB, et al. Nuclear/radiological terrorism: emergency department management of radiation casualties. *J Emerg Med.* 2007;32(1):71–85.

Center for Radiological Nuclear Training (CTOS). www.ctosnnsa.org/. Accessed April 5, 2025.

Centers for Disease Control and Prevention. *Explosions and Blast Injuries: A Primer for Clinicians.* https://stacks.cdc.gov/view/cdc/28987/cdc_28987_DS1.pdf. Accessed April 5, 2025.

Centers for Disease Control and Prevention. Radiological Terrorism: Emergency Services Clinicians Toolkit. www.cdc.gov/radiation-emergencies/hcp/radiological-terrorism-toolkit/. Accessed April 5, 2025.

DePalma RG, Burris DG, Champion HR, Hodgson MJ. Blast injuries. *New Engl J Med.* 2005;352(13):1335–1342.

Oak Ridge Institute for Science and Education. Radiation Emergency Assistance Center/Training Site. https://orise.orau.gov/reacts/. Accessed April 5, 2025.

Radiation Emergency Medical Management. Guidance on diagnosis and treatment for healthcare providers. https://remm.hhs.gov/index.html. Accessed April 5, 2025.

Smith JM, Ansari A, Harper FT. Hospital management of mass radiological casualties: reassessing exposures from contaminated victims of an exploded radiological dispersal device. *Health Phys.* 2005 Nov;89(5):513–520.

Wolf SJ, Bebarta VS, Bonnett CJ, Pons PT, Cantrill SV. Blast injuries. *Lancet.* 2009 Aug 1;374(9687):405–415.

CASE 34

# Chaos at the Country Fair

## Organophosphate Poisoning from Airborne Chemicals

Meghan Maslanka

DISASTER PRINCIPLES

- Clinical diagnosis and treatment
- Timing of medical and surgical interventions
- Strategic national stockpile
- Emergency operations plans for the healthcare environment
- Medical surge capability
- Mass-casualty incidents
- Field operations and logistics
- Mass-casualty care in the field
- Field disaster triage
- Field stabilization, treatment, and transport
- Disaster operations
- Decontamination in the field
- Scene safety and security in the field
- Chemical agents
- Recognition and clinical treatment
- MCI triage and considerations for chemical agents
- Pediatrics and chemical exposure
- Chemical safety
- Decontamination
- Nerve agents

## 1. SCENARIO OVERVIEW

A community ED receives a notification from EMS that they are en route with a patient who became ill at a country fair after someone sprayed an unknown substance into a crowd. Multiple patients are ill with symptoms of organophosphate poisoning on scene. The patient requires decontamination on arrival and pralidoxime and atropine to treat his organophosphate toxidrome.

## 2. TEACHING OBJECTIVES AND DISCUSSION POINTS

**Clinical and Medical Management**

- Perform patient decontamination
- Discussion of whether any treatment can or should be performed prior to decontamination – specifically, could a very sick patient with presumed organophosphate poisoning get a dose of antidote prior to decon as a lifesaving intervention if the provider was trained and in PPE
- Recognize organophosphate poisoning
- Treat organophosphate poisoning with pralidoxime and atropine

**Communication and Teamwork**

- Coordinate with EMS to identify HAZMAT concerns prior to patient arrival

## 3. SUPPLIES

- Radios
- Decontamination room/area and supplies
- Syringes with medications

## 4. MOULAGE

- Spray bottle (for diaphoresis, lacrimation, nasal secretions)
- Respiratory secretions (frothy)
- Emesis bag in hand
- Vomit on shirt

## 5. IMAGES AND LABS

- ECG: sinus bradycardia
- CXR: pulmonary edema

## 6. ACTORS (CONFEDERATES) AND THEIR ROLES

- Patient: actor or mannequin

## 7. CRITICAL ACTIONS

- Assess HAZMAT risks
- Decontaminate patient
- Provide airway support (oxygen, suctioning)
- Recognize organophosphate poisoning
- Treat toxidrome with pralidoxime and atropine
- Plan for possible atropine shortage
- Toxicology or poison control consult

## 8. TIMELINE WITH TRANSITION POINTS

### Time: Zero

- Report given via radio: EMS is en route with a 31-year-old male with no PMH who presents with trouble breathing and vomiting that started shortly after being sprayed with an unknown substance at a fair. Multiple other patients on scene were sprayed with the same substance and have similar symptoms. Vitals are BP 110/70, HR 55, RR 24, $O_2$ sat 93% RA, 98°F. ETA two minutes.

- Team should ask additional questions to gather additional information about the patient and scene.
  - Additional ill patients on scene (10)
  - Additional ill patients en route to this hospital (two)
  - Information about substance exposure (occurred when an individual sprayed a liquid substance onto a crowd at a fair)
  - Decontamination completed prior to transport (clothing removed, bottles of water used to wash hands and face)
  - Medications given en route (none)
- The team should plan to decontaminate the patient on arrival.
- The team should prepare for additional patients.
- The team should discuss the differential of possible HAZMAT exposures.

### Time: Two Minutes – Transition Point 1

VS: BP 105/65, HR 50, RR 26, $O_2$ sat 93% RA, 98°F

Summary of initial presentation: A 31-year-old male with no significant PMH arrives by EMS with trouble breathing and vomiting after he was one of multiple individuals sprayed with an unknown substance at a fair. His exam is notable for diaphoresis, tearing, rhinorrhea, frothy oral secretions, wheezing, and bouts of active vomiting and diarrhea.

- Initial intervention
  - Remove the patient's clothing and send him through decontamination.
  - Assess EMS personnel's exposure to the substance (PPE was worn, medics are asymptomatic).

### Time: Seven Minutes – Transition Point 2

VS: BP 90/60, HR 40, RR 30, $O_2$ sat 89% RA

- Physical exam
  - General: alert but disoriented. Intermittently vomiting, but maintaining airway.
  - Skin: diaphoretic. No rash.
  - HEENT: pupils miotic. Copious lacrimal and nasal secretions. Moderate frothy sputum.
  - Neck: trachea midline. No JVD. No injuries. No tenderness.
  - Chest: diffuse bilateral wheezing and rales
  - Heart: sinus bradycardia
  - Abdomen: no tenderness, guarding, or rebound
  - Musculoskeletal: no deformity or tenderness. No extremity edema.
  - Neuro: Glasgow Coma Scale 4E 4V 6M. Confused responses to questions. Follows commands. Moving all extremities equally.
- Team should recognize the cholinergic/organophosphate toxidrome.
- Place on oxygen
- Provide airway support (suctioning)
- Treat with pralidoxime
  - 30 mg/kg IV loading dose over 15–30 minutes, followed by 8 mg/kg/hr IV infusion.
  - Or 1–2 g IV infusion over 15–30 minutes, repeat in one hour, then Q12hr PRN.

- Treat with atropine
  - Atropine 1–2 mg IV. Double dose Q5 minutes until secretions are controlled, then start atropine drip.
- Discuss potential to run out of atropine in the hospital, especially if multiple patients arrive.
- The patient's vitals improve after three doses of atropine.

### Time: 12 Minutes – Transition Point 3

VS: BP 110/65, HR 70, RR 20, $O_2$ sat 97% on 15 L NRB

- Physical exam: The patient's vitals improve after pralidoxime and three doses of atropine. The patient's secretions are now controlled.
- Upon controlling secretions, start atropine drip at 10%–20% of the effective dose per hour.
- EMS reports that empty containers of Malathion were identified on scene.
- If the patient is not treated for a cholinergic/organophosphate toxidrome, he will go into a respiratory arrest.

### Transition Point 4: Final Actions

VS: BP 115/70, HR 75, RR 18, $O_2$ sat 99% on 15 L NRB

- Physical exam: Secretions from the eye, nose, and mouth have resolved. Diaphoresis improved. Respiratory rate and lung sounds improved. The patient's mental status is improving.
- Wean the oxygen.
- Consult poison control or toxicology, if this has not yet been done.
- Consult the medical ICU for admission.
- Prepare for additional patients.

## 9. STIMULI

- ECG: sinus bradycardia
- CXR: pulmonary edema

## BIBLIOGRAPHY

Cook M, Frey A. Pesticides and cholinergic toxicity and poisoning. In: Swadron S, Nordt SP, Mattu A, Johnson W, eds. *CorePendium*. Burbank, CA: CorePendium, LLC; updated September 14, 2020. https://www.emrap.org/corependium/chapter/recdvP3Xjhrp9vbC8/Pesticides-and-Cholinergic-Toxicity-and-Poisoning#h.12ve7wjzbu63. Accessed March 3, 2023.

CASE 35

# Postal Worker Presenting with Respiratory Failure after a Bioterrorism Attack

Michael De Luca

DISASTER PRINCIPLES

- Clinical diagnosis and treatment
- Timing of medical and surgical interventions
- Recognition and clinical treatment
- Decontamination
- National disaster management system
- Role of public health agencies in disaster medicine
- Public health surveillance
- Decontamination
- Biological disasters
- Category A bioterrorism agents
- Anthrax
- MCI triage and considerations for biological agents
- Biological safety
- Epidemiologic and medical countermeasures
- Personal protective equipment (PPE)

## 1. SCENARIO OVERVIEW

A 45-year-old male with a history of hypertension presents to the ED with shortness of breath and altered mental status. He is brought in by ambulance and accompanied by his wife, who reports he became ill with "the flu" four days ago and has not shown up to work (they both work in a mailroom at a government office) for the past two days. Today she found him asleep in bed at 4:00 PM and he would not wake up, so she called 911. He is unable to give any history due to his profound lethargy and dyspnea. He is critically ill appearing and requires immediate resuscitation and intubation. Chest X-ray demonstrates a widened mediastinum. The patient is suspected of having been a victim of a bioterrorism attack at work with inhalational anthrax and is treated with antibiotics, while providers contact infection control and hospital administration for further guidance.

## 2. TEACHING OBJECTIVES AND DISCUSSION POINTS

### Clinical Management

a. Recognition of presentation of a bioterrorism-associated illness based on history, exam, and diagnostic studies, including a chest X-ray with evidence of a widened mediastinum

b. Securing advanced airway and ensuring adequate resuscitation in critically ill patient
c. Appropriate antibiotic selection and diagnostic testing for suspected inhalational anthrax
d. Prescribing postexposure prophylactic medications
e. How important is decontamination in this situation? If there is suspicion of ongoing exposure, then may be necessary but the patient is not likely to be currently contaminated. His symptoms are caused by anthrax infection at this point, not the white powder that is likely no longer present as patient has not been at work for some time.

**Public Health Interventions**

a. Recognition of possible bioterror event
b. Notification of appropriate public health and law enforcement authorities (via hospital administration and infection control)

## 3. SUPPLIES

a. Stretcher
b. IV supplies and tubing
c. Syringes with medications
d. IV fluids
e. Noninvasive airway equipment (oxygen, oxygen tubing, NRB, oral-pharyngeal airway, nasopharyngeal airway, BVM, suction)
f. Invasive airway equipment (endotracheal tube, laryngoscope, lubricant, stylet, LMA)
g. Lumbar puncture kit
h. Thoracostomy tray
i. Telephone

## 4. MOULAGE

a. Mannequin with dried vomitus on clothes; clothing damp from diaphoresis

## 5. IMAGES AND LABS

a. Chest X-ray: widened mediastinum, bilateral pleural effusions
b. ECG: sinus tachycardia
c. Labs: BG, CBC, INR/PTT, CMP, ABG, lactate

## 6. ACTORS (CONFEDERATES) AND THEIR ROLES

a. Patient: mannequin
b. Wife: appropriately worried; relates the majority of the history to providers. She notes that patient has showered and changed clothes multiple times since he was last at work.
c. EMS: brings patient into ED and when asked by providers describes the critical state of the patient
d. Nurse: if asked, places patient on monitor, administers fluids and medications, retrieves equipment
e. Respiratory therapy: if called, assists in intubation if performed
f. Infection control/infectious disease: provides recommendations to team; liaises with local/state authorities
g. Administrator-on-call: informs providers of multiple cases reported throughout city; Convenes hospital incident command system, initiates biohazard response plan if contacted by providers; liaises with local/state authorities

h. ICU attending: listens to patient course in ED and accepts patient to ICU. Recommends multidisciplinary discussion with infection control and hospital administration.

## 7. CRITICAL ACTIONS

a. Refer to critical actions under timeline

## 8. TIMELINE WITH TRANSITION POINTS

### Time: Zero

a. Vital signs (per EMS): BP 70/40, HR 144, RR 30, $O_2$ sat 82% on NRB at 15 L/min, 38.8°C (temporal).
b. Summary of initial presentation: A 45-year-old male with a history of hypertension presents to the ED with shortness of breath and altered mental status. He is brought in by ambulance accompanied by his wife. He is unable to give any history given profound lethargy and dyspnea.
c. Physical exam
   i. General: ill appearing, diaphoretic, in respiratory distress, dry vomitus on clothing
   ii. HEENT: normocephalic atraumatic, PERRLA, dry mucous membranes
   iii. Neck: rigid
   iv. Pulmonary: tachypneic, decreased breath sounds at bilateral bases, diffuse rhonchi
   v. Cardiovascular: tachycardic, regular, no MRG
   vi. GI: soft, nontender, nondistended
   vii. Musculoskeletal: no obvious deformities
   viii. Skin: warm, wet, poorly perfused, mottled, capillary refill >3 seconds
   ix. Neuro: lethargic, opens eyes to deep painful stimuli only, does not follow commands, does not answer questions, withdraws all four extremities equally to painful stimuli
d. Initial interventions
   i. Providers don standard PPE
   ii. Place on monitor
   iii. Obtain labs through IV placed by EMS
   iv. Fluid-resuscitate
   v. Continue oxygenation with NRB while preparing for intubation
   vi. ECG presented to team
e. Wife: upset. Reports husband became ill with "the flu" four days ago and hasn't shown up to work (they both work in a mailroom at a government office) for the past two days. Today she found him asleep in bed at 4:00 PM and he would not wake up, so she called 911. She has felt fine.
f. EMS: reports vitals as indicated previously. Notes that patient is minimally responsive, required NRB for oxygenation. They were able to establish one peripheral IV and have given 500 cc of NS. Reports this is the second patient they have seen today who works in that mailroom.
g. Nurse: assist team when directed to give additional fluids, collect equipment for intubation. Places additional peripheral IV.

**Critical Actions**
- Adequate fluid resuscitation for presumed septic shock
- Recognition of need to secure patient's airway due to altered mental status and respiratory distress and preoxygenate patient in preparation of intubation
- Obtain labs, ECG, chest X-ray

- Obtaining history concerning for possible bioterrorism agent exposure (mailroom employee)
- Use of appropriate PPE (standard barrier isolation precautions for anthrax unless spore-containing powder present, in which case respirator and protective clothing needed)
- Alert lab of possibility of bioterror agent to ensure safe processing of specimens

### Time: 15 Minutes – Transition Point 1

a. Vital signs: BP 115/60, HR 107, RR 33, $O_2$ sat 85% on NRB at 15 L/min, 38.8°C (temporal).
b. Physical exam: unchanged except patient's skin warm and well perfused now. Remains tachypneic. Continues to be lethargic, but awakens to loud voice briefly.
c. EMS departs.
d. Wife remains at bedside, raises concerns about patient's breathing.
e. Course
    i. If team has ordered a chest X-ray, it shows widened mediastinum (hemorrhagic mediastinitis), bilateral pleural effusions.
    ii. If team has ordered an ECG, it shows sinus tachycardia.
    iii. If team has obtained an ABG, results are 7.18/55/60/12.
    iv. Respiratory therapy arrives in room (called by RN earlier).
    v. If team decides to intubate patient, RN and respiratory therapy bring equipment to team and ask what medications and doses team would like for intubation and sedation.
    vi. If team has not intubated patient, RN states that she is worried this patient is unable to protect his airway and that his oxygen is very low even on an NRB.

**Critical Actions**

- Optimizing hemodynamics prior to intubation as able
- Obtaining a definitive airway in a critically ill, altered patient in respiratory distress
- Initiating a correct antibiotic regiment for inhalational anthrax when meningitis has not been ruled out: IV ciprofloxacin (or levofloxacin) plus meropenem (or imipenem/cilastatin) plus minocycline (or doxycycline) along with possible adjunctive IV dexamethasone given concern for meningitis

### Time: 35 Minutes – Transition Point 2

a. Vital signs: BP 88/50, HR 130, RR 12, $O_2$ sat 99% on 100% $FiO_2$ via ventilator, 38.8°C (temporal). Vitals are status-post intubation.
b. Physical exam: if team has decided to intubate, patient is now mechanically ventilated.
c. Course
    i. Patient is successfully intubated, oxygenation improves.
    ii. Patient becomes hypotensive after intubation despite having received appropriate fluid resuscitation for his weight.
    iii. RN asks team if they would like to start a vasopressor if not already started.
    iv. If requested by team, labs have resulted. Refer to 9. Stimuli for lab results.

**Critical Actions**

- Starting appropriate postintubation sedation and pain control
- Obtaining postintubation chest X-ray
- Starting vasopressors for hypotension once patient has been adequately fluid resuscitated

### Time: 45 Minutes – Transition Point 3

a. Vital signs: BP 111/65, HR 109, RR 12, $O_2$ sat 99% on 100% $FiO_2$ via ventilator, 38.8°C (if given antipyretic, temperature now 37.5°C)
b. Physical exam: unchanged
c. Course
   i. Vitals improve after initiation of a vasopressor
   ii. Repeat chest X-ray shows ETT in appropriate position
   iii. If not already done, RN asks team if they should contact infection control/infectious disease and the administrator on call given the concern for bioterrorism.
   iv. Infection control/infectious disease recommends a lumbar puncture unless contraindicated, consideration of thoracostomies for pleural effusions (which may improve survival), and appropriate antibiotic regiment if not already done. They state they will contact local public health authorities regarding obtaining access to anthrax anti-toxins (raxibacumab, anthrax immune globulin intravenous, obiltoxaximab) from the Strategic National Stockpile.
   v. Hospital administrator states that they will enact their biohazard response plan, activate the hospital incident command system, and contact local authorities for further guidance. They have heard of additional cases at other facilities.
   vi. If providers decide to perform LP and/or thoracostomies, RN provides equipment. If LP/thoracostomies performed, fluid appears blood tinged.

**Critical Actions**

- Notification of appropriate hospital (infection control, infectious disease, emergency management) and/or local government authorities (public health department, law enforcement, state lab, Centers for Disease Control and Prevention) in accordance with local hospital policy
- Consideration of lumbar puncture to rule out anthrax meningitis and thoracostomies for pleural effusions

### Time: 60 Minutes – Transition Point 4

a. Vital signs: BP 108/65, HR 103, RR 12, $O_2$ sat 99% on 100% $FiO_2$ via ventilator, 38.8°C (if given antipyretic, temperature now 37.5°C)
b. Physical exam: unchanged (status-post bilateral thoracostomies if performed with improved bilateral breath sounds at bases)
c. Course
   i. Team contacts ICU to discuss admission. If not done, RN asks where the patient will be admitted.
   ii. ICU attending accepts patient for admission but recommends involvement of infection control and hospital administration if not already done.

iii. If not already done, infection control calls back to the ED to remind team to offer postexposure prophylaxis to anyone else exposed. This would include others at his place of work and possibly ED personnel, but caregivers would be at much lower risk of exposure if they were wearing appropriate PPE, particularly as it is unlikely that anthrax spores are still present on the patient. Anthrax pneumonia is generally not transmissible from human to human; however, there is a significant risk of infection for those who were directly exposed to the spores (i.e. coworkers).

iv. Team should inform wife of concern for anthrax as the cause of the patient's illness and acknowledge the severity of her husband's illness and poor prognosis.

v. Team should recommend that wife (as she also works in the mailroom) take a 42–60-day course of ciprofloxacin (or doxycycline, levofloxacin) and obtain the three-dose series of the anthrax vaccine adsorbed (AVA) in collaboration with local public health authorities.

**Critical Actions**

- Admit patient to higher level of care in discussion with ICU and hospital administration
- Initiation of postexposure prophylaxis for other exposed individuals

## 9. STIMULI

a. Chest X-ray 1: widened mediastinum, bilateral pleural effusions
b. Chest X-ray 2: ETT in place 4 cm above carina, otherwise unchanged
c. ECG: sinus tachycardia
d. Labs
   i. BG: 80
   ii. CBC: WBC 24, Hgb 13, hematocrit 39, platelets 200
   iii. INR 2.7, PTT 45
   iv. BMP: sodium 131, chloride 100, BUN 35, potassium 5.1, glucose 92, creatinine 2.7, $CO_2$ 10, calcium 8.5
   v. LFTs: AST 100, ALT 120, alkaline phosphatase 100, total bilirubin 1.9, direct bilirubin 0.7, albumin 2.9, total protein 5.5
   vi. ABG 7.18/55/60/12
   vii. Lactate: 4.5

## BIBLIOGRAPHY

Bower WA, Schiffer J, Atmar RL, et al. Use of anthrax vaccine in the United States: Recommendations of the Advisory Committee on Immunization Practices, 2019. *MMWR*. 2019;68(4):1–14. doi:10.15585/mmwr.rr6804a1.

Hendricks KA, Wright ME, Shadomy SV, et al. Centers for Disease Control and Prevention Expert Panel Meetings on Prevention and Treatment of Anthrax in Adults. *Emerg Infect Dis*. 2014 Feb;20(2):e130687. doi:10.3201/eid2002.130687.

Inglesby TV, O'Toole T, Henderson DA, et al. For the Working Group on Civilian Biodefense. Anthrax as a biological weapon: 2002 updated recommendations for management. *JAMA*. 2002;287(17):2236–2252. doi:10.1001/jama.287.17.2236.

Jernigan DB, Raghunathan PL, Bell BP, et al. Investigation of bioterrorism-related anthrax, United States, 2001: epidemiologic findings. *Emerg Infect Dis.* 2002;8(10):1019–1028. doi:10.3201/eid0810.020353.

Pillai SK, Huang E, Guarnizo JT, et al. Antimicrobial treatment for systemic anthrax: analysis of cases from 1945 to 2014 identified through a systematic literature review. *Health Secur.* 2015;13(6):355–364. doi:10.1089/hs.2015.0033.

Siegel JD, Rhinehart E, Jackson M, Chiarello L. 2007 guideline for isolation precautions: preventing transmission of infectious agents in health care settings. *Am J Infect Control.* 2007;35(10):S65–S164. doi:10.1016/j.ajic.2007.10.007.

Swartz MN. Recognition and management of anthrax: an update. *New Engl J Med.* 2001;345(22):1621–1626. doi:10.1016/j.ajic.2007.10.007.

CASE 36

# Bioterror Attack on the Subway

## Managing a Critically Ill Patient with Pneumonic Plague

Michael De Luca

DISASTER PRINCIPLES

- Clinical diagnosis and treatment
- Timing of medical and surgical interventions
- Recognition and clinical treatment
- Decontamination
- National disaster management system
- Role of public health agencies in disaster medicine
- Public health surveillance
- Decontamination
- Biological disasters
- Category A bioterrorism agents
- MCI triage and considerations for biological agents
- Biological safety
- Epidemiologic and medical countermeasures
- Personal protective equipment (PPE)
- *Yersinia pestis*

### 1. SCENARIO OVERVIEW

You receive the following notification over the ED radio: "We are coming to your facility with a 55-year-old female who presented in respiratory distress, with severe hypoxia, and is now intubated. Patient is tachycardic and hypotensive. We will be at your facility in five minutes." EMS arrives and relates that the patient's husband called 911 after he found her unresponsive in bed. She had been coughing up blood and experiencing high fevers for two days. The patient required intubation en route by EMS for altered mental status and hypoxic respiratory failure. Care team is informed of rumors of possible plague bioterrorism attack in the subway by EMS. Patient is critically ill, requiring fluid resuscitation and vasopressors. The patient is noted to have poor breath sounds on the left and chest X-ray demonstrates a left-main-stemmed ETT. The ETT is adjusted, resulting in exposure of care team to blood-tinged patient secretions. The patient is suspected of having been a victim of a bioterrorism attack with pneumonic plague and is treated with antibiotics. Providers contact infection control and hospital administration for further guidance. Postexposure prophylaxis is given to the care team.

## 2. TEACHING OBJECTIVES AND DISCUSSION POINTS

**Clinical Management**

a. Recognition of presentation of a bioterrorism-associated illness based on history, exam, and diagnostic studies
b. Using personal protective equipment (droplet precautions) and isolating patient
c. Managing advanced airway and ensuring adequate resuscitation in critically ill patient
d. Appropriate antibiotic selection
e. Prescribing postexposure prophylactic medications

**Public Health Interventions**

a. Recognition of possible bioterror event
b. Notification of appropriate public health and law enforcement authorities (via hospital administration and infection control)
c. Managing contaminated waste

## 3. SUPPLIES

a. Stretcher
b. IV supplies and tubing
c. Syringes with medications
d. IV fluids
e. Invasive airway equipment (endotracheal tube, laryngoscope, lubricant, stylet, LMA, BVM, suction)
f. Telephone

## 4. MOULAGE

a. Mannequin with dried blood on mouth and on clothes; clothing damp from diaphoresis

## 5. IMAGES AND LABS

a. Chest X-ray: ETT is in right main bronchus, left lung is poorly aerated, bilateral pulmonary infiltrates concerning for multifocal pneumonia
b. ECG: sinus tachycardia
c. Labs: BG, CBC, INR/PTT, CMP, ABG, lactate

## 6. ACTORS (CONFEDERATES) AND THEIR ROLES

a. Patient: mannequin
b. EMS: brings patient into ED and when asked by providers describes the critical state of the patient and relates the history of a possible bioterror attack on the subway.
c. Nurse: if asked places additional IV, administers medications
d. Infection control/infectious disease: instructs providers to isolate patient, adhere to droplet precautions, carefully manage waste, and alert laboratory of suspected pneumonic plague case; liaises with local/state authorities
e. Administrator-on-call: convenes hospital incident command system if contacted by providers; liaises with local/state authorities

f. ICU attending: listens to patient course in ED and accepts patient to ICU. Recommends multidisciplinary discussion with infection control and hospital administration.

## 7. CRITICAL ACTIONS

a. Refer to actions under timeline

## 8. TIMELINE WITH TRANSITION POINTS

a. EMS report over radio: "We are coming to your facility with a 55-year-old female who presented in respiratory distress, with severe hypoxia, and is now intubated. Patient is tachycardic and hypotensive. We will be at your facility in five minutes."

### Time: Zero

a. Vital signs (per EMS): BP 80/50, HR 139, RR 12, $O_2$ sat 92% on 100% $FiO_2$ via ventilator, 39.4°C (temporal).
b. Summary of initial presentation: EMS arrives and relates that the patient's husband called 911 after he found her unresponsive in bed. She had been coughing up blood and experiencing high fevers for two days. The patient required intubation en route by EMS for altered mental status and hypoxic respiratory failure. Care team is informed of rumors of possible plague bioterror attack in the subway by EMS.
c. Physical exam
    i. General: diaphoretic, dry blood on clothing and face, intubated
    ii. HEENT: normocephalic atraumatic, PERRLA, dry mucous membranes, dry blood in mouth
    iii. Neck: supple
    iv. Pulmonary: mechanically ventilated, no breath sounds on left side, diffuse rhonchi
    v. Cardiovascular: tachycardic, regular, no MRG
    vi. GI: soft, nondistended
    vii. Musculoskeletal: no obvious deformities
    viii. Skin: wet, poorly perfused, mottled, capillary refill >3 seconds
    ix. Neuro: 3T. Does not withdraw to painful stimuli.
d. Initial interventions
    i. Providers wear appropriate PPE (droplet precautions), isolate patient in room
    ii. Place on monitor
    iii. Obtain labs through IV placed by EMS
    iv. Fluid-resuscitate
    v. Obtain chest X-ray
    vi. ECG presented to team
e. EMS: reports history and vitals as previously. They were able to establish one peripheral IV and have given 500 cc of NS. Reports this is the fifth patient they have seen today in respiratory distress.
f. Nurse: assists team when directed to give additional fluids, medications. Places additional peripheral IV. If providers have not employed proper PPE or isolated patient, RN asks team if they should consider these actions.

**Critical Actions**

- Adequate fluid resuscitation for presumed septic shock
- Obtain labs, EKG, chest radiograph
- Obtaining history concerning for possible bioterrorism agent exposure
- Isolation of patient
- Use of personal protective equipment (droplet precautions)
- Notify laboratory of concern for possible bioterror agent to ensure safe processing of specimens

### Time: 10 Minutes – Transition Point 1

a. Vital signs: BP 80/50, HR 123, RR 12, $O_2$ sat 92% on 100% $FiO_2$ via ventilator, 39.4°C (temporal).
b. Physical exam: unchanged. Decreased breath sounds on left side.
c. EMS departs.
d. Course
   i. If team has ordered a chest X-ray, it shows ETT is in right main bronchus, left lung is poorly aerated, bilateral pulmonary infiltrates concerning for multifocal pneumonia
   ii. If team has ordered an ECG, it shows sinus tachycardia
   iii. If team has obtained an ABG, it results with ABG 7.13/50/72/10
   iv. If team decides to pull ETT back to improve ventilation of left lung, they are exposed to blood-tinged secretions when the ETT balloon is deflated. If the team does not attempt to move ETT, the RN asks the team if the tube should be repositioned.
   v. The team should start vasopressors after the patient has received appropriate weight-based fluid resuscitation. If the team does not start vasopressors, the RN asks the providers what they want to do about the blood pressure.

**Critical Actions**

- Troubleshooting difficulties with a definitive airway in a critically ill patient
- Initiating vasopressors for shock after adequate fluid resuscitation
- Initiation of a correct parenteral antibiotic regiment: an aminoglycoside (streptomycin or gentamicin) PLUS a fluoroquinolone (levofloxacin, ciprofloxacin, or moxifloxacin) given concern for bioterrorism-related pneumonic plague

### Time: 20 Minutes – Transition Point 2

a. Vital signs: BP 105/65 (if team has initiated vasopressors), HR 110, RR 12, $O_2$ sat 99% on 100% $FiO_2$ via ventilator (if team has repositioned tube), 39.4°C (temporal).
b. Physical exam: If team has decided to reposition ETT, patient now has equal breath sounds. Patient is making some spontaneous movements and gagging.
c. Course
   i. Vitals improve after initiation of vasopressors
   ii. ETT is successfully repositioned, oxygenation and breath sounds improve
   iii. If requested by team, labs have resulted. Refer to section 9. Stimuli for lab results.
   iv. Team initiates sedation and pain-control for intubated patient if not already done. RN asks team if they would like to start sedation if the team has not yet done so.

**Critical Actions**

- Starting appropriate postintubation sedation and pain-control

### Time: 25 Minutes – Transition Point 3

a. Vital signs: BP 110/67, HR 109, RR 12, $O_2$ sat 99% on 100% $FiO_2$ via ventilator, 39.4°C (temporal).
b. Physical exam: patient no longer making spontaneous movements or gagging (if sedation has been started)
c. Course
   i. If not already done, RN asks if team if they should contact infection control/infectious disease and the administrator on call given the concern for plague.
   ii. Infection control/infectious disease recommends isolating patient, appropriate PPE, appropriate antibiotic regiment if not already done, and postexposure prophylaxis for care team exposed to patient droplets (if they did not follow standard and droplet precautions). They state they will contact local public health authorities.
   iii. Hospital administrator states that they will enact their biohazard response plan and contact local authorities for further guidance.

**Critical Actions**

- Notification of appropriate hospital (infection control, infectious disease, emergency management) and/or local government authorities (public health department, law enforcement, state lab, Centers for Disease Control and Prevention) in accordance with local hospital policy
- Initiation of postexposure prophylaxis with ciprofloxacin or doxycycline (levofloxacin, moxifloxacin can also be used) for exposed hospital staff for seven days.

### Time: 40 Minutes – Transition Point 4

a. Vital signs: BP 117/60, HR 105, RR 12, $O_2$ sat 98% on 100% $FiO_2$ via ventilator, 39.4°C (temporal). (Temperature is 37.4°C if antipyretic given.)
b. Physical exam: Unchanged.
c. Course
   i. Team contacts ICU to discuss admission. If not done, RN asks where the patient will be admitted.
   ii. ICU attending accepts patient for admission but recommends involvement of infection control and hospital administration if not already done.
   iii. If not already done, infection control calls back to the ED to remind team to offer postexposure prophylaxis to care team, and to carefully manage waste generated during hospitalization. Facility approved sporicidal/germicidal agent or 0.5% hypochlorite solution is recommended for disinfection.

**Critical Actions**

- Admit patient to higher level of care in discussion with ICU and hospital administration
- Proper management of contaminated waste and patient samples, including those sent to lab

## 9. STIMULI

a. Chest X-ray: ETT is in right main bronchus, left lung is poorly aerated, bilateral pulmonary infiltrates concerning for multifocal pneumonia
b. ECG: sinus tachycardia
c. Labs
   i. BG: 80
   ii. CBC: WBC 25, Hgb 14, hematocrit 42, platelets 90
   iii. INR 1.7, PTT: 25
   iv. BMP: sodium 129, chloride 99, BUN 36, potassium 4.9, glucose 89, creatinine 2.4, $CO_2$ 11, calcium 8.7
   v. LFTs: AST 79, ALT 88, alkaline phosphatase 124, total bilirubin 1.4, direct bilirubin 0.5, albumin 2.7, total protein 5.4
   vi. ABG 7.13/50/72/10
   vii. Lactate: 5.4

## BIBLIOGRAPHY

Butler T, Bell WR, Nguyen-Ngoc-Linh, Nguyen-Dinh-Tiep, Arnold K. *Yersinia pestis* infection in Vietnam. I. Clinical and hematologic aspects. *J Infect Dis.* 1974; 129(Suppl):S78–S84. doi:10.1093/infdis/129.supplement_1.s78.

Earnest M. On becoming a plague doctor. *N Engl J Med.* 2020;383:10:e64. doi:10.1056/NEJMp2011418.

English JF, Cundiff MY, Malone JD, et al. *Bioterrorism Readiness Plan: A Template for Healthcare Facilities.* Atlanta: Centers for Disease Control and Prevention; 1999. https://emergency.cdc.gov/bioterrorism/pdf/13apr99apic-cdcbioterrorism.pdf. Accessed April 5, 2025.

Godfred-Cato S, Cooley KM, Fleck-Derderian S, et al. Treatment of human plague: a systematic review of published aggregate data on antimicrobial efficacy, 1939–2019. *Clin Infect Dis.* 2020;70(70 Suppl 1):S11–S19. doi:10.1093/cid/ciz1230.

Koirala J. Plague: disease, management, and recognition of act of terrorism. *Infect Dis Clin North Am.* 2006;20(2):273–287. doi:10.1093/cid/ciz1230.

Nelson CA. Antimicrobial treatment and prophylaxis of plague: recommendations for naturally acquired infections and bioterrorism response. *MMWR. Recommendations and Reports.* 2021;70. doi:10.15585/mmwr.rr7003a1.

Nelson CA, Fleck-Derderian S, Cooley KM, et al. Antimicrobial treatment of human plague: a systematic review of the literature on individual cases, 1937–2019. *Clin Infect Dis.* 2020;70(70 Suppl 1):S3–S10. doi:10.1093/cid/ciz1226.

Prentice MB, Rahalison L. Plague. *Lancet.* 2007;369(9568):1196–1207. doi:10.1016/S0140-6736(07)60566-2.

Siegel JD, Rhinehart E, Jackson M, Chiarello L. 2007 guideline for isolation precautions: preventing transmission of infectious agents in health care settings. *Am J Infect Control.* 2007;35(10):S65–S164. doi:10.1016/j.ajic.2007.10.007.

CASE 37

# Balancing Trauma Response and ED Preparedness during an Active Shooter Incident

Meghan Maslanka

DISASTER PRINCIPLES

- Clinical diagnosis and treatment
- Timing of medical and surgical interventions
- Recognition and clinical treatment
- Information management/communications
- Scene safety and security in the field
- Hospital preparedness
- Tactical EMS
- Active threats
- Care under fire

## 1. SCENARIO OVERVIEW

A 54-year-old woman with a history of hypertension is brought to a critical access ED in a rural town after an assailant opened fire at the local grocery store. The patient was shot near the front of the store, so was able to be safely removed from the scene and taken to the hospital by private vehicle. However, other injured victims inside the store have been unable to exit the scene due to ongoing active shooting. The patient has multiple penetrating wounds to the neck, groin, and extremities that require stabilization. The patient will require hemorrhage control and resuscitation while awaiting transport to a trauma center.

## 2. TEACHING OBJECTIVES AND DISCUSSION POINTS

### Clinical and Medical Management

- Manage life-threatening bleeding using various modalities, including pressure dressings, wound packing, and tourniquets.
- Obtain IO or IV access.
- Fully undress the patient to identify all injuries/wounds.
- Manage the airway in a patient with an expanding neck hematoma including considerations of rapid airway deterioration, possibility of needed surgical airway, etc.
- Obtain patient vitals.
- Give blood as needed for hemorrhagic shock.
- Give antibiotics for open fractures.

- Update tetanus vaccination.
- Arrange for transfer to a trauma center.

**Communication and Teamwork**

- Coordinate early transport to a trauma center.
- Discuss actions to be taken by the ED to prepare for additional patients from the scene.

## 3. SUPPLIES

- Wheelchair
- CAT tourniquet
- Triangle bandages/cravats
- Tongue depressors
- Silk tape
- Combat gauze
- 4 × 4 gauze
- Kerlex
- Coban
- Intubation supplies: BVM, ETT, stylet, Eschmann stylet (bougie), blade and handle, suction, cricothyrotomy kit
- Syringes with medications
- Blood for transfusion
- IO kit
- Central line kit

## 4. MOULAGE

- Right neck: small penetrating wound
- Right groin: large gaping penetrating wound with active hemorrhage
- Left thigh: bony deformity of the femur due to fracture, small entrance wound of the anterior midthigh, and large gaping exit wound of the posterior midthigh with heavy bleeding
- Right upper arm: small penetrating wound to the anterior mid humerus

## 5. IMAGES AND LABS

- Labs: no results prior to transfer
- CXR: normal
- Other X-rays (if obtained)
  - Abdominal X-ray: ballistic fragments in right pelvis, no fracture
  - X-ray pelvis: right-sided ballistic fragments, no fracture
  - X-ray left femur: comminuted midshaft fracture with displacement and ballistic fragments
  - X-ray right humerus: ballistic fragments, no fracture

## 6. ACTORS (CONFEDERATES) AND THEIR ROLES

- Patient: mannequin

## 7. CRITICAL ACTIONS

- Identify all ballistic wounds
- Manage active hemorrhage
- Obtain rapid IO or IV access
- Give blood for hemorrhagic shock
- Secure airway
- Prepare the ED for additional patients

## 8. TIMELINE WITH TRANSITION POINTS

### Time: Zero

VS: none available

- Summary of initial presentation: A 54-year-old female is brought to the ED by private vehicle after an active shooter incident. She arrives to the resuscitation room in a wheelchair, fully clothed, slumped over. Blood is dripping from her pants.
- Physical exam
  - General: anxious, distressed, repeatedly saying "help me," diaphoretic
  - HEENT: penetrating wound to right neck, no other wounds
  - Chest: no wounds
  - Heart: sinus tachycardia, no abnormal heart sounds
  - Abdomen: soft, nontender, nondistended, no wounds
  - Back: no visible injury, no midline tenderness or step-offs
  - Extremities
    - Right groin: large gaping wound with active hemorrhage
    - Left thigh: bony deformity of the femur due to fracture, small entrance wound of the anterior midthigh, and large gaping exit wound of the posterior midthigh with heavy bleeding
    - Right upper arm: small penetrating wound to the anterior mid humerus
  - Neuro: alert, moving all extremities, unable to assess sensation due to distress
- Initial intervention
  - Perform a primary assessment
    - Airway: phonating
    - Breathing: CTAB
    - Circulation: active hemorrhage of right groin and left thigh, unable to palpate pulses in RLE, +1 pulses in all other extremities
    - Disability: Glasgow Coma Scale 4E 4V 6M, moves all extremities spontaneously
  - Fully undress the patient
  - Control active hemorrhage
    - If holding pressure or pressure dressings are attempted, the patient continues to bleed.
    - Packing will stop bleeding from the groin wound.
    - A tourniquet will stop bleeding from the thigh wounds.
  - Attempt to obtain IV access
  - Place on cardiac monitor
  - Obtain vitals

### Time: Three Minutes – Transition Point 1

VS: BP 75/30, HR 130, RR 30, $O_2$ sat 96%, 98°F

- Nurse reports that attempts at IV access have been unsuccessful.
- Team must place an IO (in the left humerus) or central line.
- Team must initiate blood transfusion for hemorrhagic shock.
- Hypotension will worsen until access is obtained and blood is given.

### Time: Five Minutes – Transition Point 2

VS: BP 95/60, HR 110, RR 50, $O_2$ sat 92%, 98°F

- Physical exam: The patient starts to spit blood and develops stridor. She remains alert but is gurgling. A large, rapidly expanding hematoma is visible in her right neck.
- Team should recognize the need to secure an airway.
  - RSI must be performed but visualization of the airway will be difficult due to distorted anatomy and contaminated airway. If intubation is not performed immediately after recognizing the expanding hematoma, the airway will be completely occluded and cricothyrotomy will be required. If it is performed promptly and airway decontamination is performed using suction, the RSI attempt will be successful.
  - If the simulation center being used owns an advanced airway mannequin, hypopharyngeal swelling may be simulated in order to make airway attempt difficult.
  - If the team does not prepare for intubation, the patient should desaturate to 50% and become unresponsive.

### Time: Eight Minutes – Transition Point 3

VS: BP 110/70, HR 105, RR 16, $O_2$ sat 100%

- Physical exam: The patient has a secure airway. All active hemorrhage is controlled.
- Team should complete a secondary assessment.
- Team should obtain a CXR to confirm ETT placement.
- Team must coordinate transfer to a trauma center.
- If time permits prior to transfer, the team should
  - Give antibiotics for open fracture.
  - Update tetanus vaccine.
- If time permits, obtain CT imaging including arterial phase contrast enhanced images of the neck.

### Transition Point 4: Final Actions

- If the team has not yet discussed how to handle an influx of additional patients, they should be notified that ambulances are en route with three additional patients who require stabilization.
  - Discuss preparations the ED can make to handle additional patients.

## 9. STIMULI

- N/A

## BIBLIOGRAPHY

American College of Surgeons Committee on Trauma. *Advanced Trauma Life Support.* 10th ed. Chicago: Hearthside Publishing Services; 2018.

Beldowicz BC, Matthew MJ. Penetrating neck trauma. In: Mattu A, Swadron S, eds. *CorePendium.* Burbank, CA: CorePendium, LLC; updated April 26, 2021. www.emrap.org/corependium/chapter/recvkJTmh25glAi6Z/Penetrating-Neck-Trauma#h.9sbu0q7s0nr5. Accessed August 1, 2022.

Quinn J, Straube S. Penetrating extremity trauma. In: Swadron S, Nordt SP, Mattu A, Johnson W, eds. *CorePendium.* Burbank, CA: CorePendium, LLC; updated March 28, 2025. www.emrap.org/corependium/chapter/reciGsVEOIKauMelM/Penetrating-Extremity-Trauma#h.68a5jexnoj7k. Accessed April 5, 2025.

Stop the Bleed. BleedingControl.org website. 2019–2022. www.stopthebleed.org/resources-poster-booklet. Accessed July 27, 2022.

CASE 38

# Stabbed in the Crowd

## Tackling Trauma in a Live Concert Attack

Kyle Herbert and Emily Marx

DISASTER PRINCIPLES

- Clinical diagnosis and treatment
- Timing of medical and surgical interventions
- Recognition and clinical treatment
- Information management/communications
- Scene safety and security in the field
- Hospital preparedness
- Tactical EMS
- Active threats
- Care under fire
- Medical surge capacity
- Field disaster triage
- Mass gatherings

## 1. SCENARIO OVERVIEW

a. EMS brings in a 24-year-old male with multiple stab wounds from scene after being involved in local large-scale active assailant MCI. Patient was standing in line at a local concert ticket booth when he was stabbed multiple times in the back. Patient also has wounds to the bilateral upper extremities consistent with self-defense injuries. On scene, patient with Glasgow Coma Scale (GCS) 12 (E3 V4 M5). Hypotensive to upper 80s with concurrent tachycardia to 110. Patient's $O_2$ saturation initially upper 70s on scene; improvement with administration of NRB to mid-80s. Unable to ascertain breath sounds as paramedics on scene lost stethoscope in the commotion however, patient needle decompressed in field given hypotension. Active exsanguination from large volar, right midforearm laceration and a tourniquet was applied on scene. He also has left, lateral upper back and left flank wounds apparent. Patient was given red tag designation on scene and transported as priority to local level III trauma center. Patient arrives as multiple other patients from scene are being evaluated and treated. Patient's GCS on arrival has deteriorated to GCS 8 (E2 V2 M4) .

## 2. TEACHING OBJECTIVES AND DISCUSSION POINTS

a. Teaching objectives
   i. Primary assessment with ABCs, secondary assessment
   ii. Recognition and stabilization of tension pneumothorax

   iii. Recognition and stabilization of life-threatening bleeding
   iv. Recognition of when to activate massive transfusion protocol (MTP)
   v. Complete workup, imaging, labs, and procedures needed for penetrating injury victims

b. Discussion points
   i. Discuss immediate management of tension pneumothorax, indications for field needle decompression
   ii. Surgical chest tube placement
   iii. Discuss immediate management of traumatic extremity bleeding
   iv. Discuss management of resuscitating critical patient with multiple significant traumatic injuries
   v. Discuss management of critically ill, but salvageable patient in the setting of MCI protocols

## 3. SUPPLIES

a. Cardiac monitor, $SpO_2$, BP monitor, ECG
b. Noninvasive airway supplies such as NRB, HFNC, or BiPAP
c. Intubation supplies in the room for backup airway in case of decompensation: bag-valve mask (BVM), endotracheal tube (ETT), stylet, blade, suction
d. Provider PPE (gown, mask with shield, gloves)
e. Intravenous (IV)/Intraosseous (IV) material
f. Tourniquet
g. Wound dressing (hemostatic gauze, regular gauze, Kerlex, Coban, etc.)
h. Chest tube, kit, pleura-vac
i. Laceration repair tray
j. Cordis, MAC, or other large-bore central access device
k. Rapid blood infuser device

## 4. MOULAGE

a. Deep, gaping laceration to medial volar surface of right proximal forearm just distal to clavicular fossa
b. Superficial lacerations to distal dorsal lateral forearm
c. Penetrating laceration to left upper back just lateral to left paraspinal muscles at approximately C5/T1
d. Penetrating laceration to left lateral flank at approximately T8 level
e. Bilateral needle decompression catheters at midclavicular line

## 5. IMAGES AND LABS

a. Basic labs (CBC, CMP, lactic acid, coags, type and screen, etc.)
b. Bedside ultrasound (Extended Focused Assessment with Sonography for Trauma/Rapid Ultrasound in Shock and Hypotension [EFAST/RUSH])
c. Chest X-ray (CXR) 1-view to evaluate for pneumothorax (PTX)
d. RUE X-ray (XR)
e. CT chest, CT abdomen/pelvis, CTA right upper extremity (RUE)

## 6. ACTORS (CONFEDERATES) AND THEIR ROLES

a. Nurse ×1: place on monitor, IV access
b. EMS provider ×1: volunteers to stable to help nurse with initial triage of patient
c. Respiratory therapist: management of NRB, assistance with intubation set-up and postintubation vent management (if team decided to obtain definitive airway)
d. Confederate (optional role): trauma chief who walks in and says they are taking another critically ill patient to OR (after finding patient has free fluid in abdomen). Asks ED team to stabilize and resuscitate patient, coordinated with in-house specialized surgeon emergently for definitive care (vascular and/or cardiothoracic surgery)
e. Confederate (optional role): charge nurse who informs team that CT is unavailable during initial resuscitation

## 7. CRITICAL ACTIONS

a. Attach patient to monitor
b. Complete primary survey (ABCs)
c. Bleeding control
d. Secondary survey to determine all obvious injuries
e. Obtain initial vital signs
f. Ascertain GCS of 7 and decide on definitive airway for airway protection and expected medical course
   i. Ensure suction, back-up, bougie, rapid sequence intubation (RSI) medications, postintubation sedation, ETT confirmation, oral-gastric tube (OGT)
   ii. Confirmation of ETT with $CO_2$ colorimeter, auscultated breath sounds, and/or chest rise
g. EFAST
h. STAT CXR to determine PTX, ETT placement
i. Insertion of left surgical chest tube or perform simple (finger) thoracostomy
j. Repeat CXR to confirm chest tube placement
k. CT imaging
l. Ascertain tourniquet uptime and then take down for assessment of forearm wound
m. Consultation and transfer to higher level of care, specialty services

## 8. TIMELINE WITH TRANSITION POINTS

### Time: Zero

a. Vital signs: BP 74/52, HR 134, RR 33, temp 36.1, sat 88% on NRB, point of care glucose 89
b. EMS arrives and gives report.
   i. A 24 year-old male presenting with multiple stab wounds to RUE, left upper back, left flank. Needle decompressed in field for hypoxia and hypotension in the setting of thoracic penetrating wound with no major improvement in BP. Placed on NRB with $O_2$ sats low 80s. Brisk exsanguination from RUE forearm wound, tourniquet applied (20 minutes prior to arrival). Patient initially GCS 12 with deterioration in route to GCS 8. Best BP 82/62, HR 110s–130s.
c. Initial intervention
   i. Place on monitor
   ii. Large-bore IV ×2 (at least 18 G)

   iii. Initiation of blood products via MTP
   iv. Trauma labs drawn
d. Primary survey
   i. ABCs
      1. Airway
      2. Breathing
      3. Circulation: Pulse absent in RUE
      4. Disability: GCS 7 (E2 V2 M3)
      5. Exposure

**Critical Actions**

- Place on monitor and obtain initial vitals
  i. Hypotensive
- Establish IV access
- Procedural actions
  i. Determine need for definitive airway between primary and secondary survey, obtain definitive airway
  ii. Finger thoracostomy (must be done first prior to intubation)
- Order CXR to confirm ETT
- Begin blood product administration
- Begin postintubation sedation
- Optional: discuss tranexamic acid administration
- Begin preparing the ED for arrival of additional casualties and try to obtain additional information from the scene about expected numbers of patients, severity of injury, etc.

### Time: Approximately Three Minutes – Transition Point 1

a. Reassess vitals
b. Nurse sends labs
c. Secondary survey/initial physical exam
   i. General: intubated and sedated, pale
   ii. Head/face: normocephalic, atraumatic
   iii. HEENT: no injuries, pupils sluggishly reactive
   iv. Neck: unable to visualize neck due to habitus, no appreciable crepitus
   v. Chest: bilateral needle decompression catheters at midclavicular line, second intercostal space, unequal chest rise, diminished breath sounds over left chest wall
   vi. Abdomen: nondistended, nontender, no acute injuries
   vii. Pelvis: stable
   viii. Back: penetrating wound to left back at approximately T4 level, lateral to spine; penetrating wound to left flank
   ix. Extremities: large gaping laceration middle right volar forearm with obvious muscle exposure; tourniquet proximal to injury
   x. Neuro: GCS 3T
d. CXR ordered: demonstrates large left-sided PTX

**Critical Actions**

- Reassess vitals
- Determine need for surgical chest tube given needle decompression, tension PTX, and finger thoracostomy
- Place surgical chest tube
- Reassess vitals postprocedure
- Call for CXR to determine placement of ETT and chest tube while moving to RUE (CXR results will come back in Transition Point 3)

### Time: Approximately 10 Minutes – Transition Point 2

a. Reassess vitals
b. Evaluate right forearm wound
   i. Prepare dressings, combat gauze
   ii. Take down tourniquet and appreciate brisk bleeding
   iii. Replace tourniquet/hold vessel pressure proximal to wound
c. Continue MTP

**Critical Actions**

- Determine need for transfer for vascular surgery for definitive treatment
- Determine need for temporizing source control given complications associated with prolonged tourniquet application time
- Removal of tourniquet after hemostasis achieved
- Place wound under pressure dressing

### Time: Approximately 15 Minutes – Transition Point 3

a. Reassess vitals
b. EFAST
   i. Ensure no cardiac injury given thoracic penetrating wound, negative for abdominal free fluid
   ii. No slide on left despite chest-tube
   iii. Discuss FAST utility for penetrating trunk wound, utility in evaluating cardiac injury in setting of thoracic stab wound
iii. Repeat CXR for confirmation of chest tube and ETT
   i. Vitals have improved, but CXR shows that PTX has not resolved to the level expected. However, chest tube appears to be in appropriate place
iv. Confederate (charge nurse) informs team that CT is available, but angiography is not possible at this time
v. Team makes decision to go to scanner, given evidence of persistent PTX, as well as to evaluate belly for occult injury due to flank injury
vi. CT abdomen and pelvis: negative
vii. CT chest
   i. Residual left-sided PTX, possible bronchial injury

**Critical Actions**
- VS reassessment
- CT imaging
- Place second left-sided chest tube
- Expedited consultation – vascular and CT surgery

### Time: Approximately 20 Minutes – Transition Point 4

a. Reassess vitals
b. Repeat CXR
   i. Shows interval improvement in PTX
c. Consultation to local/regional transfer center for transfer to level I trauma center

**Critical Actions**
- Make decision to transfer patient for higher-level care
- Situation, Background, Assessment, and Recommendation transfer report to accepting provider

## 9. STIMULI

a. HR on monitor sinus tachycardia to 130s
b. Tachypneic RR to mid-30s
c. Hypotensive to 80s palp
d. CXR with identification of left-sided PTX of approximately 60% volume loss
e. EFAST: No left-lung slide
f. Actively exsanguinating RUE forearm wound when tourniquet taken down
g. CBC: Hgb 6.3
h. CMP: sodium 134, potassium 2.9, chloride 97, bicarb 24, Cr 1.6
i. Lactate: 5.3
j. CT chest
   i. PTX still present necessitating need for additional chest tube and suggesting possible bronchial tree injury that may require cardiothoracic surgery and/or bronch
   ii. Would require additional left-sided chest-tube
k. CTAP: Left flank laceration without intra-abdominal, retroperitoneal injury

## BIBLIOGRAPHY

Ahmad S. Mass casualty incident management. *Mo Med.* 2018 Sep–Oct;115(5):451–455. PMID: 30385995; PMCID: PMC6205284.

Malo C, Bernardin B, Nemeth J, Khwaja K. Prolonged prehospital tourniquet placement associated with severe complications: a case report. *CJEM.* 2015 July;17(4):443–556. doi: 10.1017/cem.2014.44. PMID: 26134057.

Peck MA, Clouse WD, Cox MW, et al. The complete management of extremity vascular injury in a local population. *J Vasc Surg.* 2007 June;45(6):1197–2204; discussion 1204–1205. doi: 10.1016/j.jvs.2007.02.003. PMID: 17543685.

Sharma A, Jindal P. Principles of diagnosis and management of traumatic pneumothorax. *J Emerg Trauma Shock.* 2008 Jan;1(1):34–41. doi: 10.4103/0974-2700.41789. PMID: 19561940; PMCID: PMC2700561.

SECTION 9

# MASS CASUALTY INCIDENT

CASE 39

# Botulism Bioterrorism in a Small Rural Hospital

James Aiken

DISASTER PRINCIPLES

- Clinical diagnosis and treatment
- Timing of medical and surgical interventions
- Recognition and clinical treatment
- Biological disasters
- MCI triage and considerations for biological agents
- Biological safety
- Epidemiologic and medical countermeasures
- Personal protective equipment (PPE)
- Information management/communications
- Disaster triage concepts
- Local disaster response
- Hospital preparedness program
- Role of public health agencies in disaster medicine
- Public health surveillance
- Field operations and logistics
- Mass-casualty care in the field
- Field disaster triage
- Field stabilization, treatment, and transport
- Category A bioterrorism agents
- Botulism

## 1. SCENARIO OVERVIEW

Simultaneous intentional botulism neurotoxin (BoNT) acts of terrorism on a local community restaurant salad bar and across the country. The scenario will challenge the participants to manage numerous ED presentations of patients with illnesses having common signs and symptoms of progressive neurologic deficits with varying respiratory distress acuities that overwhelm conventional operations.

### Background

Russian terrorists from the east European country of Georgia infiltrate the United States in five areas of the continent contaminating restaurant salad bars with BoNT. A restaurant in this small rural community is a target. The 10-bed ED in this scenario is located within a single 45-bed community hospital that has limited critical care capabilities: six ICU beds and four ventilators. The hospital has a full-service lab and CT capabilities. The ED is single covered with an ED group composed of five emergency physicians all living within the community. There are two general internists on staff and one intensivist on call for the region available to the ED.

On the day of the scenario, there are two patients in the ED awaiting floor beds. The ICU has four available beds. One current ICU ventilator patient is a 72-year-old patient not expected to live but a full code status. The other ventilator patient is a drug overdose with possible anoxic brain injury with uncertain prognosis.

## 2. TEACHING OBJECTIVES AND DISCUSSION POINTS

### Teaching Objectives

1. Recognize the initial assessment and stabilization of patients presenting in respiratory distress with neurologic deficits.
2. Demonstrate ability to diagnose botulism and treat BoNT poisoning.
3. Demonstrate awareness of the national emergency preparedness capabilities to respond to botulism bioterrorism.
4. Recognize the need for and employ emergency management resources as the ED transitions its operations from conventional through contingency operations to crisis management.

### Discussion Points

1. This scenario is intended to reinforce the recognition of a botulism presentation without available botulism diagnostic capabilities with the additional challenge of supporting such patients until procurement of antitoxin. The participant will demonstrate awareness of the need for advanced airway support in a setting of limited resources and recognize that patients without shortness of breath can be managed without advanced airway intervention initially.
2. Upon recognition of botulism, the participant must initiate obtaining the antitoxin from external sources. The participant will be expected to call the local public health department or poison control center for assistance in getting the antitoxin and to report the cases for investigation.
3. As more patients present, the participant must recognize the transition of conventional ED operations to contingency and beyond by calling the house supervisor for extra resources and initiate transfer processes as the hospital's ICU capabilities become overwhelmed.
4. At a later time, the ED will learn via public health that reports of botulism epidemics in other communities has raised the suspicion of bioterrorism and that the local and state offices of emergency preparedness and FBI will become involved.
5. This development mandates launching the hospital incident command system (HICS) and understanding how that changes the features of the mounting disaster response.
6. As more respiratory distress patients arrive, the participant will be motivated to communicate his predicament of lack of critical care capacity for incoming respiratory failure patients. The emergency manager may prompt a discussion on crisis standards of care. Should the 72-year old already on a ventilator in the ICU be reassessed for discontinuation of care to allow access to an incoming patient with a greater chance of survival? (This is not considered a critical treatment decision.) How about the younger patient? Who makes those decisions (treating physician versus independent panel of physician, nurse, clergy and perhaps a community participant who may have participated in the hospital's crisis standards planning)? What are the guidelines for such decisions? (Sequential Organ Failure Assessment [SOFA] versus Acute Physiology and Chronic Health Evaluation [APACHE]?). When does the hospital initiate recovery processes and decision making.

## 3. SUPPLIES

- Oxygen delivery masks
- Pulse ox equipment
- Intubation equipment: endotracheal tubes, laryngoscopes, Eschmann bougies, laryngeal mask airways, BVM
- Suction
- $ETCO_2$
- IV equipment
- Thermometers
- ECG
- Cardiac monitor
- Customary emergent airway management drugs
- Standard provider PPE

## 4. IMAGES AND LABS

- Full lab capacity
- Venous blood gas/arterial blood gas
- Does not have botulism antitoxin detection capabilities.
- Chest X-ray
- CT
- Bedside ultrasound

## 5. ACTORS (CONFEDERATES) AND THEIR ROLES

Six patients (number can be adjusted according to desired scope of the disaster and length of scenario) aged 15 to 92 years of age with varying levels of respiratory distress and neurologic deficits. They share the common experience of having eaten at the local restaurant within the last four hours. Another patient who ate at the restaurant has gastroenteritis.

**Confederates**

- Initially two ED nurses; the hospital is fully staffed with nurses that day.
- One hospital respiratory technician
- CEO who normally serves as HICS incident commander
- Chief medical officer

## 6. MOULAGE

No makeup necessary

## 7. TIMELINE

### Time: Zero – Patient 1

EMS calls regarding transport of a 44-year-old male complaining of difficulty swallowing, shortness of breath, double vision, and bilateral arm weakness for the past two hours. He denies pain, fever, vomiting. Vital signs are POx 90% on RA, pulse rate 100. BP 118/62 R 24 and appears shallow. He is alert and oriented but appears anxious and obeys all commands. POx improves to 92% on 100% ventimask.

### Time: Two Minutes – Patient 2

EMS calls regarding a 66-year-old female with Phx of stroke being transported for complaints of slurred speech, double vision, inability to raise both eyelids, difficulty swallowing, and uncoordinated bilateral hand strength.

Vital signs are BP 166/ 102 P 98 R 18 POx 88% on RA. Paramedics find her oriented with ptosis and disconjugate gaze, slurred speech, bilateral upper arm drift on stroke exam, equal normal lower extremity motor exam. POx improves to 92% on ventimask.

### Time: Five Minutes

Patient 1 arrives.

- Vital signs, POx and appearance are confirmed. Patient afebrile.
- General: fatigued, answers confusional questions appropriately with slurred speech.
- HEENT: no infection. + ptosis. EMS claims ptosis is new.
- Neck: supple, nontender, no JVD, stridor
- Chest: poor air movement, clear to auscultation
- Heart: regular rate, no murmurs
- Abdomen: soft nontender
- Extremity: all pulses present. Minimal spontaneous upper extremity movement. No swelling.
- Neuro: diminished right lateral rectus movement and ptosis, bilateral smile deficit. Bilateral upper extremity motor weakness and drift with diminished deep tendon reflexes. Lower extremity neuro exam normal. No meningeal signs.
- Skin: no rash

#### Desired Interventions

- Continued oxygen support. ABG (if ordered): $PaO_2$ 62/ $PaCO_2$, 50/$HCO_3$ 35 PH 7.30
- IVs +/- fluids
- Monitor: sinus rhythm
- CXR: furnished if ordered: normal
- Head CT: negative
- Bedside echo negative
- Labs unremarkable. Blood sugar 93.

### Time: Seven Minutes

Patient 2 arrives appearing somnolent but arousable to answering correct orientation questions.

- BP 160/100. P 86/R 12 afebrile. POx 91% on 100% ventimask
- HEENT: bilateral ptosis, deconjugate gaze, pupils 7 mm with sluggish reaction. Other cranial nerves are intact.
- Neck: supple, no JVD, stridor
- Chest: clear
- Heart: irregular rate
- Abdomen: soft, nontender

- Extremities: pulses irregular but intact. No swelling.
- Neuro: bilateral ptosis, weak smile and tongue movement. EOMI above. Weak bilateral upper extremity motor exam in all muscle groups. DTRs diminished in upper extremities.
- On Eliquis and unknown blood pressure medications

**Desired Interventions**

- Continued oxygen support. ABG (if ordered): $PaO_2$ 62/ $PaCO_2$ 55/$HCO_3$ 40 PH 7.30
- IVs +/- fluids
- Monitor: atrial fibrillation
- CXR: furnished if ordered: normal
- Head CT: negative if ordered
- Labs unremarkable other than blood sugar 110. Normal INR PT PTT
- Bedside echo if ordered negative

### Time: Seven Minutes – Patient 3

EMS calls for the transportation of a 25-year-old male with a Phx of asthma complaining shortness of breath, difficulty swallowing, double vision, vertigo, upper extremity paresthesias, and difficulty raising shoulders. Patient is alert and obeys commands. Mother worried over hoarseness. BP 105/50, P 88, R 20 POx on RA 90%. Improves to 96% on 5 L $O_2$. Patient received solumedrol and albuterol treatments en route given past history of asthma.

### Time: 10 Minutes

Stimulus: Patient 2's POx and $ETCO_2$ deteriorating. Patient 2 now with bilateral ptosis, muffled voice, and drooling. She is exhibiting bilateral leg weakness.

Participant should recognize need for advanced airway management in the face of neurological deterioration.

### Time: 11 Minutes

Stimulus: Patient 1 is also exhibiting respiratory deterioration manifested by poor excursion and global muscle weakness. Provider should recognize need for advanced airway management for Patient 1 and need for extra medical providers capable of intubation and critical care. The response to this request should be delayed enough that the provider must simultaneously intubate Patient 1 while obtaining an initial assessment of Patient 3 via a nurse and directing the staff to set up for intubating Patient 2. If the participant does not ask for more ED staff and available physicians, an ED nurse may prompt him.

### Time: 15 Minutes

Patient 3 arrives and exhibits the vital signs and neurologic deficits as noted by EMS. He is not short of breath with supplemental oxygen, after receiving aerosol treatment.

- HEENT: throat clear
- Neck: supple, no stridor
- Chest: clear, good movement. No wheezing.
- Heart: regular rate, no murmur
- Abdomen: soft nontender
- Extremites: pulses present, no swelling

- Neuro: pupils 7 mm and sluggish. Left eyelid slight ptosis. Diminished bilateral deltoid motor tone against resistance. DTRs diminished relative to lower extremities.

**Desired Interventions**

- Continued oxygen support and pulse oximetry.
- IVs +/- fluids
- Monitor: sinus rhythm
- CXR: furnished if ordered: normal
- Head CT: negative if ordered
- Labs unremarkable

Patients 1, 2, and 3 are successfully intubated. There are no more hospital ventilators. A nurse is bagging Patient 3.

### Time: 20 Minutes – Patients 4, 5, and 6

EMS call regarding transport of 55-year-old husband, 53-year-old wife, and 15-year-old son with near simultaneous complaints of weakness especially facial muscles, difficulty swallowing, double vision (wife), ptosis (husband), and upper arm motor weakness. Husband and wife are complaining of shortness of breath. All three patients, although fatigued, are alert and afebrile. They have been healthy prior to this event otherwise.

Stimulus: Participant should now recognize an evolving cohort of very similar and unusual presentations. If the provider does recognize these presentations as botulism, he should be self-motivated or by a coworker's suggestion to report this to public health. The provider will then be told by public health of reports of similar outbreaks across the country. This should trigger a call to hospital administration who will then stand up their HICS. An emergency physician and the intensivist have arrived.

### Time: 25 Minutes – Patients 4, 5, and 6 Arrive

Patients 4 and 5 are in respiratory distress requiring 100% oxygen with manual assist. They soon deteriorate, now requiring emergent intubation. Their physical exams are unremarkable other than neurological deficits and respiratory insufficiency. Their workups are similar to prior presentations with unremarkable labs, normal CXRs. Patients 4 and 5 should be presented as needing emergent intubation prior to head CT for expected demise. Patient 6 exhibits the neurologic deficits reported by EMS but is in minimal respiratory distress. His POx is 94% on 100% ventimask.

Stimulus: Participant should recognize the rapid progression of conventional ED operations through contingency to crisis. The participant should initiate mobilization of other resources including more ED staff and ICU intensivist, maximizing hospital potential patient transfers (participant should be informed that there are delays in finding transfer destinations), situation awareness for other possible victims, obtaining botulism antitoxin (the provider will learn that the Centers for Disease Control and Prevention is parceling antitoxins across the country, so there will be a delay), and more ventilators (not going to happen anytime soon).

The additional ED physician asks about the status of the hospital's crisis standard of care plan (unless the participant initiates that discussion.) The hospital completed the planning processes but did not assign critical care allocation and withdrawal of care panel members.

At this point, the son mentions that he and his parents had lunch at a restaurant as did the other patients for his birthday. A survey of Patient 3 and family members of Patients 1 and 2 reveal that all had eaten at the same restaurant.

## Time: 30 Minutes – Patient 7

EMS calls for transport of a 32-year-old patient with vomiting and epigastric pain for four hours. VS: BP 140/60 P 102 R: 16 POx 96% RA. No shortness of breath, neuro deficits other remarkable findings are reported.

The additional emergency medicine physician assumes airway management of Patient 4, while the participant stabilizes Patient 5. The intensivist admits Patients 1 and 2 to the ICU. The hospital now has no other ventilators.

Stimulus: HICS planning chief and hospital chief medical officer arrive in the ED. They confirm that public health is suspecting botulism and that there have been several other instances across the country. Bioterrorism is suspected. The state office of public health is sending personnel to the community, and the state office of emergency preparedness emergency operations center has been stood up.

A facilitated discussion should be conducted with the participant on how emergency response changes in the event of an act of terrorism (e.g. federal lead agencies, federal assets available, and the forensic characteristics that come into play) and what assets the hospital should be requesting (botulism antitoxin, ventilators, federal medical personnel, destination hospitals for anticipated transfers).

## Time: 35 Minutes – Patient 7 Arrives

Vital signs unchanged. Patient still vomiting and complaining of abdominal pain. He ate at the same restaurant as the other patients. He is found to have a T 101°F. He is lethargic but oriented. IV fluids were initiated by EMS.

- HEENT: no infection or jaundice
- Neck: supple
- Chest: clear
- Heart: regular rate, no abnormal heart sounds
- Abdomen: epigastric tenderness, no rebound or other surgical findings
- Extremities: no swelling
- Neuro: intact

### Desired Intervention

The participant should recognize that Patient 7 is probably not a case of botulism given the lack of neurological deficits and presence of fever. Discretion is allowed as to how detailed this workup needs to be and should be reported as unremarkable. Patient should be observed with continued fluids and antiemetics.

Stimulus: Patient 3's neurologic deficits are deteriorating. He now has lower extremity weakness but is maintaining POx saturations of 94% on 100% ventimask. The participant should decide not to intubate at this point given lack of resources and anticipated future demand, but he requires ICU admission.

Stimulus: HICS incident commander reports that botulism antitoxin is being flown in from the Strategic National Stockpile. Will arrive in two hours. The incident commander is conducting a meeting to discuss whether to employ the hospital crisis standards plan. The preexisting ICU patient is still not expected to survive hospitalization and ICU is now saturated with no available hospital bed. HICS will obtain a community situational awareness report for possible additional botulism cases.

What can be done to decompress the ED? The ICU? How are decisions to be made regarding allocation of critical resources? The incident commander assigns the chief medical officer to recruit who will determine future allocation and/or withdrawal of resources.

#### Patient 7 Is Improving and Is Discharged

Stimulus: antitoxin has been delivered to the hospital. A facilitated discussion should ensue to the effectiveness of antitoxin (does it cure or prevent further progression?). Participant should elect to intubate Patient 7. Which of the patients in this scenario should receive the antitoxin?

A situation awareness report from EMS does not indicate more calls suggestive of botulism. The restaurant has been identified as the source of botulism.

### Time: 40 Minutes

No further patients suggestive of botulism. Wrap-up discussion should include recovery decision making and lessons learned. This discussion should emphasize the importance of prior planning and drilling of disaster plans to include crisis standards of care.

## BIBLIOGRAPHY

Arnon SS, Schechter R, Inglesby TV, et al. Botulinum toxin as a biological weapon: medical and public health management. *JAMA*. 2001;285(8):1059–1070. doi:10.1001/jama.285.8.1059. [published correction appears in JAMA 2001 Apr 25;285(16):2081].

Chatham-Stephens K, Fleck-Derderian S, Johnson SD, et al. Clinical features of foodborne and wound botulism: a systematic review of the literature, 1932–2015. *Clin Infect Dis*. 2017;66(suppl_1):S11–S16. doi:10.1093/cid/cix811

Rao AK, Lin NH, Griese SE, Chatham-Stephens K, Badell ML, Sobel J. Clinical criteria to trigger suspicion for botulism: an evidence-based tool to facilitate timely recognition of suspected cases during sporadic events and outbreaks. *Clin Infect Dis*. 2017;66(suppl_1):S38–S42. doi:10.1093/cid/cix814

Rao AK, Sobel J, Chatham-Stephens K, Luquez C. Clinical guidelines for diagnosis and treatment of botulism, 2021. *MMWR Recomm Rep*. 2021 May 7;70(2):1–30. doi:10.15585/mmwr.rr7002a1

Rathish B, Pillay R, Wilson A, et al. Comprehensive review of bioterrorism. [Updated March 27, 2023]. In: *StatPearls* [Internet]. Treasure Island, FL: StatPearls Publishing; 2025 Jan-. www.ncbi.nlm.nih.gov/books/NBK570614/.

CASE 40

# Tularemia Outbreak in a Resource-Limited Setting

James Aiken

DISASTER PRINCIPLES

- Clinical diagnosis and treatment
- Timing of medical and surgical interventions
- Recognition and clinical treatment
- Biological disasters
- MCI triage and considerations for biological agents
- Biological safety
- Epidemiologic and medical countermeasures
- Personal protective equipment (PPE)
- Information management/communications
- Disaster triage concepts
- Local disaster response
- Hospital preparedness program
- Role of public health agencies in disaster medicine
- Public health surveillance
- Field operations and logistics
- Mass-casualty care in the field
- Field disaster triage
- Field stabilization, treatment, and transport
- Category A bioterrorism agents
- Tularemia

## 1. SCENARIO OVERVIEW

Simultaneous intentional tularemia acts of terrorism on a local community and across the country. The scenario will challenge the participants to manage numerous ED presentations of patients with illnesses having common signs and symptoms of the various tularemia presentations that overwhelm hospital conventional operations.

### Background

Al Qaeda terrorists, in response to the US assassination of their leader Ayman al-Zawahiri, spray multiple farming communities in the Midwest with weaponized *Francisella tularensis* (FT) on the same day. A farming community in Western Kentucky is subjected to aerosol exposure seven days ago with FT bacteria by low flying airplanes masquerading as pesticide planes. The eight-bed ED in this scenario is located within a 65-bed critical access community hospital that has limited critical care capabilities: six ICU beds and three functional ventilators. This is the communities' only hospital for a 50-mile radius. The hospital has a full-service lab and CT capabilities. The ED is single covered with an ED group of five emergency physicians all living within the community. There are two general internists on staff and one intensivist on call for the region available to the ED. On the day of the scenario, there are four patients in the ED awaiting floor beds. The ICU has two available beds. One current ICU patient is a 68-year-old man on a ventilator. He is expected to die. The hospital generally transfers their patients in need of higher level of care to Paducah, 65 miles away.

## 2. TEACHING OBJECTIVES AND DISCUSSION POINTS

### Teaching Objectives

1. Recognize the initial assessment and stabilization of patients presenting with various presentations of infections ranging from ulcerative glandular to pneumonia and sepsis.
2. Demonstrate ability to diagnose and treat tularemia.
3. Recognize the various stages of an evolving disaster and the contingency measures required to adjust healthcare operations to mounting demand for care including employment of hospital incident command system (HICS).
4. Recognize the need for and employ emergency management resources as the ED transitions its operations from conventional through contingency operations to crisis management.
5. Demonstrate awareness of the national emergency preparedness capabilities to respond to tularemia bioterrorism.
6. Recognize the particular features and processes of a healthcare facility/ED entering into recovery from a mass casualty disaster.

### Discussion Points

1. This scenario is intended to reinforce the recognition of tularemia presentations without available FT diagnostic capabilities with the additional challenge of supporting such patients in the setting of diminishing capabilities and transfer options.
2. Tularemia has once again been a reportable disease since 2000. On the scale presented, the participant's suspicion of bioterrorism of this Category A potential agent is paramount. What are the categories of bioterrorism agents? What makes FT a Category A weapon of bioterrorism?
3. As more cohorts present, a discussion should occur of how to transition conventional ED operations to contingency and beyond. This discussion should include who to call (house supervisor, chief medical officer [CMO], etc.) and for what purpose (for extra resources and staff, hospital bed decompression, and to initiate ED transfer processes as the hospital's ICU capabilities become overwhelmed).
4. A discussion on the recognition of the possibility of bioterrorism should ensue as the news of other similar medical presentations come in from other communities. Discuss the escalation of communications with external agencies particular to terrorism. Who do you call and who makes the call? The local, state, and federal offices of emergency preparedness and the FBI will become involved.
5. This development mandates launching the HICS and understanding how that changes the features of the mounting disaster response. How can the ED best employ their HICS? What can the ED expect from the HICS.
6. As more patients arrive, the participant will be motivated to communicate his predicament of lack of critical care capacity for incoming respiratory failure patients. The facility/emergency

manager may prompt a discussion on crisis standards of care in the event of no external transfer options. Should the 68-year-old already on a ventilator in the ICU be reassessed for discontinuation of care to allow access to critical care capabilities for an incoming patient with a greater chance of survival? How should these decisions be made? What are the ethical considerations involved?

7. Discuss when and how to initiate operational recovery from the disaster. How does this process segue with the community hot zone?

## 3. SUPPLIES

- Oxygen delivery masks
- Pulse ox equipment
- Intubation equipment: endotracheal tubes, laryngoscopes, Eschmann bougies, laryngeal mask airways, BVM
- Suction
- The ED has one ventilator, ICU has three. One BiPAP machine.
- $ETCO_2$
- IV equipment
- Thermometers
- ECGCardiac monitor
- Customary emergent airway management drugs
- Standard provider PPE

## 4. IMAGES AND LABS

- Full lab capacity
- Venous blood gas/arterial blood gas COVID rapid testing available
- Apart from cultures, the lab does not have FT detection capabilities.
- Chest X-ray CT
- Bedside ultrasound

## 5. PHARMACY

Full-service antibiotic inventory

## 6. ACTORS (CONFEDERATES) AND THEIR ROLES

Ten patients (number can be adjusted according to desired scope of the disaster and length of scenario) aged 15 to 62 years of age with varying levels of glandular disease, respiratory distress, and sepsis interspersed with critically ill patients not found to have tularemia. The patients infected with tularemia share the common experience of having been outside at a state fair on the day of the spraying a week ago.

### Confederates

- Single emergency medicine MD coverage with two ED nurses initially; the hospital is only partially staffed with nurses that day given a high sick call-in.

- One hospital respiratory technician
- CMO; can double as HICS incident commander
- CEO makes a delayed appearance
- Facility manager

## 7. MOULAGE

Reddened masses to neck and groin. Can use pictures in the absence of actors or simulation mannequins.

## 8. STIMULI

- Pictures of patients with ulcerative glandular disease
- Pictures of tularemia CXR
- Picture of community-acquired pneumonia CXR
- Picture of congestive heart failure

## 9. TIMELINE AND TRANSITION POINTS

### Time: Zero – Patient 1

EMS calls regarding transport of a 35-year-old male complaining of fever and shortness of breath for the past two days. He has a dry cough and occasional vomiting.

Vital signs are POx 90% on RA, pulse rate 100 BP 118/62 R 24He is alert and oriented but appears anxious and obeys all commands. POx improves to 96% on 100% ventimask.

### Time: Two Minutes – Patient 2

EMS calls regarding a 66-year-old female with Phx of congestive heart failure being transported for complaints of shortness of breath, productive cough, pleuritic chest pains and fever for three days. Vital signs are BP 98/58 P 116 R 26 POx 88% on RA, which improves to 92% on nonrebreather.

On initial field assessment the paramedics report that the patient is oriented but in obvious respiratory distress.

### Time: 10 Minutes – Patient 1 Arrives

Vital signs, POx, and appearance are confirmed. BP 122/62; P 110; R 28 T 100°F POx 95%

- Gen: Fatigued, in moderate respiratory distress
- HEENT: Pharynx erythematous without exudate
- Neck: multiple cervical lesions/adenopathy (Figure 40.1), otherwise supple, no JVD, stridor
- Chest: poor air movement, bilateral expiratory wheezing and crackling. (Figure 40.2)
- Heart: regular rate, no murmurs
- Abdomen: soft nontender
- Extremity: all pulses present. No swelling or adenopathy.
- Neuro: intact, oriented.
- Skin: no rash or other lesions

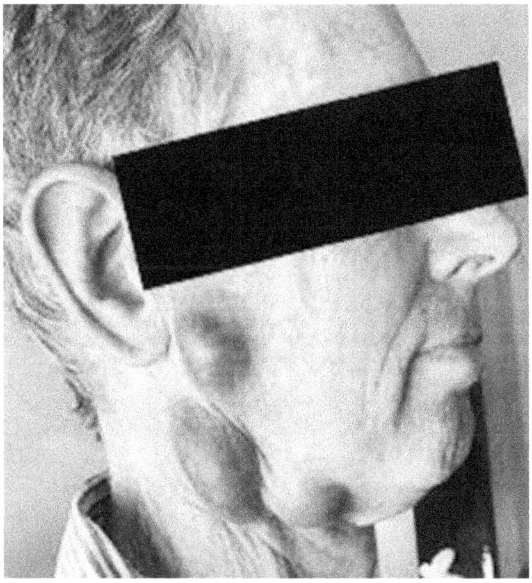

**Figure 40.1** Tularemia adenopathy: Patient 1.

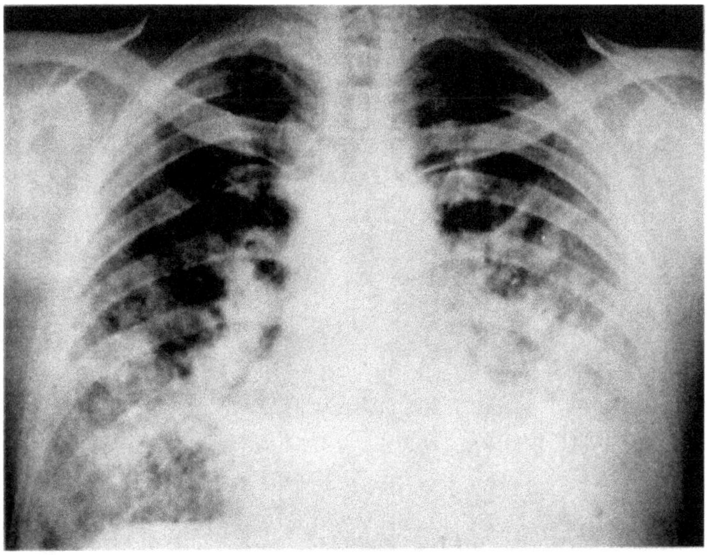

**Figure 40.2** Tularemia pneumonia: Patient 1.

**Desired Interventions**

Continued oxygen support. ABG (if ordered): $PaO_2$ 62/$PaCO_2$, 50/$HCO_3$ 35 PH 7.30 Place on $ETCO_2$

- IVs +fluids
- Monitor: sinus rhythm
- CXR: furnished if ordered: abnormal as pictured. Typical tularemia pneumonia. Bedside echo, if ordered, negative. No right ventricular strain.
- Labs: WBC 18 000 with shift, lactate 2.6 otherwise unremarkable

## Time: 15 Minutes

Patient 2 arrives appearing somnolent but arousable to answering orientation questions correctly. BP 160/100. P 86/ R 12 T 102°F. POx 94% on 100% ventimask

- HEENT: pharynx erythematous without exudate. Ears clear.
- Neck: supple, no JVD, stridor
- Chest: right mid rales and e a changes
- Heart: irregular rate normal heart sounds
- Abdomen: soft, nontender
- Extremities: pulses irregular but intact. No swelling, adenopathy.
- Neuro: somnolent but easily arousable
- Phx: atrial fibrillation, hypertension
- Meds: Eliquis and unknown blood pressure medications

**Desired Interventions**

Continued oxygen support. ABG (if ordered): $PaO_2$ 62/$PaCO_2$ 55/$HCO_3$ 40 PH 7.30 IVs + fluids, may give cautiously

Monitor: atrial fibrillation
CXR: furnished if ordered: community-acquired pneumonia (Figure 40.3)
Labs: WBC 17 000 with shift. Lactate 1.8; normal troponin and INR, BNP 630.

Bedside cardiac echo if ordered negative. IVC 50% collapsible. No right ventricular strain. Antibiotics

## Time: 22 Minutes – Patient 3

EMS calls report on a 25-year-old male with a Phx of asthma complaining sore throat, shortness of breath, fever, vomiting, and dry cough for four days. Has run out of inhaler from continued use.

BP 112/55, P 102, R 26 POx on RA 90%. Improves to 96% on 5 L $O_2$. Patient received solumedrol and albuterol treatments en route given past history of asthma.

## Time: 26 Minutes

Stimulus: Patient 1 is in respiratory distress and deteriorating. The patient appears to be weakening. POx now 92 on 100% on 15 L nonrebreather and $ETCO_2$ if employed, shows 52.

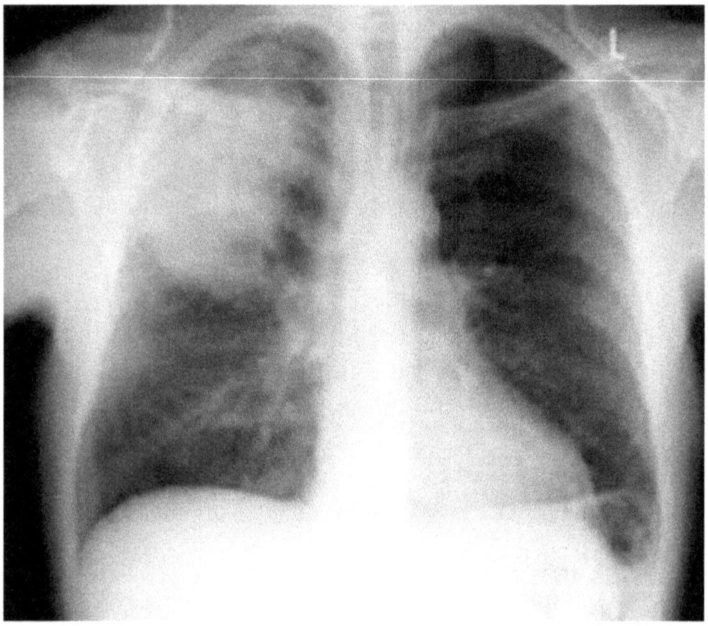

**Figure 40.3** Community-acquired pneumonia: Patient 2.

Participant should recognize need for advanced airway management. BiPAP is available but have patient tire quickly if used to stimulate decision to intubate.

## Time: 30 Minutes

Stimulus: Patient 2 is also exhibiting respiratory deterioration manifested by increased respiratory rate and decreased POx to 90% by provider should recognize need for advanced airway management for Patient 2. The patient may elect BiPAP, but the hospital has only one available machine. The provider must decide how to allocate resources for his two deteriorating patients with a third incoming.

## Time: 35 Minutes

Patient 3 arrives. He is not short of breath with supplemental oxygen, after receiving aerosol and steroid treatment, but appears ill.

BP 112/52 P 98 R 22 T 100.4°F POx 98 on 5 L.
HEENT: exudate to throat (Figure 40.4)
Neck: supple, no stridor. Right cervical lesion seen in Figure 40.4.
Chest: clear, good movement. Expiratory wheezing to all fields
Heart: regular rate, no murmur
Abdomen: soft nontender
Extremities: pulses present, no swelling or other adenopathy.
Neuro: intact. No meningeal signs

### Desired Interventions

Continued oxygen support and pulse oximetry. IVs +/- fluids
Continued aerosol treatments
Monitor: sinus rhythm
CXR if ordered: normal
Labs unremarkable. Strept screen not available. Antibiotics.

## Time: 45 Minutes – Patients 4 and 5

EMS call regarding transport of a 28-year-old husband and 32-year-old wife. The husband (Patient 4) is complaining of fever, dry cough, and shortness of breath. The wife (Patient 5) is complaining of several ulcerative lesions and masses to her neck and groin. The husband is in extremis and is becoming confused. His BP is 100/50; P 120; R 32; POx 88% on room air that improved to 92% on 15 L rebreather mask. The wife's vital signs are BP 112/62; P 88; R 20; POx 95% on room air.

## Time: 50 Minutes

The provider needs to be stimulated to address the airway needs of Patient 1 and 2 while Patients 4 and 5 are en route. Patient 1's condition should be described to encourage intubation of him with the sole BiPAP machine transferred to Patient 2.

## Time: 55 Minutes – Patients 4 and 5 Arrive

Patient 4 is in respiratory distress requiring 100% oxygen with manual assist. He soon deteriorates, now requiring emergent intubation.

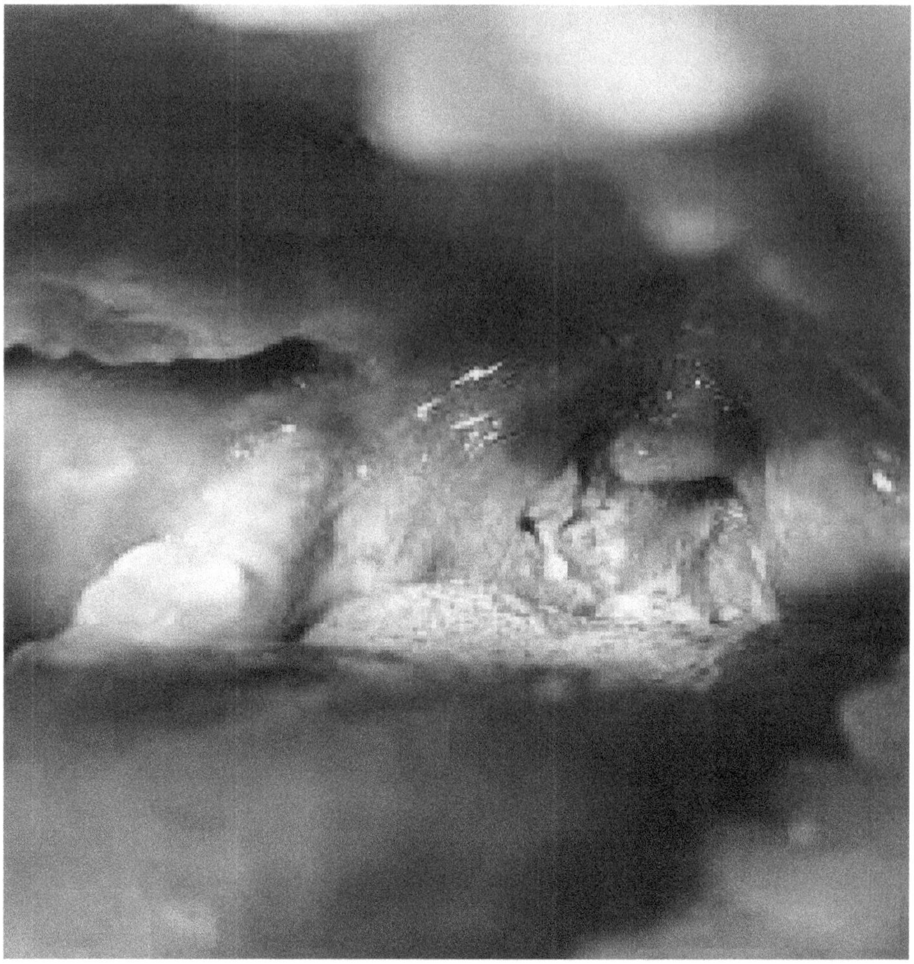

**Figure 40.4** Typical pharyngeal exudate that could be seen in tularemia: Patient 3.

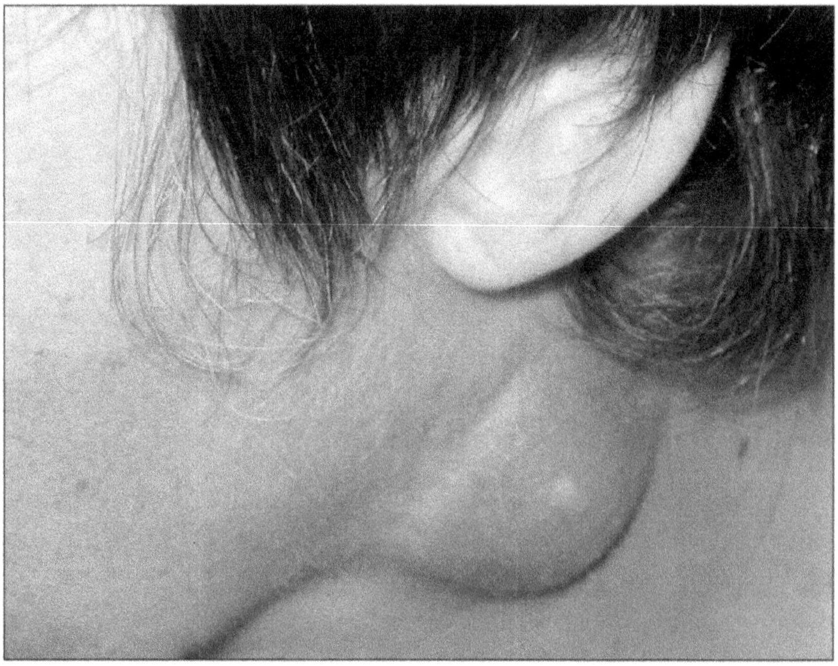

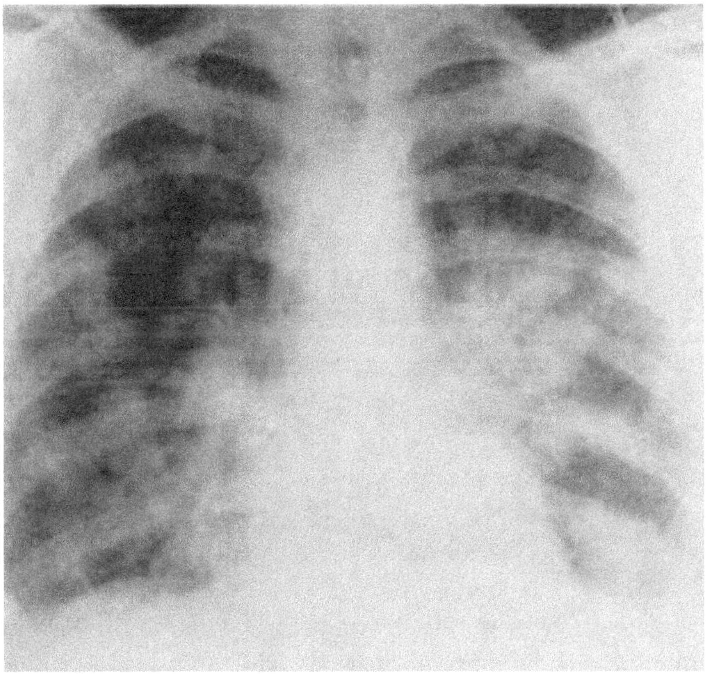

**Figure 40.5** Tularemia pneumonia: Patient 4.

### Patient 4

BP 90/58 P120 R 30 T 101°F
In extremis
HEENT: throat clear
Neck: no JVD or stridor
Chest: Bilateral rales, poor air movement (Figure 40.5)
Heart: normal hear sounds
Abdomen: soft nontender
Ext: no swelling or adenopathy
Neuro: no meningeal signs.

### Desired Interventions

This patient clearly requires intubation.
Fluids, vasopressors
Antibiotics
If bedside ultrasound employed: hyperdynamic cardiac function with collapsed IVC WBC 19 000 with shift. Lactate 3.2 other unremarkable.

### Patient 5

Vital signs are BP 112/62: P 88; R 20; T 100°F POx 95% on RA.

HEENT: pharynx erythematous without exudate
Neck: enlarged adenopathy similar to Patient 1 (Figure 40.6)
Chest: scattered faint expiratory wheezing. Good air movement.
Abdomen: soft nontender
Ext: bilateral inguinal adenopathy
CXR: negative
WBC 14 000
Lactic 1.8

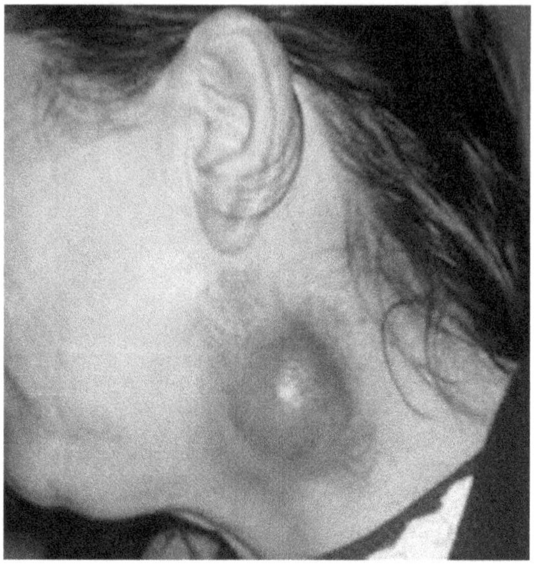

**Figure 40.6** Cervical adenopathy seen in tularemia: Patient 5.

Stimulus: The ED receives a call from the state office of public health asking whether the ED has been seeing any unusual presentations of pneumonia and glandular diseases. The office is also asking whether any such patients attended a regional state fair a week ago. Patients 5 and 3 replied affirmatively. Patient 2 says no. The public health officer says they are very concerned about weaponized FT act of terrorism.

Participant should now recognize an evolving cohort of very similar and unusual presentations. If the provider does recognize these presentations as tularemia, he should also begin the process to call another emergency medicine provider into the ED and alert ICU of potential mass presentations. The provider will then be told by public health of reports of similar outbreaks across the country. This should trigger a call to hospital administration. The CMO advises the ED to stand by. He plans to initiate a limited HICS in the absence of the hospital CEO. Participant should be encouraged to request immediate floor acceptance of his four holding patients. How could this be accomplished? The CMO tells the participant to have patients sent upstairs. He will work with nursing leadership to accommodate.

### Time: 75 Minutes

Patient 1 is intubated on the sole ED ventilator. Patient 2 is tolerating BiPAP and being watched closely for fatigue. The ICU intensivist agrees to come in and will take Patient 1 to the ICU. The ED is now saturated. The provider turns his attention to Patient 3 and should be prompted to intubate.

Stimulus: Participant should recognize the rapid progression of conventional ED operations through contingency to crisis. The provider should understand the need to call in extra emergency physicians and alert ICU of the situation. The participant should discuss the need to initiate mobilization of other resources including potential patient transfers, community situation awareness for other possible victims, and inventorying resources (antibiotics for FT, advanced airway equipment, etc). Participant is encouraged to call HICS with their thoughts.

### Time: 90 Minutes – Patient 6

EMS calls regarding a 62-year-old patient with fever, shortness of breath and dry cough for three days. Has a past history of COPD. VS: BP 140/60 P 102 R: 16 POx 92% RA, which improved to 96% on 100% rebreather.

An additional emergency medicine physician arrives and assumes airway management of Patient 3, while the participant communicates with administration. The intensivist admits Patients 1 and 2 to the ICU, but more ICU nurses will need to be called in.

Stimulus: HICS planning chief and hospital CMO arrive in the ED. They confirm that public health is suspecting tularemia and that there have been several other instances across the country including Paducah. Bioterrorism is suspected. The state office of public health is sending personnel to the community, and the state office of emergency preparedness emergency operations center (EOC) has been set up.

A facilitated discussion should be conducted with the participant on how emergency response changes in the event of an act of terrorism (e.g. federal lead agencies, federal assets available, and the forensic activities that come into play) and what assets the hospital should be requesting (medications, ventilators, federal medical personnel, destination hospitals for anticipated transfers).

## Time: 110 Minutes – Patient 6 Arrives

VS: BP 140/60 P 102 R: 16 POx 92% on 100% rebreather. He looks ill. He is found to have a T 101°F. He is lethargic but oriented. IV fluids were initiated by EMS.

HEENT: no infection or jaundice
Neck: supple
Chest: clear (Figure 40.7)
Heart: regular rate, no abnormal heart sounds
Abdomen: epigastric tenderness, no rebound or other surgical findings
Extremities: no swelling
Neuro: intact. No meningeal signs
WBC 23 000
Lactate 3.6
Other labs including cardiac markers and D-dimer, if ordered, are unremarkable

### Desired Intervention

Fluids and antibiotics are ordered for Patient 6. The ED provider suspects that Patient 2 might not have tularemia but can elect to give antibiotics. (However, a discussion should be triggered on the need to maintain stewardship of antibiotics considering that the triage nurse is reporting that 10 patients are checking in with similar complaints of fever, sore throat, neck masses and cough. One has additional eye infection.)

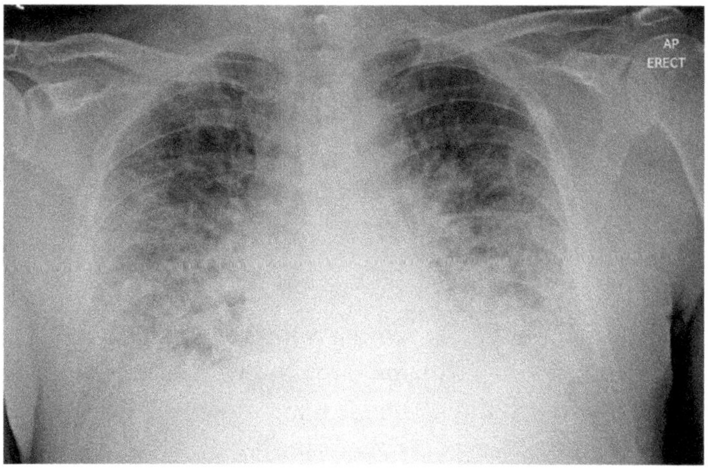


**Figure 40.7** Tularemia pneumonia: Patient 6.

Stimulus: Patient 4 should be intubated. Patient 6's respiratory condition is also deteriorating. He is clearly fatigued with diffuse inspiratory and expiratory wheezing and rales. The participant should be encouraged to intubate him. Patient 2 still requires the BiPAP. This depletes the hospital of ventilators.

### Time: 130 Minutes – Patient 7

EMS calls regarding transport of an 85-year-old male with PHx of coronary artery disease with complaints of fever, cough, shortness of breath, chest pains, and vomiting. BP 210/130 P 88 R 18 POx 94% on RA.

Stimulus: The hospital CEO has arrived and assumed the role of incident commander and has convened a planning meeting. Branch chief level HICS has been established. Afterwards, the CMO reports to the ED to provide a situational awareness briefing. The ICU is now saturated with no available hospital beds. All elective services have been suspended and calls to medical staff to decompress the floors are being made. More patients are checking in having arrived on their own. The preexisting elderly ICU patient is still not expected to survive hospitalization. The CEO and CMO have decided not to consider termination of treatment of this patient at this time, but the next planning meeting has crisis standards on the agenda pending consultation with the state office of health and hospitals. Search is underway for destination hospitals for patient transfer.

What can be done to decompress the ED? What does it mean to invoke crisis standards? Does it mean triage critical care to those patients with the best chance to survive (how do you make that comparative assessment?) going forward and/or termination of critical care for those with diminished outcome expectations compared to those now presenting for critical services.

Participant should be prompted to recommend opening alternative treatment areas for the less critical. Triage can also be instructed to add attendance at the state fair last week to their screening and cohort accordingly. Triage can also be directed to establish cohort areas for triaging tularemia suspected patients. Only those requiring respiratory support should be brought back to the ED. HICS has not located destinations for potential patient transfers due to simultaneous overwhelming demand for services in regional hospitals.

### Time: 143 Minutes – Patient 7 Arrives

Vital signs: BP 260/132 P 102 R 28 POx 94 on 100% rebreather. Patient is afebrile. The patient appears in respiratory distress but is oriented and obeys commands. The patient did not attend the state fair.

HEENT: clear
Neck: + JVD, no adenopathy
Chest: diffuse crackling and wheezing (Figure 40.8)
Heart: irregular rate (ECG reveals atrial fibrillation)
Abdomen: soft nontender
Ext: 3+ bilateral pitting edema
Lab: WBC 14 000
Troponin mildly elevated; BNP 2340

#### Desired Intervention

Can the participant distinguish nontularemia presentations with similar symptoms? Or should the provider give all such patients antibiotics? If the participant treats the patient for hypertensive crisis with pulmonary edema, the patient improves but is tiring. If the patient is treated with antibiotics and fluids, the patient becomes even more critical requiring advanced airway support.

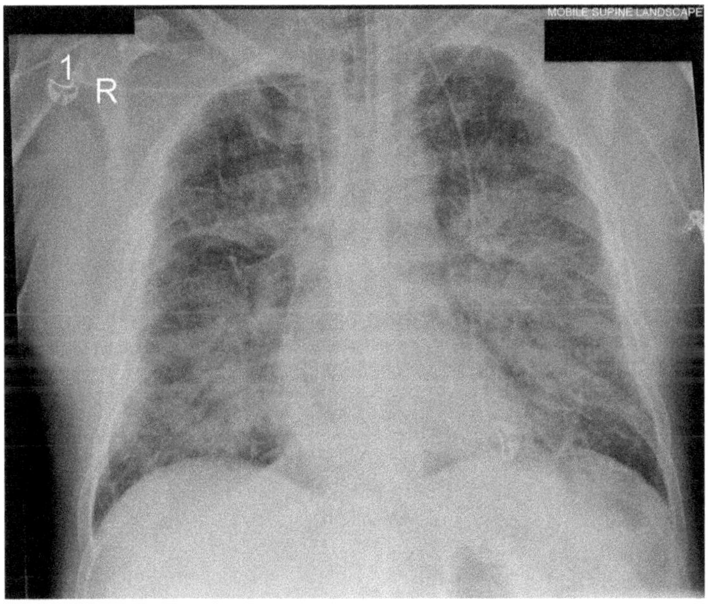


**Figure 40.8** Congestive heart failure: Patient 7.

### Time: 145 Minutes – Patients 8 and 9

EMS calls for transport of 65-year-old mother and 32-year-old daughter with near simultaneous onset of fever, cough, and shortness of breath. The mother has metastatic lung cancer and has a six-month prognosis. Mother's vital signs are BP 98/60 P 112 R 30, POx 90% on 100% rebreather. Her lungs sound "congested." The daughter's vital signs are BP 106/76 P 100 R 24 POx 96% on 5 L nasal cannula (EMS has run out of rebreather masks). She appears more stable than her mother.

### Time: 160 Minutes – Patients 8 and 9 Arrive

The mother is in respiratory distress. Her POx is 92% on 100% ventimask with inadequate chest wall excursions. Both patients are febrile. The daughter's POx is 96% on 5 L $O_2$. She appears ill but not in need of advanced airway support. The ED is now saturated. Both patients should receive fluids and antibiotics for tularemia.

**Desired Intervention**

Participant should elect to intubate the mother given expected demise. Instructor can have a nurse who is active in hospital emergency preparedness question whether this patient with a limited life expectancy should receive critical care in the setting of diminishing critical care capacity. As there are no ventilators available, nurse assistants are mobilized to bag.

### Time: 163 Minutes

Stimulus: HICS has identified a receiving hospital to accept a critical patient. Which one should be sent? An alternative treatment area has been established.

### Time: 175 Minutes

EMS calls regarding a 45-year-old male daily user of tobacco with a Phx of sarcoidosis on steroids with a two-day history of progressive fever, cough, and shortness of breath. He worked for a state fair vendor. VS: BP 134/76 P 111 R 28. POx 92 on 5 L. He is getting albuterol inhalation therapy en route.

Stimulus: The CMO calls the ED to report that the state EOC is reporting diminishing regional ED presentations of critical tularemia patients. State air med companies are being contracted to widen the radius of potential patient transfer. Extra personnel are arriving at the hospital. No more ventilators can be expected. The CMO reports that the hospital EOC leadership had declined to activate a crisis standard plan. The hospital had not done such planning in the past.

### Time: 182 Minutes – Patient 10 Arrives

VS: BP 88/50. P 120, R 32 T 104°F The patient is confused and clammy. He is not able to answer questions regarding state fair attendance. He has diffuse rales and wheezing. No other pertinent findings. He should be intubated immediately with fluids and broad-spectrum antibiotics. Another nurse assistant is recruited to bag the patient.

### Time: 190 Minutes

Stimulus: regardless of the state report of diminishing regional critical ED presentations, how should this ED and hospital plan for continued expected demand for services or to initiate recovery. How does the hospital staff to handle high stress, high volume demand for care? There should be provider awareness that healthcare recovery always lags behind the hot zone perspective especially for epidemics/pandemics and acts of terrorism.

The scenario can be terminated here with a final discussion on the particular features of the impact of bioterrorism on health care, the need for prior planning and training, the need for robust HICS capabilities and the awareness to employ innovative thinking in the actual response (cohort/forward triage, alternative treatment sites, alternative staffing scheduling to ensure staff wellness, spiritual support, etc.).

## BIBLIOGRAPHY

Adalja AA, Toner E, Inglesby TV. Clinical management of potential bioterrorism-related conditions. *N Engl J Med.* 2015;372:954–962. doi:10.1056/NEJMra1409755.

Celli J, Zahrt TC. Mechanisms of *Francisella tularensis* intracellular pathogenesis. *Cold Spring Harb Perspect Med.* 2013 Apr 1;3(4):a010314. doi:10.1101/cshperspect.a010314. PMID: 23545572; PMCID: PMC3683997.

Kelson M, Burnett J, Girgis S, Bakr M. Tularemia: the resurgence of a diagnostic challenge and clinical dilemma in the United States. *Cureus.* 2022 July 27;14(7):e27363. doi:10.7759/cureus.27363. PMID: 36046284; PMCID: PMC9417589.

Rathish B, Pillay R, Wilson A, et al. Comprehensive review of bioterrorism. [Updated April 5, 2022]. In: *StatPearls* [Internet]. Treasure Island, FL: StatPearls Publishing; 2022 Jan-. www.ncbi.nlm.nih.gov/books/NBK570614/. Accessed April 11, 2025.

Thomas LD, Schaffner W. Tularemia pneumonia. *Infect Dis Clin North Am.* 2010;24(1):43–55.

CASE 41

# Stampede Survival

## Treating Traumatic Asphyxiation and Mass Casualty Injuries

Christopher Hayden

DISASTER PRINCIPLES

- Clinical diagnosis and treatment
- Information management/communications
- Timing of medical and surgical interventions
- Recognition and clinical treatment
- Field operations and logistics
- Field disaster triage
- Field stabilization, treatment, and transport
- Stampede injuries
- Mass gatherings

### 1. BACKGROUND

A human stampede or crush occurs when a large number of people, often at an event or gathering, attempt to rapidly egress from an area through a limited number of exits. These exits become choke points preventing orderly egress and this can result in many injuries. Injuries from this type of event fall into two broad categories: trampling injuries and crush or asphyxiation injuries. The former occurs if people fall to the ground and are stepped on whereas the latter typically occur as people are pressed against a hard surface or are so compressed by those around them that they cannot breathe. This is referred to as traumatic asphyxiation. These events tend to occur in indoor venues and can be challenging not only because of the number of potential casualties involved but also because EMS response can be hampered by the same ingress/egress issues that cause the injuries in the first place.

### 2. SCENARIO OVERVIEW

A local county fair has been set up for the weekend. At the time of the incident there were around 300 people enjoying an indoor event. A fire was ignited by flammable material near a hot light and, although the blaze was small, some in the crowd began to panic and push their way toward the only open door.

The patient is a 26-year-old female who was trying to exit with her husband when they became separated. He saw her become compressed against a wall and then fall to the ground in the flow of traffic toward the only open door. Report from EMS crew is a female patient who is minimally responsive with Glasgow Coma Scale (GCS) of 11 (E3 V4 M4) vitals with blood pressure 86/P heart rate 136 with $O_2$ saturation of 88% on NRB mask at 15 LPM and nasopharyngeal airway. There is a small amount of bleeding from the nose with multiple bursas across the patient's chest. At this time unable to assess breath sounds due to the environment with no other interventions having been performed.

The hospital the patient is being transferred to has an eight-bed ED located within a single 50-bed community hospital with limited critical care capabilities. There are two ICU beds and ventilators. The hospital has a full-service lab and CT capabilities. The ED is single coverage with six ED physicians, three of whom live in the community. There are three general internists with two midlevel providers on staff. The ICU is open and managed by the admitting internist and an intensivist who can be consulted as needed. The hospital administration has received rudimentary training on hospital indecent command and maintains joint commission emergency management standards. The local fire department chief is the emergency manager. On the day of the scenario there are four patients in the ED: two are awaiting transfer, one awaiting a floor bed, and one whose workup has just begun. The ICU has no beds available and one ventilator for use if needed.

## 3. TEACHING OBJECTIVES AND DISCUSSION POINTS

### Teaching Objectives

1. Perform basic trauma assessment and stabilization in the patient with respiratory distress.
2. Demonstrate ability to diagnose traumatic asphyxiation
3. Demonstrate ability to treat traumatic asphyxiation
4. Recognize the need for immediate transfer to a trauma center.
5. Demonstrate consideration of additional pathology from a structure fire including CO and cyanide poisoning.

### Discussion Points

1. This scenario is intended to reinforce the recognition of the severe chest trauma following traumatic injury in a small rule hospital with limited resources and a transport time by ground of two hours to the nearest hospital. The participants will demonstrate awareness to anticipate the need for advanced airway support in the setting of limited resources. The participants will demonstrate awareness to anticipate the need for chest tube placement or performance of finger thoracotomy to aid with respiratory distress in a patient with blunt chest trauma in a resource limited area.
2. As more patients present to the ED, the provider should recognize the need to obtain additional medical support and should activate the hospital's incident command system.
3. Upon recognition of multisystem trauma and need for major intervention, the participant should initiate the transfer process. This could include air medical or critical care ground. The EMS providers who brought the patient are not qualified by their training to transport the patient.
4. The provider should also, when the patient is stabilized, evaluate all patients in the waiting room via rapid triage and arrange their care to include transfer to another facility as required.

## 4. SUPPLIES

- Standard PPE
- Oxygen delivery mask
- Pulse oximeter
- BVM
- Intubation equipment: endotracheal tubes, laryngoscopes, boogies, backup airway (various supra-glottic airways), and cricothyrotomy kit
- Chest tube set-up or ability to perform finger (simple) thoracostomy

- Suction
- $ETCO_2$
- IV equipment
- Thermometers
- ECG
- Cardiac monitor
- Standard ED medications including medications for rapid sequence intubation

## 5. IMAGES AND LABS

- Point of care testing glucose
- CBC
- Type and screen
- CMP
- Lactic acid
- VBG
- PT/INR
- PTT
- Urine and serum HCG
- Urinalysis
- Urine tox
- Chest X-ray
- CT
- Bedside ultrasound

## 6. ACTORS

a. Patient's husband (around the patient's age) who is frantic but able to answer questions
b. Three nurses in the emergency department
c. Respiratory therapist
d. CT tech who doubles as the X-ray tech
e. Two EMT-Basics able to assist as needed

## 7. MOULAGE

The patient should have a bluish color or darkening of the skin around the neck and face. There should be some petechiae around the face and the eyes should have subconjunctival hemorrhages, chemosis, and bruising around the eyelids.

## 8. TIMELINE

### Time: Zero – Patient 1

EMS calls regarding transportation of a 26-year-old female with complaints of shortness of breath, chest pain, with nausea, following a stampede of people at the local fair. The patient's blood pressure is 86 by palpation, heart rate is 136 and she is saturating 88% on a nonrebreather mask at 15 LPM with a nasopharyngeal airway that was placed due to the patient's decreased GCS.

### Time: Five Minutes

Patient 1 arrives.

- Airway intact and patient is attempting to speak while lifting her head off the bed, therefore protected.
- Breathing is shallow and there are diminished breath sounds in bilateral lungs.
- There are 2+ pulses in both upper and lower extremities.
- Patient's GCS is 11.
- Patient is rolled and able to clinch her cheeks with no blood noted; therefore, rectal is deferred at this time.
- Vital signs: Pow blood pressure is confirmed, low pulse ox confirmed with point of care glucose 168
- Gen: Patient is in distress, mumbles her answers but keeps saying "my chest hurts" and "I cannot breathe." Swelling is noted to her face and eyelids with bruising and petechiae noted to her chest and face.
- HEENT: Eyelids and face are swollen. There are subconjunctival hemorrhages, chemosis, and petechia noted to bilateral eyes with no blood behind the TM or CSF drainage.
- Neck: Jugular venous pressure is present, darkening of the skin is noted, with no stridor or tracheal deviation at this time.
- Chest: Darkening of the skin is noted from around the middle of the chest. There is bruising noted to bilateral chest with crepitus felt with palpation. The patient has minimal air movement and breath sounds are diminished bilaterally.
- Heart: tachycardia with no murmurs present
- Extremities: all pulses present with bruising noted to multiple areas of both the upper and lower extremities with no obvious fractures appreciated.
- Neuro: Patient is moaning, she is responsive to pain, and at times yelling her chest hurts and she cannot breathe. The is not able to participate in full neuro exam due to agitation and she is unable to open her eyes because of pain and swelling.
- Skin: bruising noted to multiple areas of the patient body with petechiae noted to the chest, face, and eyes.

**Critical Actions**

- Complete primary and secondary survey in a prompt fashion (five minutes)
- Place patient on the monitor and obtain vital signs
- Start two large-bore IVs
- Initiate blood products
- Trauma labs to include pregnancy test
- Point of care blood sugar
- Start Extended Focused Assessment with Sonography for Trauma (EFAST)
- Recognize the patient is too unstable for your facility and have the nursing staff call the transfer center to start transfer

### Time: Seven Minutes

Patient becomes more confused and is pulling her mask off her face. She is flailing her arms and is yelling she cannot breathe.

**Critical Actions**

- On bedside E-FAST you notice right sided pleural effusion with no lung sliding, RUQ clear, LUQ clear, bladder clear and uterus is normal without overt signs of pregnancy.
- Prepare patient for intubation.
- Make sure you have the proper equipment, and that the equipment is working.
- Place endotracheal tube.
- Check placement with $ETCO_2$ as well as normal assessment methods.
- Place patient on the vent with lung protective strategy.
- Consider proper sedation strategies for patients with hypotension.
- Order chest X-ray and blood gas and have the nurses place an NG tube.
- Place chest tube or perform finger thoracostomy.
- If blood not started need to initiate blood therapy.

### Time: 15 Minutes

Patient's oxygen saturation is increased and there is better air movement. Patient is stable on sedation and pain management. Patient's husband is questioning what is next and calling family members to advise of the patient's current predicament.

**Critical Actions**

- At this time, the participant should recognize the patient is suffering from traumatic asphyxiation complicated by a hemothorax.
- Transfer should be arranged, and helicopter crew is on their way to get the patient.
- Vitals reassessed and now with BP 136/86 HR 110, oxygen saturation 95% with better air movement in the right lung.
- Initiate triage system for patients in the waiting room using a standard methodology such as Simple Triage and Rapid Treatment.

### Time: 30 Minutes

- Helicopter transport has arrived.
- Patient report is given with proper information labs are still pending.
- Additional patients assigned to ED are currently being worked on by other staff who are available.
- Additional transport units should be en route to aid with extra patients as needed.
- Scenario ends.

## BIBLIOGRAPHY

American College of Surgeons Committee on Trauma. *Advanced Trauma Life Support.* 10th ed. Chicago: American College of Surgeons; 2012.

Anft M. When humans stampede. *Johns Hopkins Magazine.* 2010, December 8. https://magazine.jhu.edu/2010/12/08/when-humans-stampede/. Accessed April 10, 2025.

Hsieh YH, Ngai KM, Burkle FM Jr, Hsu EB. Epidemiological characteristics of human stampedes. Disaster Med Public Health Prep. 2009 Dec;3(4):217–223. doi:10.1097/DMP.0b013e3181c5b4ba. PMID: 20081418.

Hubble MW, et al. Chapter 14: Chest trauma. In Hubble MW, Hubble JP, eds. *Principles of Advanced Trauma Care*. Albany, NY: Delmar/Thompson Learning, 2002.

Netherton S, Milenkovic V, Taylor M, Davis PJ. Diagnostic accuracy of eFAST in the trauma patient: a systematic review and meta-analysis. *CJEM*. 2019 Nov;21(6):727–738. doi:10.1017/cem.2019.381. PMID: 31317856.

Ngai KM, Burkle F, Hsu A, Hsu E. Human stampedes: a systematic review of historical and peer-reviewed sources. *Disaster Med Public Health Prep*. 2009;3:191–195. doi:10.1097/DMP.0b013e3181c5b494.

SALT mass casualty triage: concept endorsed by the American College of Emergency Physicians, American College of Surgeons Committee on Trauma, American Trauma Society, National Association of EMS Physicians, National Disaster Life Support Education Consortium, and State and Territorial Injury Prevention Directors Association. *Disaster Med Public Health Prep*. 2008 Dec;2(4):245–246. doi:10.1097/DMP.0b013e31818d191e. PMID: 19050431.

Svenson JE, O'Connor JE, Lindsay MB. Is air transport faster? A comparison of air versus ground transport times for interfacility transfers in a regional referral system. *Air Med J*. 2006 July–Aug;25(4):170–172. doi:10.1016/j.amj.2006.04.003. PMID: 16818167.

Tintinalli JE, Stapczynski JS, Ma O, et al. *Tintinalli's Emergency Medicine: A Comprehensive Study Guide*. 9th ed. New York: McGraw Hill Education; 2020. Kindle Edition.

CASE 42

# Terror at Mardi Gras

## Mass Casualties after a Truck Ramming Incident

Larissa H. Unruh and James P. Phillips

DISASTER PRINCIPLES

- Clinical diagnosis and treatment
- Timing of medical and surgical interventions
- Scene safety and security in the field
- Disaster triage concepts
- Mass-casualty incidents
- Field operations and logistics
- Mass-casualty care in the field
- Field disaster triage
- Field stabilization, treatment, and transport
- Disaster operations
- EMS disaster operations
- Transportation disasters
- Fireground safety

### 1. SCENARIO OVERVIEW

Patient 1: A 23-year-old man with unknown past medical history is participating in a parade for Mardi Gras in New Orleans when he hears screams behind him and the roar of a loud engine. A large pickup truck had pulled out of a parking garage and accelerated to approximately 40 miles per hour while swerving into the parade route. He lost consciousness immediately when the truck struck him on his right side, throwing him several feet onto the concrete sidewalk. There are an unknown number of additional victims on the scene. Participant(s) are ALS ambulance on scene.

Patient 2: A 37-year-old woman with no past medical history was also watching this parade from some bleachers that are set up along the parade route. When she sees the truck swerve into the crowd she attempts to get down from the bleachers. Upon jumping off the bleachers she hears a crack, feels a sharp pain in her right lower leg and ankle region, and sees an obvious deformity to her lower leg/ankle. She is awake and alert but unable to walk and endorses severe pain when first responders arrive.

Patient 3: A 63-year-old man on blood thinners for atrial fibrillation was at the parade with this family. He trips as he is trying to vacate the area and strikes his head on a street sign. When first responders arrive, his wife tells them that he did lose consciousness briefly when he fell. There is a notable laceration on his forehead that is briskly bleeding. He is awake but appears confused.

## 2. TEACHING OBJECTIVES AND DISCUSSION POINTS

**Clinical and Medical Management**

- Scene safety assessment
- Airway assessment
- Breathing assessment
- Circulation assessment and hemorrhage control
- Secondary survey
- Stabilize C-spine

**Communication and Teamwork**

- Early call for police/security backup
- Crowd control
- Delegation of tasks
- Alert hospital of arrival
- Transport to hospital

## 3. SUPPLIES

- C-collar
- Tourniquet
- Limb immobilizers
- Intubation equipment
- Finger pulse ox
- Portable monitor
- BVM
- IO line
- IV supplies
- Manual blood pressure cuff
- Normal saline
- Chest tube/needle decompression supplies

## 4. MOULAGE

- Bruising to right ribs
- Flail chest right side
- Deformity to right upper leg with large ecchymosis of anterolateral thigh
- Laceration on scalp with profuse active bleeding

## 5. IMAGES AND LABS

- None

## 6. ACTORS

- Patient: unresponsive
- Bystander crowd: some try to be helpful; most are spectators taking photos and videos
- Police: perimeter control crowd
- Receiving ED on phone when calling to transport patient

## 7. CRITICAL ACTIONS

- Scene safety
- Crowd control
- ABC assessment and stabilization
- Full assessment with skin exposure
- C-collar placement
- Quick transport

## 8. TIMELINE

### Time: Zero

Location: on scene
Patient 1: VS: BP 102/54, HR 122, RR 44 (shallow), $O_2$ sat 88%, temp: unavailable
Patient 2: VS: BP 136/88, HR 106, RR 12, $O_2$ sat 98%, temp: unavailable
Patient 3: VS: BP 164/102. HR 128 (irregularly irregular), $O_2$ 100%, temp: unavailable

- Patient 1. Summary of initial presentation: a 23-year-old male pedestrian struck on the right side by a truck going approximately 40 miles/hour
- Patient 2. Summary of initial presentation: a 37-year-old female with severe right lower leg and ankle pain presents with obvious lower leg deformity after jumping down from bleachers
- Patient 3. Summary of initial presentation: a 63-year-old man on blood thinners with briskly bleeding laceration to forehead, who lost consciousness after tripping and striking head on a metal pole

**Patient 1: Physical Exam**

- General: nonresponsive, eyes closed
- HEENT: PERRL
- Neck: trachea midline, normal appearance
- Chest: decreased breath sounds on right, paradoxical rib movement on R side underlying area of ecchymosis and crepitus under clothing
- Heart: tachycardic, regular rhythm, weak pulses
- Abdomen: bruising on right flank
- Skin: pale, cool, diaphoretic
- Neuro: Glasgow Coma Scale (GCS) 3
- Extremities: pulses present in all four. No movement to painful stimulation.

**Patient 2: Physical Exam**

- General: in obvious pain
- HEENT: PERRL, no deformities to head
- Neck: normal ROM, no pain on evaluation
- Chest: mildly tachypneic, good air movement
- Heart: tachycardic, very weak right-sided pedal pulse
- Abdomen: soft and nontender
- Skin: right foot is pale and cool to touch
- Neuro: GCS 15
- Extremities: obvious deformity to the right-sided lower limb with extensive bruising, unable to bear weight, screams in pain with even slightest movement of the extremity. Foot is cool, with decreased pulse on the right side.

**Patient 3: Physical Exam**

- General: older man, appears confused, has a bleeding laceration on forehed
- HEENT: briskly bleeding 3.5 cm laceration to forehead, no crepitus
- Neck: reports midline tenderness
- Chest: clear lungs
- Heart: tachycardic, irregularly irregular
- Abdomen: soft and nontender
- Skin: warm, dry, well perfused
- Neuro: GCS 14, confused about event
- Extremities: no obvious deformity, moving all extremities

**Patient 1: Initial Intervention**

- Ensure scene safety, police on scene
- Be alert for coordinated attack with potential for subsequent attacks once responders are on scene.
- Airway assessment: Patient is not protecting airway. First, open airway with jaw thrust or oral airway device while protecting C-spine. Decide to intubate and ventilate.
- Breathing assessment: listen for bilateral breath sounds, note decreased breath sounds on right – place needle thoracostomy or chest tube
- Circulation: note hemorrhage at scalp laceration. Perform bleeding control measures.
- Apply C-collar, maintain C-spine precautions throughout.
- Place IO or IV line.

**Patient 2: Initial Intervention**

- Ensure scene safety, police on scene
- Be alert for coordinated attack with potential for subsequent attacks once responders are on scene.
- Airway assessment: Patient is protecting airway – no intervention needed
- Breathing assessment: listen for bilateral breath sounds. Note equal breath sounds with good air movement.
- Circulation: note right foot has very weak pedal pulse, bruising, quick splint of the extremity for transport.
- Place IO or IV line. Pain control.

**Patient 3: Initial Intervention**

- Ensure scene safety, police on scene
- Be alert for coordinated attack with potential for subsequent attacks once responders are on scene.
- Airway assessment: Patient is protecting airway – no intervention needed
- Breathing assessment: listen for bilateral breath sounds. Note equal breath sounds with good air movement.
- Circulation: briskly bleeding forehead laceration. Perform bleeding control measures.
- Place IO or IV line.

Security/police: ensure scene safety and maintain a perimeter

### Critical Actions

**Patient 1**

- Identify patient not protecting airway and in respiratory distress
    - Open airway with physical maneuver followed by oral airway and BVM. Recognize need to intubate before transport. Must protect C-spine throughout.
- Fully expose patient and recognize flail chest

- Performs thoracostomy to decompress possible tension pneumothorax
- Identifies that the head laceration requires immediate hemorrhage control

**Patient 2**

- Identify patient's lower extremity deformity, note that it is pale and cool to touch with decreased pulse. Splint.
- Pain control

**Patient 3**

- Identify patient's head laceration and perform bleeding control
- Perform neurol exam, identify confusion and assign appropriate GCS

## Time: Five Minutes – Transition Point 1

Patient 1: VS (if all actions addressed): BP: 105/62, HR 120, RR 20 (bagged), $O_2$ 92

If bleeding not controlled or thoracostomy not performed, patient's vitals become more unstable until cardiac arrest occurs.

- Physical exam: head laceration bleeding controlled. The patient has been intubated or is being bagged, thoracostomy needle/tube is in place. C-vollar intact.
- Once IO established, begin giving IV fluids
- Move patient to gurney and then into ambulance. Backboard is most appropriate.
- Once in route, call hospital to alert them to transport
- Intubate patient if not previously performed.

**Patient 2**

VS (if all actions addressed): BP: 128/82, HR 108, RR 12, $O_2$ 98

- Physical exam: lower extremity splinted; patient more comfortable with pain medication
- Once IO established, begin give pain medication
- Move patient to gurney and then into ambulance.
- Once in route, call hospital to alert them to transport

**Patient 3**

VS (if all actions addressed): BP: 160/102, HR 122, RR 12, $O_2$ 98

- Physical exam: bleeding head wound with appropriate hemorrhage control.
- IO/IV established
- Move patient to gurney and then into ambulance.
- Once in route, call hospital to alert them to transport

### Critical Actions

**Patient 1**

- Quickly moving to transport once patient is stabilized
- Spine precautions
- Definitive airway established prior to transport
- Ensure transport to trauma center
- Provide prearrival notification to ED

**Patient 2**

- Quickly moving to transport once patient is stabilized
- Pain control before reaching hospital
- Lower limb stabilized.
- Ensure transport to trauma center
- Provide prearrival notification to ED

**Patient 3**

- Quickly moving to transport once patient is stabilized
- Hemorrhage control
- Ensure transport to trauma center
- Provide prearrival notification to ED

### Patient 1: VS (If Actions Missed)

If not intubated: HR 180 and RR 55 and BP 85/45, $O_2$ Sat 78%

If laceration not addressed: HR 144 and BP: 95/50.

If thoracostomy not addressed, HR 190, RR 60, BP 70/30, $O_2$ sat 80% on 100% $O_2$, hard to bag, %, tracheal deviation to left if recognized through C-collar.

- Physical exam: profuse bleeding from head, patient becomes more unstable
- Give hints if parts unaddressed.
- Unable to transport until patient stabilized.

### Patient 2: VS (If Actions Missed)

If limb not stabilized and pain not addressed: HR 120 and RR 16 and BP 152/94, $O_2$ sat 100%

- Physical exam: Patient becomes more agitated
- Give hints if parts unaddressed

### Patient 3: VS (If Actions Missed)

If laceration not addressed: HR 140 and BP: 120/90.

If thoracostomy not addressed, HR 190, RR 60, BP 70/30, $O_2$ sat 80% on 100% $O_2$, hard to bag, %, tracheal deviation to left if recognized through C-collar.

- Physical exam: profuse bleeding from head, patient becomes more unstable, and more altered.
- Give hints if parts unaddressed.
- Unable to transport until patient stabilized.

## 9. STIMULI

- Monitor showing vital signs

## BIBLIOGRAPHY

Phillips JP, Young JF, Brady WJ. Preparation and response to a targeted automobile ramming mass casualty (TARMAC) attack: an analysis of the 2017 Charlottesville, Virginia TARMAC attack. *Am J Disaster Med.* 2019;14(3):219–223.

CASE 43

# Trampled in New Orleans

Kyle Herbert

DISASTER PRINCIPLES

- Clinical diagnosis and treatment
- Information management/communications
- Timing of medical and surgical interventions
- Recognition and clinical treatment
- Field operations and logistics
- Field disaster triage
- Field stabilization, treatment, and transport
- Stampede injuries
- Mass gatherings

## 1. SCENARIO OVERVIEW

a. EMS brings in a 48-year-old female from scene. Patient 1 was at a second line parade for a major festival in New Orleans when reported gunshots rang out, which caused a stampede of approximately 300 people. Patient was seen falling to the ground and was subsequently stepped on by multiple people and possibly one horse. Patient 2, patient's husband, was able to drag her from under bystanders; however, he also suffered blows to his head, neck, and arms during the incident. EMS notes that on arrival, patient was lying on back, unresponsive, in a tank top with obvious large bruise consistent with hoof print to left anterior chest wall. Patient 2 is at her side, initially unconscious with pulse; obvious slow oozing laceration to right frontal scalp. Patient 2 regains consciousness and appears alert and oriented, initially. Patient 1 without palpable pulse on initial assessment, compressions immediately initiated. Rhythm on monitor showed ventricular fibrillation. Patient subsequently shocked ×2 with return of spontaneous circulation (ROSC) after second defibrillation. Laryngeal mask airway (LMA) placed in field prior to transport for airway protection, C-collar placed for C-spine precautions. Patient 2 accompanies EMS to ED; patient's scalp wound wrapped by EMS in transit, hiding extent of wound.

## 2. TEACHING OBJECTIVES AND DISCUSSION POINTS

### Teaching Objectives

a. Complete appropriate workup, imaging, labs, and procedures needed for blunt cardiac trauma patients

b. Postcardiac arrest care
c. Emergent pericardial effusion treatment
d. Prepare emergency department for arrival of multiple casualties given the description of the event.

**Discussion Points**

a. Trauma algorithm for in-field resuscitation of cardiac arrest due to blunt trauma
b. Immediate recognition and management of commotio cordis in cardiac arrest due to direct chest wall blunt trauma
c. Importance and utility of bedside echocardiogram in the setting of blunt chest wall trauma
d. Performing emergent pericardiocentesis

## 3. SUPPLIES

Standard PPE

a. Cardiac monitor, $SpO_2$, BP monitor, ECG
b. Intubation supplies in the room for backup airway in case of decompensation: BVM, ETT, stylet, blade, suction
c. Provider PPE (gown, mask with shield, gloves)
d. Pericardiocentesis kit
e. Cordis, MAC, or other large-bore central access device
f. Blood products and transfusion platform

## 4. MOULAGE

a. Patient 1
    i. Scattered abrasions and minor lacerations to head/face
    ii. Large left anterior chest wall and peristernal bruising/abrasion (in the rough shape of a hoof)
    iii. Scattered ecchymosis to bilateral upper extremities
    iv. Scattered ecchymosis to anterior abdomen
    v. Wound to dorsum of left forearm with proximally placed tourniquet
    vi. Obvious dinner-fork deformity to left distal forearm
b. Patient 2
    i. Scalp wound head dressing initially hiding wound until after patient is sedated
    ii. Approximately 3–4 cm linear gaping laceration to right forehead, just below scalp line
    iii. Scattered nonspecific ecchymosis to face, neck, bilateral upper extremities

## 5. IMAGES AND LABS

a. Patient 1
    i. Basic labs (CBC, CMP, lactic acid, coags, type and screen, troponin, BNP, VBG, etc.)
    ii. Chest X-ray 1-view
    iii. Left forearm X-ray
    iv. Bedside ultrasound (Extended Focused Assessment with Sonography for Trauma [EFAST])
    v. CT head, CT cervical spine, CT chest (with contrast), CT abdomen/pelvis (with contrast)
b. Patient 2
    i. Basic labs (CBC, CMP, lactic acid, coags, type and screen, VBG, etc.)
    ii. Bedside ultrasound (EFAST)
    iii. Chest X-ray
    iv. CT head, CT C-spine, CT chest, CT abdomen/pelvis

c. Patient 3
   i. Right wrist and forearm X-ray

## 6. ACTORS (CONFEDERATES) AND THEIR ROLES

a. Nurse: obtain IV access, place on monitor, obtain labs, administers rapid-sequence intubation (RSI) medications and other needed intravenous therapies
b. Medical technician: obtain IV access, place on monitor
c. Respiratory therapist: management of LMA, assistance with intubation setup and postintubation ventilator management (if team decides to obtain definitive airway)
d. Confederate 1 = Patient 2: rushes in during resuscitation, frantic, distracting team
   i. Medical tech initially attempts to redirect patient
   ii. Becomes agitated and strikes medical tech, turning them into Patient 3
e. Confederate 2 = Patient 3: struck in face by Patient 2 during agitated episode
   i. Knocked to the ground, but does not lose consciousness
   ii. Falls backward on outstretched RUE with subsequent pain to right wrist
f. Confederate 3: Security presents and restrains Patient 2 (after medical technician becomes Patient #3) and aids with subsequent sedation

## 7. CRITICAL ACTIONS

a. Patient 1
   i. Attach patient to monitor
   ii. Obtain initial vital signs
   iii. Complete primary survey (ABCs)
   iv. Ascertain Glasgow Coma Scale (GCS) and decide on definitive airway for airway protection
      1. Ensure suction, backup, bougie, RSI medications, postintubation sedation, ETT confirmation, OGT
      2. Confirmation of ETT with $CO_2$ colorimeter, auscultated breath sounds, and/or chest rise
   v. Identification of hypotension in setting of trauma, initiation of transfusion
   vi. EFAST exam with identification of positive pericardial tamponade
   vii. Pericardiocentesis
   viii. Resuming EFAST after procedure (if stopped to perform procedure), with identification of absent left-sided lung-sliding
   ix. Placement of left-sided surgical chest tube
   x. Consultation of cardiothoracic surgery
   xi. Take down forearm tourniquet, assess and dress wound, splint left forearm
   xii. Decision to obtain further/advanced imaging (if patient stabilizes)
b. Patient 2
   i. Attempt to appropriately redirect
   ii. Decision to chemically sedate after violent action
   iii. Attach patient to monitor + end-tidal $CO_2$
   iv. Obtain initial vital signs
   v. Complete primary survey (ABCs): expose patient's wound to reveal laceration
   vi. Place C-collar
   vii. EFAST exam: determine negative exam
   viii. Obtain CXR and advanced CT imaging
   ix. Transfer patient to medical hold for observation once imaging negative

c. Patient 3
   i. Evaluate injury and elicit snuff box tenderness to right wrist
   ii. Obtain XR imaging of right wrist/forearm
   iii. Place empiric right thumb spica splint and provided follow-up instructions
   iv. Provide PO pain medication
   v. Discharge home (or other appropriate nonclinical disposition)

## 8. TIMELINE WITH TRANSITION POINTS

### Time: Zero

a. Vital signs: BP 83/62, HR 145, RR 18, temp 36.1, sat 95% on NRB, POC glucose 114
b. EMS arrives with report
   i. A 48-year-old female presenting after stampede with obvious blunt trauma to chest. In Vfib arrest on scene with ROSC after shocking ×2. LMA placed in field. Continued hypotension, tachycardia, decreased mentation in route; IVF and norepinephrine initiated.
c. Initial intervention
   i. Place on monitor
   ii. Large-bore IV ×2 (at least 18 G)
   iii. Trauma labs drawn
d. Primary survey
   i. ABCs
      1. Airway: LMA in place
      2. Breathing: equal chest rise, lungs coarse bilaterally
      3. Circulation: 1+ pulses throughout
      4. Disability: GCS 3
      5. Exposure: remove all clothing

**Critical Actions**
- Place on monitor and obtain initial vitals
- Establish IV access
- Initiate PRBC administration
- Procedural actions
   i. Determine need for definitive airway and obtain
   ii. Optional: intubation strategies while hypotensive
- Begin antiarrhythmic infusion (i.e. amiodarone) in the setting of ventricular fibrillation arrest

### Time: ~Five Minutes – Transition Point 1

a. Repeat vitals: persistent hypotension despite volume repletion
b. Secondary exam
   i. General: intubated and sedated
   ii. Head/face: normocephalic, atraumatic
   iii. HEENT: no injuries, pupils sluggishly reactive
   iv. Neck: unable to visualize neck due to habitus, no appreciable crepitus

v. Chest: bilateral needle decompression catheters at midclavicular line, second intercostal space. Horse-shaped bruising and small divot appreciable to left anterior chest wall, just lateral to sternum, at approx. ribs 4/5. Unequal chest rise, diminished breath sounds over left chest wall.
vi. Abdomen: nondistended, bruising appreciable to abdomen
vii. Pelvis: stable
viii. Back: shallow 3 cm laceration to left back at approximately T4 level, lateral to spine
ix. Extremities: large, gaping laceration middle right volar forearm with obvious muscle exposure; tourniquet proximal to injury
x. Neuro: GCS 3T

**Critical Actions**

- Reevaluation of vital signs
- Decision to defer CT imaging given persistent hypotension
- Proceed with EFAST

### Time: ~Seven Minutes – Transition Point 2

a. Repeat vitals: persistent hypotension
b. EFAST with evidence of pericardial effusion, impending tamponade physiology
c. Patient 2 barges in during EFAST (after team discovers cardiac tamponade on Patient 1). He is hysterical and interfering with resuscitation. Subsequently strikes medical technician, turning them into Patient 3
d. Restrain and chemically sedate Patient 2 and move to nearby stretcher, briefly assess Patient 3 and move to chair quickly, and return to Patient 1
e. Perform emergent pericardiocentesis

**Critical Actions**

- Demonstrate appropriate EFAST technique
- Effectively deal with interfering family member and unexpected new patients
- Reorganize team to provide adequate observation of new patients
  i. Team should decide how Patients 2 and /3 will be monitored while Patient 1's resuscitation continues
- Determine need for, and perform, pericardiocentesis

### Time: ~15 Minutes – Transition Point 3

a. Repeat vitals
   i. Only mild improvement in vitals (BP/HR) following PRBCs and pericardiocentesis
   ii. Patient's $O_2$ sats also remain lower than expected, respiratory tech meeting some increased resistance bagging (ventilator not available)
b. Resume EFAST with identification of absent left-sided lung sliding
c. Perform left surgical chest tube placement

**Critical Actions**
- Triage issues leading differential for persistent hypotension plus evidence of respiratory compromise
- Resume EFAST
- Identification of pneumothorax by ultrasound
- Determine need for, and perform tube thoracostomy

### Time: ~25 Minutes – Transition Point 4

a. Repeat vitals
   i. Patient's BP improves gradually to low normotensive range, mechanical ventilation becomes easy
b. Chest x-ray ordered to confirm placement of ETT, pericardial catheter, chest tube
c. CT imaging (if ordered)
   i. CT head and C-spine: negative
   ii. CT chest: redemonstration of multiple bilateral rib fractures, mildly displaced sternal fractures, bilateral pulmonary contusions (L>R), residual pericardial effusion
   iii. CT abdomen/pelvis: negative
d. Consult to CT surgery: patient taken to OR

**Critical Actions**
- Reassessment of postprocedure vitals
- Determine need for CXR to confirm interventions
- Discussion of pros and cons of obtaining CT imaging on critical patient
- Clinical summary followed by final disposition with appropriate consultation technique

### Time: ~30 Minutes – Transition Point 5

a. Reassess Patient 2
   i. Perform vitals = stable
   ii. Perform ABCs = stable, GCS 11–13 (dependent on sedation medication used)
   iii. Place C-collar
   iv. Perform EFAST
   v. Obtain x-ray and CT imaging (head, C-spine)
   vi. Wound care
   vii. +/– Appropriately provide update on patient's wife (Patient 1)
   viii. Appropriately disposition
b. Reassess Patient 3
   i. Perform targeted exam with discovery of right snuff box tenderness
   ii. Obtain focal x-ray imaging
   iii. Place in thumb spica
   iv. Appropriately disposition

**Critical Actions**

- Placement of C-collar on Patient 2
- Discussion of pros/cons of providing update of Patient 1's condition in setting of spouse's condition
- Identification of the significance of persistent snuff box tenderness despite negative wrist x-ray
- Placement of thumb spica splint and appropriate follow-up counseling
- Appropriate disposition of both patients
  i. Patient 2: observation
  ii. Patient #3: discharge home

## 9. STIMULI

a. Patient 1
   i. EFAST with pericardial effusion, evidence of impending tamponade physiology
   ii. Follow-up EFAST with negative left-sided lung-sliding
   iii. CXR findings: adequate ETT, pericardial catheter, and chest tube placement, sternal fracture, multiple broken ribs bilaterally, evidence of developing pulmonary contusions
   iv. CT chest findings: redemonstration of multiple bilateral rib fractures, mildly displaced sternal fractures, bilateral pulmonary contusions (L>R), residual pericardial effusion
   v. Lactate 6.1
   vi. ABG: pH 7.28, $PaO_2$ 95, $PaCO_2$ 44, $HCO_3$ 17, $O_2$ sat 95%
   vii. Hemoglobin 10.2
b. Patient 3: negative right wrist XR with persistent snuff box tenderness

## BIBLIOGRAPHY

Dogrul BN, Kiliccalan I, Asci ES, Peker SC. Blunt trauma related chest wall and pulmonary injuries: an overview. *Chin J Traumatol.* 2020 June;23(3):125–138. doi: 10.1016/j.cjtee.2020.04.003. Epub 2020 Apr 20. PMID: 32417043; PMCID: PMC7296362.

Link MS. Commotio cordis: ventricular fibrillation triggered by chest impact-induced abnormalities in repolarization. *Circ Arrhythm Electrophysiol.* 2012;5(2):425–432. doi:10.1161/CIRCEP.111.962712.

Spodick DH. Acute cardiac tamponade. *N Engl J Med.* 2003 Aug 14;349(7):684–690. doi: 10.1056/NEJMra022643. PMID: 12917306.

Willner DA, Grossman SA. Pericardiocentesis. [Updated March 9, 2022 ]. In: *StatPearls* [Internet]. Treasure Island, FL: StatPearls Publishing; 2022 Jan-. www.ncbi.nlm.nih.gov/books/NBK470347/. Accessed April 8, 2025.

CASE 44

# Mass Casualty Triage and Early Stabilization Following a Bus Crash

C. Clare Charbonnet and Michael Weiner

DISASTER PRINCIPLES

- Clinical diagnosis and treatment
- Conventional standards of care
- Disaster triage concepts
- Timing of medical and surgical interventions
- Local disaster response
- Hospital preparedness program
- Emergency operations plans for the healthcare environment
- Information management/communications
- Medical surge capacity
- Mass-casualty incidents
- Field operations and logistics
- Mass-casualty care in the field
- Field disaster triage
- Field stabilization, treatment, and transport
- Disaster operations
- EMS disaster operations
- Transportation disasters
- Vehicle extraction

## 1. SCENARIO OVERVIEW

You are the single attending working the late shift at an academic hospital and trauma center. Three residents are staffing with you during this shift. Halfway through your shift, your charge nurse informs you that the local dispatch center has called. A vehicle traveling at high speed on the freeway lost control in the snow and struck a commuter bus, which rolled onto its right side. Dispatch estimates that your hospital will receive between 15 and 20 victims from the scene, starting in the next 10 minutes.

## 2. TEACHING OBJECTIVES AND DISCUSSION POINTS

a. Understand the essentials of preparing for a mass casualty incident.
b. Rapidly activate a mass casualty event and communicate a plan with team members both in the ED and in other departments.

c. Assign roles to team members.
d. Recognize and manage reverse triage, in which walking wounded patients with minor injuries will arrive by private vehicle rapidly.
e. Perform the fundamentals of the Simple Triage And Rapid Treatment (START) triage protocol.
f. Correctly use rapid assessment tools.
g. Use early stabilization measures to enable the team to manage a large number of victims.
h. Constantly reassess current victims pending available resources.

## 3. SUPPLIES

a. START triage tags ×15
b. Suture kit ×1 (alternatively, stapler ×1)
c. Packet of 0-0 silk thread ×2
d. Pelvic binder ×1
e. Tourniquet ×2
f. Thoracostomy needle ×2
g. Endotracheal tube ×1
h. Size 4 Macintosh blade ×1
i. Chest tube and insertion kit ×2
j. Ultrasound machine
k. Unit of packed red blood cells ×8
l. 2500 units of prothrombin complex concentrate ×1

## 4. MOULAGE

a. Parietal scalp laceration for Passenger 1
b. Ecchymosis on right side of chest and RUQ of Passenger 3
c. Ecchymosis on right wrist for Passenger 5
d. Subtle small contusion at edge of left hairline of Passenger 6
e. Ecchymosis of pelvis for the Passenger of the other vehicle
f. Deformity of right ankle with exposed broken bone, ecchymosis, and small amount of dark blood for Passenger 8. Foot should be faintly blue.
g. Shard of glass protruding from left leg just above the knee with large amount of red blood for Passenger 9
h. Large ecchymosis in LUQ for Passenger 11
i. Moderate amount of blood overlying depressed skull fracture for Passenger 12
j. If possible, rightward tracheal deviation for Passenger 13
k. Deformity of proximal right lower leg with exposed broken bone, ecchymosis, and a small amount of dark blood for the Driver of the other vehicle

## 5. IMAGES AND LABS

a. Extended Focused Assessment with Sonography for Trauma (EFAST) exam that is positive in RUQ and has no lung sliding on right side for Passenger #3
b. CXR with right-sided pneumothorax for Passenger 3
c. X-ray of comminuted right distal ulna fracture for Passenger 5
d. Head CT with 6 mm left-sided SDH and another head CT with an 11 mm left-sided SDH with midline shift for Passenger 6

e. PXR with open-book fracture for the passenger of the other vehicle
f. X-ray of right trimalleolar fracture for Passenger 8
g. EFAST exam that is positive in LUQ for Passenger 11
h. CXR with left-sided tension pneumothorax (PTX) for Passenger 13
i. X-ray of right tibia and fibula fractures for the Driver of the other vehicle

## 6. ACTORS (CONFEDERATES) AND THEIR ROLES

a. See Table 44.1 for a list of victims in the order in which they arrive at the ED.
b. An emergency medicine attending physician is elected from among the learners.
c. The remainder of learners are emergency medicine residents.
d. Eight ED nurses
e. Four ED medics
f. Flight paramedic and flight nurse from the helicopter
g. Two-person paramedic teams for each of the nine ambulances (can be reused once they drop off a patient)
h. Trauma surgery providers
i. Operating room and/or interventional radiology providers
j. Husband of Passenger 12 (and son-in-law of Passenger 11)

## 7. CRITICAL ACTIONS

a. Verbalize activation of a mass casualty incident and establish Incident Command.
b. Contact appropriate ancillary services including blood bank, pharmacy, radiology, trauma surgery, the operating room, and hospital leadership.
c. Assign team roles including attending (leader) and triage provider.
d. Communicate the need for using START triage algorithm (see Figure 44.1) rather than standard triage algorithms.
e. Designate parts of the ED to minor, delayed, critical, and expectant acuity patients.
f. Appropriately triage patients. In anticipation of reverse triage in which lower acuity walking wounded will arrive before the most critical patients, delay rooming minor acuity patients.
g. Identify life and limb threats as part of initial trauma examinations.
h. Perform immediate stabilization procedures for patients whose definitive care can be delayed (e.g. needle decompression, pelvic binder, tourniquet, etc.).
i. Determine that Passenger 3, the Passenger of the other vehicle, and Passenger 11 should be emergently transported to the operating room or interventional radiology.
j. Perform frequent reassessments of minor acuity patients. Room them as needed based on reassessment or as space becomes available in the ED.
k. Black tag Passenger 12. Explain injuries and prognosis to her husband when he arrives.

## 8. TIMELINE AND TRANSITION POINTS

### Time: Zero Minutes

a. Dispatch contacts the ED to notify the team of an MVC in which a vehicle struck a bus, which then rolled over onto its side. Ambulances are bringing people from the scene. Based on information from first responders on the scene, dispatch estimates the ED will receive 15–20 patients.

**Table 44.1** Actors in the order in which they arrive at the ED

| Actor | Description | Relationship | Injury | START triage vital signs | | | START triage color | Method of arrival | Arrival after time zero (minutes) | Associated stimulus | Critical actions | Course if critical action is performed | Course if critical action is not performed |
|---|---|---|---|---|---|---|---|---|---|---|---|---|---|
| | | | | Respiratory rate | Capillary refill | Mental status | | | | | | | |
| Bus driver | 55 yo M with PMH CAD, HTN, HLD, and DM2 with neck and upper back pain | | Paraspinal muscle spasm | 16 | <2 | Following commands | Minor (green) | EMS | 8 | | | | |
| Bus passenger 1 | 25 yo M with history of asthma complaining of pain and cut on his right parietal scalp | | Parietal scalp laceration with significant bleeding | 18 | <2 | Following commands | Minor (green) | Private vehicle | 9 | | Hold direct pressure or primarily repair scalp laceration with sutures or staples | Bleeding is controlled and patient's BP remains within normal limits. | Bleeding continues and patient becomes tachycardic to 110 and hypotensive to 90/60. |
| Bus passenger 2 | 40 yo F with pain and stiffness on the right side of her neck | | Paraspinal muscle spasm | 20 | <2 | Following commands | Minor (green) | Private vehicle | 10 | | | | |
| Bus passenger 3 | 63 yo M with GERD, HTN, and HLD with severe right-sided chest and abdominal pain | | Anterior fractures of right ribs 6–9 with flail chest and hemopneumothorax, liver laceration | 32 | 6 | Agitated | Critical (red) | HEMS | 10 | EFAST exam positive in RUQ and no lung sliding on right side. CXR with right-sided PTX. | Perform EFAST exam, intubate and place chest tube, transfer to OR/IR, consider administration of uncrossed blood | Stabilizes to BP 100/65 only if intubated, effectively sedated, and there is intervention on the PTX. Stabilizes to BP 110/70 if blood is transfused. | If intubated without prompt intervention on the PTX, the patient codes. If no blood is transfused within 15 minutes, BP falls to 80/40. |
| Bus passenger 4 | 38 yo F with bipolar disorder and GERD but no complaints | Mother of Passenger 5 | None | 18 | <2 | Following commands | Minor (green) | Private vehicle with Passenger 5 | 15 | | Keep together with son | | Patient becomes agitated about not knowing her child is. |
| Bus passenger 5 | 10 yo M with right forearm deformity | Son of Passenger 4 | Closed comminuted right distal ulna fracture | 24 | <2 | Crying but following commands | Minor (green) | Private vehicle with | 15 | X-ray of comminuted | Keep together with mother | | Patient cannot provide mother's name or phone |

**Table 44.1** *(cont.)*

| Actor | Description | Relationship | Injury | START triage vital signs: Respiratory rate | Capillary refill | Mental status | START triage color | Method of arrival | Arrival after time zero (minutes) | Associated stimulus | Critical actions | Course if critical action is performed | Course if critical action is not performed |
|---|---|---|---|---|---|---|---|---|---|---|---|---|---|
| | | | | | | | | Passenger 4 | | right distal ulna fracture | | | number. Perform family reunification. |
| Bus passenger 6 | 88 yo F with PMH of CAD, CHF, COPD, afib on Eliquis, CKD, DM2 with headache, neck pain, diffuse back pain, and left shoulder pain | | 6 mm left-sided subdural hematoma | 24 | <2 | Following simple commands but very hard of hearing | Minor (green) | EMS | 18 | Head CT with 6 mm left-sided SDH and another head CT with an 11 mm left-sided SDH with midline shift | Obtain head CT and diagnose SDH, then reverse her Eliquis | Repeat head CT shows a stable bleed, and patient's mental status remains stable. | Patient becomes somnolent. Repeat CT shows a 11 mm SDH with midline shift. |
| Bus passenger 7 | 18 yo M with history of anxiety with left-sided chest pain, refusing to ambulate | | Nondisplaced anterior fractures of left rib 5–6 without PTX | 30 | <2 | Redirectable | Critical (red) | EMS | 19 | | | | |
| Passenger of other vehicle | Unrestrained 19 yo F with severe abdominal and pelvic pain; speaks only Spanish | | Open book pelvis fracture | 26 | 6 | Redirectable | Critical (red) | EMS | 24 | PXR with open-book fracture | Apply pelvic binder, transfer to OR/IR, consider administration of uncrossed blood, obtain Spanish translator | With application of binder, BP is 95/65. With transfusion, BP improves to 105/70. | BP falls to 60/30. If still no intervention within five minutes, patient codes. If no Spanish translator is obtained, patient becomes agitated. |
| Bus passenger 8 | 26 yo F with severe right ankle pain and obvious | Partner of Passenger 9 | Open right trimalleolar fracture with compromised vasculature. If HCG is ordered, she is | 26 | <2 | Following commands | Delayed (yellow) | EMS with Passenger 9 | 28 | X-ray of right trimalleolar fracture | Reduce fracture emergently to restore circulation. | Right leg is salvaged. | Right foot becomes dusky and more painful. If fracture is not reduced during |

| | | | | | | | | | | | | |
|---|---|---|---|---|---|---|---|---|---|---|---|---|
| | deformity; unable to walk | | incidentally found to be pregnant. She does not want her partner to know. | | | | | | | | Later, if learner orders HCG, they can tell the patient she's pregnant in private. | | the simulation, the patient's foot dies. |
| Bus passenger 9 | 32 yo right-handed M with shard of glass protruding from anterior left leg just above the knee with pulsatile bleeding | Partner of Passenger 8 | Laceration of left femoral artery; does not know his partner is pregnant because she does not know | 24 | 3 | Following commands | Critical (red) | EMS with Passenger 8 | 28 | | Apply two tourniquets high on left leg; do not tell him his partner is pregnant without her permission | If one tourniquet is applied, bleeding slows but does not stop. Two stops the bleeding. | If no tourniquets are applied within 10 minutes, BP drops to 60/40. After 15 minutes, the patient codes. If only one tourniquet is applied, BP drops to 75/45 after twenty minutes and patient complains of being cold and short of breath. |
| Bus passenger 10 | 42 yo M with lower thoracic and upper lumbar pain | | Acute endplate fracture of T12 with anterior spondylolisthesis, acute transverse process fractures T3–4 | 16 | <2 | Following commands | Minor (green) | Private vehicle | 30 | | Maintain spine precautions | Patient has no lower extremity deficits. | Patient reports weakness and numbness in his lower extremities. |
| Bus passenger 11 | 93 yo F with dementia, HTN, CKD, DM with no complaints | Mother of Passenger 12 | Grade IV splenic laceration | 22 | 4 | Demented | Critical (red) | EMS | 35 | EFAST exam positive in LUQ | Perform EFAST exam, consider blood transfusion, transfer to OR/IR | Patient remains stable. | Patient becomes somnolent and BP drops to 80/40. If diagnosis is not made in 30 minutes, patient codes. |
| Bus passenger 12 | 68 yo F with HTN and RA with large contusion on forehead | Daughter of Passenger 11 | Depressed skull fracture and subdural hematoma with herniation | 0 | 3 | Obtunded | Expectant (black) | EMS | 38 | | Black tag the patient | Patient loses pulses. This outcome is appropriate in this scenario. | If learner attempts resuscitation, patient does not code but she is |

Table 44.1 (*cont.*)

| Actor | Description | Relationship | Injury | START triage vital signs: Respiratory rate | Capillary refill | Mental status | START triage color | Method of arrival | Arrival after time zero (minutes) | Associated stimulus | Critical actions | Course if critical action is performed | Course if critical action is not performed |
|---|---|---|---|---|---|---|---|---|---|---|---|---|---|
| | | | | | | | | | | | | | pronounced brain dead in the ICU later. |
| Bus passenger 13 | 53 yo M with PMH AUD and HTN with shortness of breath and left-sided chest pain | | Anterior fractures of left ribs 3–5 with rightward tracheal deviation and crepitus due to tension PTX | 28 | <2 | Following commands | Delayed (yellow) | EMS | 42 | CXR with left-sided tension PTX | Perform needle decompression | RR normalizes and patient remains stable. | If needle decompression is not performed within five minutes, RR increases to 34 and BP drops to 90/60. If decompression is not performed within 10 minutes, $SpO_2$ drops to 85% and BP drops to 75/45. If no intervention by 20 minutes, patient codes. |
| Driver of other vehicle | Unrestrained 20 yo M with right leg deformities | | Open comminuted right tib/fib fractures without compromised circulation | 24 | 4 | Intoxicated | Critical (red) | EMS | 48 | X-ray of right tib/fib fractures | Assess circulation to extremity | | |

Abbreviations: AUD, alcohol use disorder; CAD, coronary artery disease; CHF, congestive heart failure; EFAST, Extended Focused Assessment with Sonography for Trauma; HEMS, helicopter EMS; HLD, hyperlipidemia; PTX, pneumothorax; RA, rheumatoid arthritis; yo, year old.

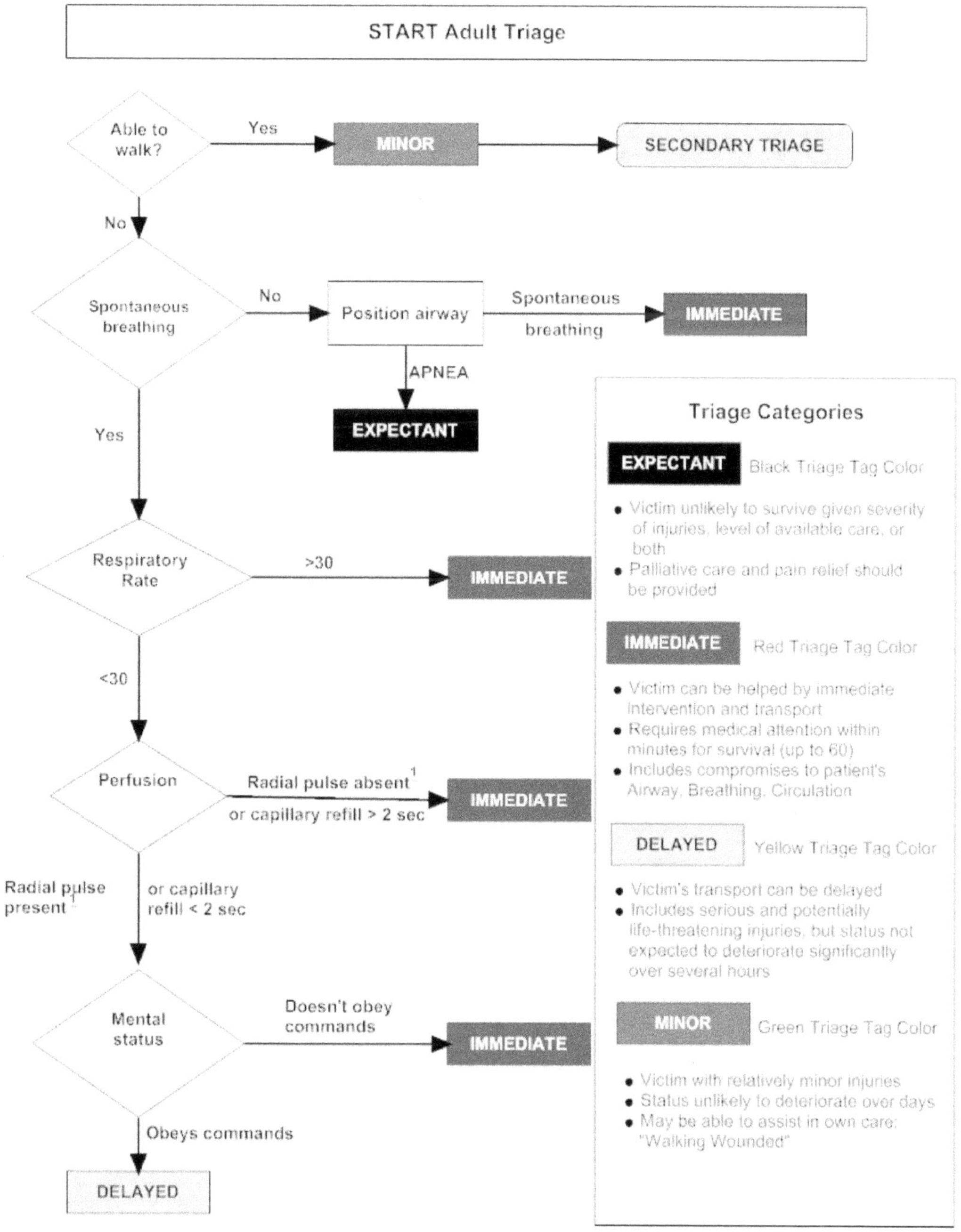


Adopted from http://www.start-triage.com

REMM RADIATION EMERGENCY MEDICAL MANAGEMENT
REMM.hhs.gov

**Figure 44.1** START triage algorithm.
US Department of Health and Human Services. Chemical Hazards Emergency Medical Management [Internet]. Available from: https://chemm.hhs.gov/startadult.htm.

### Time: Eight Minutes

a. First patient arrives. Other patients will arrive based on the timing listed in Table 44.1.

### Time: 65 Minutes

a. Husband of Passenger 12 arrives and wants to see his wife.

# Index

For EU product safety concerns, contact us at Calle de José Abascal, 56–1°,
28003 Madrid, Spain or eugpsr@cambridge.org.

www.ingramcontent.com/pod-product-compliance
Lightning Source LLC
LaVergne TN
LVHW081532060526
838200LV00048B/2058

* 9 7 8 1 0 0 9 2 7 9 0 1 7 *